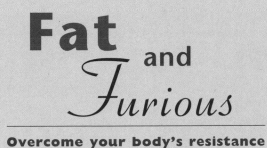

Fat and *Furious*

Overcome your body's resistance to weight loss now!

Does this sound like you?

❏ You would have better odds at winning the lottery than losing ten pounds.

❏ The clothes in your closet range from thin, medium, to *OH MY GOD.*

❏ You would really like to be the weight listed on your driver's license.

❏ You have eaten so much tuna trying to lose weight, you are constantly being followed by whining cats carrying can openers.

❏ You have such a large collection of diet books that you could open your own bookstore.

❏ You've been to Jenny Craig so often that you consider her extended family.

❏ If one more person even hints that you need to lose weight, you will be on the 11 o'clock news in a fashionable orange jumpsuit for inflicting bodily harm.

❏ You are seduced at night by a handsome German guy named *Häagen-Dazs.*

❏ A carjacker would have a better chance of stealing your car than your secret stash of Snickers in your glove box.

❏ You have an inner critical voice so shaming it would make Mommie Dearest look like Mother Teresa.

If you answered yes to any of these questions, this is the book for you!

What people are saying about Fat & Furious...

Instead of a "one size fits all" diet, alternative medicine understands that everyone requires a unique plan to shed weight and regain their health. Use the information in this book and make the commitment to positive change. Your health, not just your waistline, depends on it!

– Burton Goldberg, publisher, *The Alternative Guide to Weight Loss*

Loree Taylor Jordan debunks the theory that "eat less, exercise more" is the only way to lose weight. This book explains how dietary factors, stress, toxicity, nutrient insufficiencies, food sensitivity reactions, insufficient rest, emotional factors, hormonal imbalances, and various metabolic dysfunctions all need to be considered to achieve your goal of losing body fat.

– David Ramsey, DC, director of The New Life Health Center

Ms. Jordan takes a bold approach to discussing underlying metabolic dysfunction. Although hypothyroid can be elusive, some detective work can often clinch the diagnosis and lead to appropriate treatment.

– Ralph J. Luciani, DO, MS, Ph.D., MD (H), founder and medical director of the Albuquerque Clinic

This very through, entertaining, and informative book is all about balance! It addresses balancing the hormones as the key to weight loss success. Ms. Jordan takes a no-nonsense approach to finding health care providers who will step outside the box to assist their patients.

– C. Richard Mabray, MD, author of *Lose Weight, Not Your Health*

Fat and Furious *addresses the often overlooked endocrine-based problems of unwanted weight. Obesity is a chief complaint in my medical practice. The subject is confusing to the public and poorly understood by the medical profession. This book could not have come at a better time!*

— Ron Manzanero, MD, specializing in alternative therapies and integrative practice

Every patient who has been told that their thyroid is normal should take this book to their physician. The new guidelines from the American Association of Clinical Endocrinologists will increase the number of people diagnosed with hypothyroid from 60 to 100 million. Frustrated patients and physicians alike MUST read this book!

— Howard Hagglund, MD, author of *Why Do I Feel So Bad (When the Doctor Says I'm O.K.)?*

The public needs a book like this to learn the foundations of good health. Poor diet, stress, nutritional deficiencies (minerals, vitamins, essential fatty acids), organ dysfunction (digestion, adrenal, liver, kidney, etc.), and toxic accumulation will lead to hormone disorders (thyroid, PMS, menopausal), metabolic, and weight problems.

— David Overton, PA-C, author of *Functional and Nutritional Blood Chemistry: What the Numbers Really Mean*

Fat and Furious *addresses many of the issues I face every day in my medical practice. Patients are overwhelmed with stress, struggling with hormonal imbalances, and handling anxieties and disappointments by using food to dull frightening emotions. This comprehensive book empowers the reader.*

— David Parrish, MD, multi-specialty practice in endocrinology

Loree Taylor Jordan addresses the shame and humiliation of those caught in the trap of misdiagnosis by mainstream doctors. The effects of misdiagnosis or inadequate treatment of people with thyroid disorders are devastating. Thyroid disease and thyroid hormone resistance can cause patients who have exercised faithfully, eaten wholesome diets, and taken supplements to fail in their attempts to lose weight and become healthier. This book gives hope to those at their wit's end with frustration.

– Dr. Gina Honeyman-Lowe, co-author of
Your Guide to Metabolic Health

Many doctors will brush off patients with "normal" laboratory results. Congratulations to Ms. Jordan for her determination to break through the barrier of ignorance prevalent in the medical community.

– Neal Rouzier, MD, author *of Natural Hormone Replacement for Men and Women: How to Achieve Healthy Aging,*
Director of the Preventive Medicine Clinics of the Desert

Losing weight is not a final destination—it's an ongoing journey, one that we continue throughout our lives. I know that you'll be glad to have Loree beside you on this journey. After I read Fat and Furious, *I certainly was.*

– Mary Shomon, patient advocate and
author of *Living Well with Hypothyroidism*

Fat and Furious *will assist readers in learning about their own metabolism and hormones.*

– John Hipps, MD, author of
The Country Doctor: Alive and Well

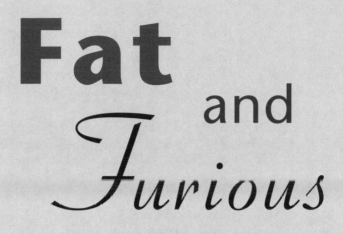

Fat and *Furious*

Overcome your body's resistance to weight loss now!

Loree Taylor Jordan, CCH, ID

MADISON PUBLISHING ✦ CALIFORNIA

Madison Publishing
P.O. Box 231
Campbell, CA 95009
(408) 379-6534

Illustrations by Steve Ferchaud
Book design by Sara Patton

ISBN #0-9679878-9-x
Library of Congress #2003114237

Printed in the USA

The information in this book is for educational purposes only and should not be used to diagnose or treat diseases. If you have a serious health challenge you should consult a competent health practitioner or doctor. It is your responsibility and privilege to gain knowledge and wisdom about your own body so that you may enjoy optimal health. Educational materials produced by the author's company, LTJ Associates, are an independent effort.

Contents

FEEDING THE HUNGRY HEART 1

Chapter 1   The Payoff for Staying Fat 3

The Reasons for Losing Weight 4

The Reasons for *Not* Losing Weight
(The Payoff for Staying Fat) 8

Chapter 2   Oh . . . The Games We Play 12

Using Food for the Wrong Reasons 13

Beating Yourself Up with Limiting Beliefs 18

Chapter 3   Feelings Buried Alive Never Die 24

Healing the Child Within 25

Denying Feelings 26

Repressing Feelings 27

Going Into the Dark 29

Chapter 4   The Feelings Behind the Fork 37

Food Responsibility 38

Chapter 5   The Shame Game 42

The Critic 45

Negative Beliefs and Food Abuse 46
by Deirdra Price, Ph.D.

Using Shame as Leverage 49

Beware of Finger-Pointers in White
Lab Coats... 52

Chapter 6   Recovery of Your Self-Esteem 58

Self-Esteem Tools 60

METABOLIC MAYHEM.. 67

Chapter 7   My Day of Reckoning 69

Chapter 8   If Your Diet Doesn't Fit You,
How Can Your Clothes? 80
                by Robban A. Sica, MD

What Types of Diets Have You Tried? 80

An Effective Diet Has Nothing to Do
with Starvation or Deprivation 82

Biochemical Individuality 83

Carbohydrate Sensitivity and
Insulin Resistance 84

So What's Wrong with the Food Pyramid? 85

Thyroid Function and Metabolic Rate 89

The Delicate Hormone Balance......................... 90

Balancing Adrenal Function 91

What About Female Hormones? 91

What About Male Hormones? 93

Adequacy of Trace Minerals 94

Digestion and Absorption 95

Toxicity 95

Food Allergy 96

Metabolic Type and Blood Type 98

The Body-Mind Connection 101

Chapter 9   Medical Doctors Speak Out About
Metabolic Imbalance 105

Metabolic Rehab Is Necessary for Many
to Overcome an Impaired Metabolism 105
by Gina Honeyman-Lowe, DC

It's All About Balance 111
by C. Richard Mabray, MD

Pursue Your Bliss and Strive for Emotional
Balance 116
by David Parrish, MD

Hormone Havoc is Prevalent 118
by David Overton, PA-C

Obesity is a Common Complaint 120
by Ron Manazero, MD

Many Doctors Will Brush Off Patients
with "Normal" Laboratory Tests 122
by Neal Rouzier, MD

Hypothyroidism: An Undertreated Illness 127
by Ralph J. Luciani, DO

How to Determine If You Have a Slow
Metabolism 129
by Dr. Joseph Debé

Chapter 10 Real People, Real Case Studies 132

Clinical Patients 132
by Neal Rouzier, MD

Hormone Havoc 134
by David Overton, PA-C

Patients Deserve to be Treated with Dignity
and Respect, Not a Five-Minute Diagnosis 145
by John G. Hipps, MD

Chapter 11 Replacing Hormones Naturally 150

My TSH Levels are "Normal," but I Think
I'm Hypothyroid 151
by Mary Shomon

Treating Hypothyroidism Naturally 151

A Hypoallergenic Treatment for
Hypothyroidism 152
by Som N. Sok

Natural Thyroid in Practice 153
by Howard Hagglund, MD

The Patient Experience 156
by Mary Shomon

Perimenopause and Menopause:
Natural Solutions 158

Female Hormone Replacement Naturally 158
by Ralph J. Luciani, DO

Chapter 12 Can Stress Make You Fat? 164

Cortisol, the Stress Hormone 164

Adrenal Fatigue Is the Price of Stress 168
by James Wilson, DC

Chapter 13 But I Can't Live Without My Chocolate! 172

Insulin Resistance and Syndrome X 172

Sugar or Alcohol: Choose Your Poison 173

Carbohydrate Addiction 175

The Two Insulin Phases 177

Insulin Resistance: Glucose Transport
Disorder 179

Symptom X: The Hidden Disease You
May Already Have 182
          by Jack Challem

Children, Sugar Addiction, and Obesity 188

Parents as Role Models 190

DETOXIFY YOUR BODY! 193

Chapter 14 Detoxify Your Colon 195

Autointoxication 195

What Is Autointoxication? 196

Medical Opinion 197

Alternative Opinion 198

Internal Toxemia 199

Death Begins in the Colon 199
          by Dr. Bernard Jensen

A Lesson from Lucy 200

Nutritional Abuse 200

Fiber Foods 201

Constipation Defined 202

Primary Causes of Constipation 203

Differences of Opinion 206

Denial Is Not a River In Egypt (More About
Loree Than You Ever Cared to Know!) 207

Medical Objections to Colon Cleansing 208

Chapter 15   You Want to Cleanse My *What,*
Put Water *Where*? 210

The Real Scoop on Colon Cleansing:
The Colonic Queen Tells All 211

Real Men Get Colonics 213

For Bulimics 213

Powerpoopin' 214

Chapter 16   Removing Parasites Can Reverse
Weight Gain 219

Did You Say Parasites? 219

What You Absolutely Have to Know
About Parasites 220

Should I Get Tested for Parasites? 222

Sources of Parasitic Infestation 224

Parasites Can Eat Human Bodies 229

More About Parasites 229

Been There, Done That 231

A Word About Tapeworms 232

Removing Parasites from Our Bodies 232

Chapter 17   Staying in the Cleansing Flow:
Water, Kidneys, Lymph 237

The Cleansing Power of Water 238

Water, Not Sodas 239

Live Water vs. Dead Water 241

The Kidneys 242

The Lymphatic System 243

Cellulite 244

Chapter 18   Love Your Liver: Flushing Away the Pounds 246

The Role of the Gallbladder 249

You Need to Detoxify Your Liver and
Gallbladder 249

A Word About Gallstones 249

Cholesterol Deprivation Can Cause
Gallstones 251

Toxic Emotions 253

**PHYSICAL MASTERY:
EXERCISE, DIET, AND NUTRITION 255**

Chapter 19   Training Day with Mr. Universe 257

Chapter 20   Exercise, Training, and Metabolism 277

An Interview with Ladislav Pataki, Ph.D. 278

A Celebrity Legend 282

Monitoring Your Metabolism 283

Overexercising to Lose Body Fat Quickly
is Not an Option 284

Chapter 21   A Word About Diet 288

Chapter 22   Balancing Body Chemistry for Weight Loss 291

Acid/Alkaline Balance in Weight Loss 291

High Alkalinity in the Body 293

Acid Alkaline Self-Test: Have You Checked
Your pH Today? 294

Enzymes Assist the Metabolic Process 296

What are Enzymes? 297

Chapter 23   Nature's Pharmacy 300

Bowel Detoxification 300

Blood Sugar and Glandular Balance 303

Glandular Support for Women 311

Glandular Support for Men 312

Kidneys, the Urinary System 313

Liver Cleansing and Support 315

Lymphatic System Cleansing 318

Parasites 319

Stress Support for the Nervous System 321

Vital Nutritional Support 323

Weight Loss 326

**PUTTING IT ALL TOGETHER:
LET THE MAGIC BEGIN 331**

Chapter 24   On the Lighter Side 333

Greta's Dream Diet 334

Donuts Are a Girl's Best Friend 335

Kids: Don't You Just Love Them? 337

Chapter 25   I Love *Me*! Self-Honoring Behaviors 339

Personal Relationships.....................................339

Emotional/Feelings 341

Physical/Fitness 341

Confidence Boosters 343

Chapter 26   Follow the Yellow Brick Road 345

Toto, We're Not In Kansas Anymore 345

Take a Leap of Faith 346

Love Yourself Now . . . Live Your Life Now
. . . Stop Waiting Until 348

Be Willing and Open to the Process of
Support 350

Searching for Dr. Right! 351

This Too Shall Pass 352

Attitude of Gratitude 353

Afterword 356

Resource Guide..357

Recommended Reading 372

References 379

This book is dedicated to those of you who are still struggling . . . with the zipper of your jeans or the pain in your heart.

Acknowledgments

I especially want to thank all the health professionals who contributed their incredible knowledge to *Fat and Furious.* Their generosity and cooperative spirit has made this book possible.

My wholehearted appreciation goes to Jack J. Challem; Ed Corney; Ann Louis Gittleman, MS; Howard Hagglund, MD; John Hipps, MD; Dr. Gina-Honeyman-Lowe; Ralph J. Luciani, MD; C. Richard Mabray, MD; Ron Manzanero, MD; David Parrish, MD; L. Pataki, Ph.D.; Deirdra Price, Ph.D.; Neal Rouzier, MD; Robban A. Sica, MD; and Melissa Diane Smith.

I would also like to thank Char Balanesi, my personal assistant, for her tireless dedication and coordination efforts in bringing *Fat and Furious* to the finish line! Char persevered with precision at times when this book project was as challenging as a corporate merger. I am grateful for her patience on days when I didn't have *any!*

Thank you to my fabulous dream team: Kathi Dunn of Dunn+Associates (who I swear can see inside my head) for her incredible cover design; Sara Patton for her talented interior design; Steve Ferchaud, who is an incredible cartoonist; Susan Kendrick for her cover copy writing; and last but not least Despina Gurlides and Anna van Raaporst-Johnson for their copy editing.

You are all, truly, the wind beneath my wings.

Fear less, hope more;
eat less, chew more;
whine less, breathe more;
talk less, say more;
love more, and all
good things will be yours.

– Swedish proverb

Foreword

■ ■ ■ ■ ■ ■ ■ ■ ■ ■

There are very few of us who can say, truthfully, that our self-image is not tied up with how much we weigh.

I'm not saying that there aren't a hundred terrific reasons to lose weight—better health and longevity, in particular—but so often what it comes down to is that we want to lose weight so we can simply feel good about ourselves. We want to feel attractive. We want to feel *normal*. We don't want others to look at us with pity, disdain, or worse yet, to not even look at us at all.

So we diet. And we exercise. And we cut out the fat . . . or the carbs . . . or the calories . . . or meat. Or we take fat-blaster pills and carb-blocker pills and appetite suppressants and thermogenics. Or we go round and round on the merry-go-round of fad diets—downing apple cider vinegar this week, cabbage soup next week, and peanut butter after that. Or we read fashion magazines and are told that the magic answer is what all the size 2 celebrities are doing—so we "Zone," we "do Atkins," we do "South Beach," and Pilates, and bosu balls, and yoga in 100-degree rooms, and to keep us company, there's Dr. Phil hollering in the background, and "figgerin' out whether it's workin' fer us."

With all the tools and information out there, how is it that so many people try so many different ways to lose weight, yet fail to lose the weight? In *Fat and Furious*, Loree Taylor Jordan suggests that it's attitude—the relationship with ourselves and with our bodies—that makes the difference.

And she's right.

Many of us have a dysfunctional relationship with the idea of weight and the failure to lose it. This becomes so ingrained that the number on the scale each morning dictates whether we're going to have a confident, "feeling great about myself" day, or a self-loathing, depressing, just plain rotten day!

I've had days ruined simply because the scale was not my friend that morning. I'll mope around all day, telling myself I'm a blob, and beating myself up emotionally. The end result? I *ensure* that I will have a bad day. And when you're moping around, I promise you, you *look* like a blob! And the next day, when the very same me climbs on the scale and gets good news, I'm on top of the world, feeling great. I stand taller, take a little extra time with hair and makeup, and walk around as if I'm fabulous. And guess what? I'm no different from day to day! But if you saw me on one of those "good" days, you'd say, "Hey, she looks good!" Why? Because I am *feeling* good about myself.

It's all about attitude.

Attitude will get you everywhere, or it will get you nowhere. And rethinking your attitude is a key feature of Loree's refreshing approach. *Fat and Furious* is not a lame pep talk about how if only you eat less and move more all your weight problems will be solved. Sure, diet and exercise are part of the equation, but they are not the end-all. Loree talks realistically about the other equally important issues you need to explore in order to lose weight. For example, Loree hones in on the "inner exercise" we all need to do to figure out what might be keeping us in unhealthy eating patterns. And when it comes to diet, Loree rightly considers cutting out self-criticism as *far more important* than cutting back on carbohydrates or calories.

Loree also gets into a topic that is particularly near and dear to my heart: the medical issues—in particular, thyroid disease— that can contribute to weight problems and sabotage weight loss efforts. Loree and I both share the struggle of having gained weight with a thyroid condition, and the frustration of trying to get that weight off. We both agree that thyroid conditions aren't an excuse for weight gain, but they certainly make it easier to gain, and harder to lose. Thyroid disease means that what is already a challenge for most people—losing weight—becomes even harder. But Loree and the practitioners she has consulted offer suggestions that may help even out the playing field.

One of the most amazing things about Loree is how she is so unflinchingly honest about the struggles she has faced. We all muddle through life's challenges, but Loree has tackled more than her fair share, and with unusual grace and courage. She brings that same grace and courage to *Fat and Furious*. When you carry around a heavy heart and mind, there is often a heavy body to match. So there's no doubt in my mind that Loree's willingness to be so open in sharing her own life's struggles is part of her successful approach to weight loss.

In the end, Loree is also willing to tell us that she hasn't lost all the weight she wants to, yet, but she *has* figured out what's working for her, and she's on the right path. And in sharing this, Loree is perhaps sharing the most important thing of all to learn and remember: Losing weight is not a final destination, it's an ongoing journey, one that we continue on throughout our lives.

I know that you'll be glad to have Loree beside you on this journey. After I read *Fat and Furious*, I certainly was.

– Mary Shomon
October 2003

Mary Shomon is the founder of several popular websites on thyroid disease, including www.thyroid-info.com and thyroid.about.com. She is also the author of a number of bestselling books and guides, including Living Well With Hypothyroidism: What Your Doctor Doesn't Tell You ... That You Need to Know; Living Well with Autoimmune Disease; The Thyroid Diet Guide; *and* The Thyroid Guide to Fertility, Pregnancy, and Breastfeeding Success. *She publishes a newsletter for thyroid patients called "Sticking Out Our Necks."*

Preface

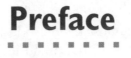

*Believe, when you are most unhappy, that there
is something for you to do in the world.*

— Helen Keller

I think when most babies cried for breast milk I cried for
Oreos. I was never overweight as a child, but I had a desire for
sweets at a very young age. I developed very young; that is a
polite way of saying that I had breasts in the fourth grade. I
always looked more physically mature than my years. When I
was 10 years old, I looked 16. I remember I was at my father's
company picnic one summer, wearing a bathing suit like all
the other girls, and a teenage boy tried to make the moves on
me. My father just about had a coronary and told this young
man in no uncertain terms that I was only 10 years old for
Pete's sake, and to beat it.

The reason I am sharing this with you is to point out that I
became aware of my body—the attention my physical appearance attracted—at a very young age. Even though I was not
overweight, I started *dieting* at the age of 12, trying to fit in
with the teenage girls. Because I saw everyone else was dieting,
I thought it was the thing to do. I remember the Dr. Stillman
diet was popular at the time. This diet was big on protein; I ate
hard-boiled eggs and cottage cheese until I thought I would
puke. This diet also required lots of water, water, and then
more water. I swear I thought my teeth would float right out
of my head!

This kind of radical dieting continued through high school:

eating sweets and then starving for days as a way of repenting for my sugar sins. I was always waking up from a sugar coma. As a teenager, I worked at a pizza parlor as a cashier. Since I was able to eat there for free, I would eat a small pizza around 4:00 P.M. in the afternoon, and then starve until 4:00 P.M. the next day. When I wasn't on this crazy diet, I was eating a school lunch (with Oreos for dessert, of course) and then going without food for 24 hours until the next day, when I would repeat this same routine. I was known around high school as the Oreo kid, because I always had Oreos in my school locker.

When I was 16 years old, my family had a terrible blow: my mother was diagnosed with breast cancer. Of course, I went into denial that my mother could actually die from this disease. Right on the heels of this diagnosis and her radical mastectomy followed my parents' divorce after 19 years of marriage. All of these life-changing events, and the resulting stress, were just about unbearable for me. I found solace in eating, which numbed my emotions. I would have been better off crying and letting out the feelings that I felt were drowning me. After two years—during which I took care of her—my mother finally lost her battle to the disease. On October 12, 1973, she passed away quietly in her sleep.

An 18-year-old woman needs her mother. To say that I was devastated is an understatement. I was numb and in shock. I could barely function. I had to go on and accept what was handed to me, but I felt cheated to have lost my mother at such a young age. When I was a bride walking down the aisle to my husband-to-be, I was smiling, but there was emptiness and an ache in my heart. My mother wasn't there to share my special wedding day.

Since I did not want children right away after marriage, I used the birth control pill for several years. The pill added about 15 pounds that I just could not get rid of, no matter what I did. My new husband was not happy with the extra pounds either, and had no problem telling me about it. So again, I began starving myself with radical dieting, but I didn't drop those extra 15 pounds until I got off the pill.

I was so hooked into having a perfect body that I was willing to try anything and everything to lose weight, and believe me when I tell you that I did! I don't know if you remember the HGC hormone shots (the urine of pregnant woman) that came out in the '70s. This program consisted of getting shots every day and staying on a 500-calorie diet. A rabbit would have had a better chance at gaining weight than anyone trying this diet. I know you are saying to yourself, "Oh no, she didn't!" Well I did, only this story gets worse.

My girlfriends and I found a doctor who would sell us the HGC, as well as all the accompanying supplies (syringes and needles), so we could give the shots to ourselves. Now if this does not scream desperation with a capital "D" I don't know what does. To stand there every morning and stick a needle into my own ass . . . now that is crazy! All my girlfriends were doing it too, so I guess insanity loves company.

Well, the ass-shot diet worked! I was down to a sickly weight of 108 pounds. After a few weeks my body adjusted to a more comfortable 115 pounds. Now comes the part that you are not going to believe. Usually when you lose weight on a radical fad diet, it is hard to keep it off. Well, the good news is that I did keep the weight off for two years. My undoing was that I decided to have a child. A great decision for me personally, but not great for my figure.

The minute the sperm met the egg it was instant obesity for me. I wish I could say that I only gained 25 pounds, but I would be lying. I had a huge 10-pound baby son and gained a lot of weight and excess water. Let's see: 10-pound baby, 25 pounds of water, 20 pounds of fat, well . . . you do the math. It is pretty humiliating when your ob-gyn asks you to put your *piano legs* up on the stirrups. I swear, if someone stuck me with a pin I would have caused a flood. I dropped 25 pounds of water three days after my son was born. However, I still felt as if I had a body as wide as the state of Texas, with flab hanging everywhere, when I came home with my beautiful son, Brandon. So I kept dieting, dieting, and dieting, until I was back in a bikini in a few months.

My second son, Christopher, was born 22 months after Brandon. I did not gain as much weight the second time around, but I was not a slender pregnant mother either. Getting the weight off the second time proved to be a real challenge. There I was with 30 extra pounds, a nursing infant, and a very active toddler. It was difficult to get out and exercise, so radical dieting seemed to be the only logical recourse. I weaned Christopher at the age of six months (a decision I regretted later) so I could begin starving myself with my radical approach to dieting.

I took dieting to the extreme, fasting one solid month on just water! Yes, you read that right: just plain water, nothing else. My in-laws watched me as if I was going to keel over any minute. Actually I felt pretty good once I got used to not eating.

Is there a pattern here? I was a radical dieting maniac out of control. My behavior suggested I had no common sense. I was either eating all the contents of the refrigerator, or eating an ice cube for dinner, with no sense of moderation. It was always all or nothing! All this overeating and starving really affected my metabolism. Believe me, it gets worse. I even repeated the Stillman diet, even though I thought I could never eat a hard-boiled egg again if my life depended on it.

I also got into the diet pill trap. Because I worked in a dental office I had access to diet pills through one of the drug companies. Not only was I becoming a diet pill junkie, I was distributing them to my friends as well. I felt terrible all the time — shaky, irritable — and if you looked at me the wrong way I could snap you like a twig. PMS could not hold a candle to me on a diet pill day. No wonder I was so good at collecting payments at the dental office; I think the patients were afraid of me. I was going days without eating, acting like an anorexic on speed. I was losing weight, wasn't I? The sad fact is that I was doing all this for a mere 10 to 15 pounds. Well, I got the weight off again and back to my slender 115 pounds, but it was a two-year ordeal, or should I say hell?

In 1983, my husband left me. If I knew then what I know now, I would have rejoiced, changed the locks, and hired an attorney; but hindsight is 20/20. I was such an emotional wreck that I would go days without eating. I was very depressed, and all I could do was cry. When I did try to eat, I felt sick to my stomach. After about three months I decided I could not go on like that. I became proactive in my own healing process. I sought counseling to deal with my emotions around a crumbling marriage.

I decided to take up running to get the endorphins flowing and get out of my funk. I had two beautiful sons who needed their mother. However, I was so physically depleted I felt like I was going to pass out from running. I remember running around the track and an older gentleman was resting after his run, watching me. As I was gasping for air and sucking wind around the track, I asked him, "How long before you start liking this?" He said to me, "Do this for a couple of weeks and you will be hooked." I did, and I was hooked. I ran for years after that and was in my best shape ever. Women who think they can't get in shape after they have children are shortchanging themselves. I was in better shape after kids than before. I looked and felt so great that my husband was begging me to let him move back in, which I did. Well, this husband issue is a whole other story, believe me, but for brevity's sake, I will say that I was still too codependent to let him go at that point.

During this time that I was running, I also became somewhat of a zealot for holistic nutrition. I developed a passion for natural healing, massage therapy, and nutrition. The dental field was just not my passion, and in 1986, I left it to create my own holistic health practice. With my busy schedule, exercise was put on the back burner, and I began to put weight back on. It was only about 20 pounds or so, but to me it felt like 100!

Natural nutrition put a whole new slant on my weight issue and radical dieting. When I worked in the dental office, no one cared if I had a little weight on me. But as a health mentor, being overweight was not a positive attribute. Even though I was practicing what I was preaching, I still had extra weight that was hanging on for dear life. As you will see, I did not understand a key issue in fat reduction. I had ruined my fat-burning metabolism with all my starving and radical dieting. I just didn't understand this at the time.

In 1988, after another marital separation (okay, I was still in codependent denial), this time for a year, I was diagnosed with Epstein Barr virus, also known as chronic fatigue syndrome, and confined to bed for about six months. Well, was this a surprise? I was under tremendous physical stress trying to look like a cover model for *Vogue* (dieting and dieting), and under emotional stress, plus running my own business and raising two sons.

My body had just collapsed completely. I was told by the doctor to eat every three hours during this time. Without running to offset this calorie intake, I put on weight very easily. I swear, just breathing air was making me gain weight. Well, you have to understand that I had no metabolism at this point— I think it died when I was eating hard-boiled eggs at age 12— so everything I ate went right to fat.

I was very sick, and my life consisted of getting IV's at the doctor's office for six hours, giving myself shots (this brought back horrible ass-sticking memories, let me tell you), taking herbs and supplements, and lying in bed. Taking a shower was a major ordeal. I swear, my carpet had more energy than I did for those six months! Little did I know that my *thin days* were behind me. It would be 14 years before I would learn about the lasting effects on my metabolism of that illness and all of my radical dieting. This will all be explained later in detail.

Later that year, as I recovered, I became a vegetarian. Even though I was eating clean (with no meats or dairy), I was consuming a lot of nonfat carbohydrates. It was nonfat, right? I was still gaining weight. What I did not realize at this time was that I was setting myself up for a carbohydrate intolerance and blood sugar problems. As I mentioned in the beginning of my story, I have had a weakness for sweets my whole life, and even though I was not eating what I call hard-core sugar sweets, I was getting it secondhand through carbohydrates. I was eating a lot of rice, beans, pasta, bread, etc. I was still putting my body through glycemic hell without realizing how intolerant my body had become to carbohydrates.

Despite my very active life, my weight was increasing to what I felt was an intolerable level. Even though I thought I was dieting, my body was not cooperating with me. I was a fat-making machine. My same old diet tricks weren't working anymore. I was so furious and frustrated that nothing was working! Was I sitting on my butt? No! I was working out with a trainer provided by the gym and getting fatter by the minute. My trainer was loading me with carbs and then shaming me for not losing weight. Hell if I knew, I was doing everything he said and *eating* everything he said. I did not know then, I was carbohydrate intolerant. Just being in the same room with a white potato, let alone eating one, would send me to fat prison with no hope of a pardon. A trainer who treats everyone the same has got the brains God gave a barbell. We are all metabolically different and need to be treated as such. We will talk later about how to find a personal trainer who is right for you and your special needs.

From 1989 through 1993, I suffered from some extremely stressful setbacks. In 1989, my newly purchased home was wrecked in the Loma Prieta earthquake. In 1991, my holistic health business was completely burned to the ground by an arsonist, and I lost everything I had worked years to obtain. As my stress level increased, so did my weight. I used food to cope. Forget a glass of wine to relax—give me some Oreos! I used to joke and say that every natural disaster was equal to at least 20 pounds. Even though I have a sense of humor and I joked about these events, it was taking its toll on me and my ever-expanding body.

To really tip the scale towards "oh no, how much more can I take?" my emotionally and verbally abusive marriage was on the final stretch of insanity. It had become intolerable for me. After two separations and much counseling, my marriage was sinking like the *Titanic,* with no lifeboat in sight. I felt completely hopeless at this point in my life, and to make matters worse, my self-esteem was in the toilet. I hated my life and the way I looked. A doctor suggested that I try antidepressants. I told him I didn't need an antidepressant; I needed a *divorce.* In January of 1995, after 21 years of marriage, I filed for a divorce. Oh great, I thought, now I will be *divorced and fat!*

My soon-to-be-ex-husband and I sat down with a yellow legal pad to divide our assets. I remember him saying to me that even though we had been through a lot together, he "deserved to have someone thin." After all the years of lost hopes and dreams, tears, being parents, marriage partners, all that mattered to him was having a wife who was *thin!* Oh, don't get me started!

The next year was a complete blur for me, trying to readjust to my new single situation. I had to move, sell my dream home, and move on with my life. Did I mention crying here? There was a great deal of crying that year. I was now on my own, with a broken heart, the mother of two teenage sons. Being the parent of teenagers can be brutal, especially if you are doing it alone. I wanted peace of mind. *I wanted my life back with my fit body to match.* I managed to lose some weight after the divorce, but not enough to get into my small sexy clothes. Not that I was thinking of men at this point, but I wanted to feel attractive and good about myself. I had felt so unnoticed and unseen for so many years in my marriage, I wanted to turn heads. No, if the truth be told, I wanted to break necks.

They say that when the student is ready the teacher will appear. Well, he appeared all right, in the form of a 200-pound-plus Czechoslovakian world-class champion athlete. In April of 1997, Ladislav Pataki, Ph.D., walked into my life. I met him at the office where I have my holistic health practice. I expressed my complete frustration with my lack of success in trying to lose weight. This was the beginning of a great friendship, both personally and professionally, and tremendous support for me.

Dr. Pataki began to teach me what I had done to my body, with all my radical dieting and fasting. I had trained my body to store fat. I now realized that I had created the very issue in my body I was trying so hard to avoid—being overweight. I learned that when you are starving all the time, your body goes into alarm and actually stores fat. I had stopped my metabolism from working on its own. Many of you have done the same thing to your body's metabolism. You have dieted yourself into obesity! Some metabolism issues are self-induced and some are just plain metabolic dysfunction (such as thyroid).

Dr. Pataki is one of a number of teachers I had in my "metabolic transformation and trusting the process" experience. I will share these teachings with you here and now so you too can stop riding this crazy dieting train we have all ridden. I mean, sticking a syringe needle in your own ass to lose weight—that is about as insane as it gets!

Many of you have picked up this book because you are sick

of being *fat*; this "F" word, along with other "F" words, is always on the tip of your tongue. You know what other "F" words I am talking about: *fed up, furious, frustrated, failure, frumpy.* Many of you have been humiliated, as I have, by well-meaning family and friends who think they owe it to you to let you know you are fat! They somehow think it has escaped your attention that you are now wearing clothes six sizes larger! God forbid that you would tell them you have a whole department store of sizes in your closet, ranging from size 6 to 16! *We get it,* people! We don't need you judging us daily that we are lazy, or we don't care about ourselves, or if we would just exercise and watch what we eat, we would lose weight. If one more person says to me, "If you would just exercise more [let's see *them* run 13 miles] or [blah, blah, blah . . .] I know you would lose some weight" you may see me on the 6 o'clock news appearing in an orange jumpsuit at my court arraignment for inflicting bodily harm! We wrestle with the bathroom scale and the zipper of our jeans like a fireman struggles with a three-alarm fire every day of our lives.

If you feel that you've tried every diet known to mankind and you are desperate, fat, and furious, please know that I truly understand how you feel. As the saying goes, "Been there, done that!" This book does not give you excuses or absolve you of self-responsibility, nor does it shame you into losing weight. I honestly know you have tried. *Fat and Furious* is written to give you experience, strength, and hope. This book is written to assist you in getting really honest with yourself, and give you answers with compassionate understanding. There may be a real metabolic issue you are unaware of which is truly not your fault.

As I open my heart and share my personal experiences, feelings, and struggles, I am not some doctor standing at a podium barking statistics, I am you, and you are me. We have shared experiences of shame and guilt. My friend, do not allow your value to be measured by a number on the scale. I know you have tried your whole life to wrestle the bear to the ground—or the zipper on your pants—to come out alive and victorious. My promise to you is that you will be victorious. You will become you. You will become one with your body and soul in a way you could have never imagined. We will laugh together, we will cry together, we will grow together. Welcome to the journey, my friend. Welcome home!

If you want to understand others, look into your own heart.
— Johann Schiller

The deepest need of man is to overcome his separateness to leave the prison of his aloneness.
— Eric Fromm

Feeding the Hungry Heart

*There's only one corner of the universe
you can be certain of improving, and
that's your own self.*

– Aldous Huxley

*It's a long road, but I know
I'm gonna find the end.*

– Bessie Smith

The great enemy of the truth is very often not the lie — deliberate, contrived, and dishonest; but the myth — persistent, persuasive, and unrealistic.

– John F. Kennedy

If you truly want to understand something try to change it.

– Kurt Lewin

CHAPTER 1

■ ■ ■ ■ ■ ■ ■ ■ ■

The Payoff for Staying Fat

The most sincere love of all is the love of food.

– George Bernard Shaw

One of the primary issues to examine when we deal with weight issues is: What is the person's emotional attachment to fat? I know you are screaming at me saying, "But I want this fat to be gone in the worst way!" Yes, I honestly believe you; but what is the unknown emotional undercurrent that may be keeping you fat? If you think that your subconscious is not capable of self-sabotage, think again.

On the one hand you are desperately searching for the Holy Grail in the diet industry, looking for every new diet in the universe. You are pumping yourself up with all the reasons you have to succeed this time. This is not idle talk this time. No, you are on a mission. You are a dieting maniac running with the hordes, following the latest diet guru's advice. You are so determined and regimented you would make a drill sergeant look like a wimp and a weenie. You will go after every fat roll and cellulite dimple like a heat-seeking missile. Your scale is standing at attention, ready for weigh-ins. You will succeed. Damn, you're good!

On the other hand, as you will see later in this chapter, you can play games with yourself. You tell yourself and everyone around you that you are determined to get the weight off, but there are emotional payoffs for staying fat. It is my goal, and hopefully yours, to truly do some soul-searching and discover what is really brewing emotionally at a soul level. You will have to do some homework because you can't change what you don't acknowledge.

THE REASONS FOR LOSING WEIGHT

Let's look at some of the reasons that you tell yourself you just have to succeed at all costs to lose the weight. Do any of these reasons sound familiar? Maybe with someone you know intimately?

To look better. There is no denying it—you would be more attractive without the excess weight. Maybe you're not so bad now, but without those extra pounds hanging around you would be so hot!

To gain self-confidence. Boy, when you get thin, the world better watch out. You'll be a dynamo. Nothing will be able to stop you then. You will be able to go anywhere and get exactly what you want. Don't anybody even think about raining on your parade!

To be healthier. No more worrying about all those diseases and health conditions that you thought being overweight would make you a target of. You don't want to walk around with a bull's-eye on your chest, just waiting to keel over from your arteries hardening. You'll be the perfect specimen of health. You are going to outlive everybody.

To get attention. When you go out to lunch with friends, you can tell them you're on a diet. They'll feel sorry for you and ask you all about it. "What kind of diet is it? How does it work? How much have you lost?" If you didn't have this on-again off-again weight issue, you might not have anything to say.

For a big event. It could be a party, a vacation, a class reunion, a wedding, a date, or any occasion where you want to look your best. You plan to lose the weight right before you go, so you won't have a chance to gain it all back.

For relationships. You want to be attractive to the opposite sex or wish to rekindle your present relationship. Or maybe you just got divorced and want to go out there and show the single world that you are really hot!

For that special someone. This is your big chance. If you blow it with this person, there may never be another. Besides, you want to please him or her. You want to show this person how sexually attractive you really are—without the blubber rolls. Without this fat you are really hot! Really!

For the doctor. Either he already told you that you have to lose weight, or you have an appointment scheduled and you know the drill. You know he's going to make you get on the scale, and you can just see his eyebrows rising.

To get a new job or promotion. You're going to breeze into that office looking like a million bucks and get that promotion or that new job. As a matter of fact you are going to look so good that they are going to beg you to take the position, and offer you more money.

To be better in sports. Having 20 or 30 fewer pounds to lug around might make it easier. You feel so bloated and tired you can't even get started.

To look younger. The fat is making you look older before your time. When people see a picture of your face, they think you're pretty young, but when they see a picture of your whole body, they guess that you're 15 years older.

It's summer. Summer is here, with summer sports, sun-bathing, and bikinis. Your throat is closing up in absolute panic just thinking about it. How can you go to the beach with all those semi-naked bodies? Oh my God, you are screaming to yourself, do you think anyone will notice if I show up wearing my bedspread? Big sweaters and baggy sweat pants are not going to be of much help here. Now what?

For new clothing. Every new fashion magazine or catalog is a new quest for thinness—a new diet waiting to happen. You want to be a walking fashion statement. You want to wear all those skinny teeny weenie clothes in your closet that you have saved for years (probably from the eighth grade—you know the ones I am talking about).

Out of habit. Life is an endless diet. You are a diet junkie. You wouldn't know what to do with yourself if you gave up the quest for thinness. If you weren't always on a diet, just think of how fat you would get. You don't even think about going on a diet any more—just like breathing, you just do it. It is automatic.

To prove you can. Whether you're proving it to yourself or to other people, someone is going to know you can do it. Everyone is beginning to think you can't, after all these years. It is starting to be too much for your pride. You'll show them.

To win a bet. A creative way to get thin and a little richer at the same time. Your family figures it will be less expensive than a funeral when you drop dead from a heart attack. Family and friends will bribe you to thinness. Surely winning money will motivate you, right?

To start eating again. You fantasize about how you'll look when you've lost all that weight. And where do you picture yourself? In an ice cream parlor, sitting down to the biggest banana split ever made. When you're thin, you'll be able to eat anything you want without feeling guilty. Pizzas every night with pitchers of beer. Oh, wow! You can't wait!

To end the misery. Life isn't worth living if you have to live as a fat person. Every day you feel worse about yourself. You hate the way you look, and your life. You're such a loser because you're not doing anything about it. You'll do anything to stop feeling so suicidal.

Life is going to be wonderful. You'll finally cross the river to Happy Land where all the thin people live. Everything over there is just great. Your life will be perfect. Our perception is that thin people have everything because they are not struggling with their weight. As if thin people don't have tragedies and pain in their lives.

You are absolutely furious with the nagging. Boy, you are just sick and tired of comments from family, friends, spouse, etc. It would be worth losing your fat just to shut everybody up.

Please take out your journal and start getting in touch with your deeper inner self. Go as far back in your life as you can remember. My suggestion is that you don't try to edit your thoughts; just write. You will find associations between weight and your feelings that you never even thought of before. I guarantee it. I will help guide you with some suggestions of dark hiding places in your soul that need to be examined.

Exercises

List all the reasons that have really motivated you to lose weight in the past. Write about them. Explain in as much detail as you can.

All these reasons have one thing in common: They aren't good enough. If they were, you would have already lost all your fat and kept it off. I am telling you that the body can only do what the subconscious will comply with. If you have a hidden agenda or a payoff for staying fat, all the reasons in the world won't be enough for you to lose weight.

THE REASONS FOR <u>NOT</u> LOSING WEIGHT
(The Payoff for Staying Fat)

Now let's look at why you may not have wanted to lose weight in the past.

Your health. Losing and gaining weight—again and again—can actually cause health problems. Better to stay as you are than to get on that yo-yo syndrome.

You're attractive enough already. Okay, maybe you could stand to lose a few pounds, but it's not like you are obese or anything. You don't have to lose weight to prove it. If they don't like you the way you are, who needs them?

The weight will just come back. Once you lose it, there's no way to keep it off. So why make yourself miserable trying? It's hopeless. You don't have any willpower. Where did you put that pizza delivery phone number?

Discipline is hard. What a drag! There are enough problems in life without discipline. Besides, you don't think discipline is exactly your strong point. What if you try and fail again?

People would leave you. Friends would be so envious of your beautiful new body that they wouldn't want to have anything to do with you. You'd rather keep the weight on than make them feel uncomfortable.

To save money. You would have to buy a whole new wardrobe. Everything you own would be hanging around your knees. At today's prices it'll cost a small fortune, and you don't have the money to do that right now. Better wait until you get a raise.

To prove them wrong. If they've shaken their heads and told you, as I used to tell people, that all you have to do is follow the diet and you'll be thin, then you can prove to them that it's not as easy as they think. You have a far more serious problem here than they'd imagined, and you're going to let them know it.

To punish someone. If someone doesn't like that you're fat, they've handed you the perfect weapon. Any time they step out of line, you can just head for the refrigerator. This is a very passive-aggressive move that says I will act like I care about your needs, but I will do what I want.

To feel rooted and strong. If you are living large, you can throw your weight around, and people pay attention. If the weight were gone, you might feel vulnerable and unprotected. This is a serious reason; many rape victims will put on weight to be less vulnerable to being violated again.

To be less vulnerable. The armor that protects you will be gone, exposing those tender, sensitive places inside you to everyone. The feelings you've been stuffing down may pop to the surface. Dealing with them would be scary and uncomfortable. Better to keep the fat where it is. Why rock the boat?

If you are married, it's safer to be fat. What if the whole town was after your sexy body? You don't want to upset your spouse, do you? You might become promiscuous!

You can say people reject you for your fat, and not for who you are. It's another great excuse. If someone doesn't like you or leaves you, you can say they're leaving your fat body and not the real you.

You don't deserve to be thin. On some unconscious level you might feel undeserving. Self-loathing can be a vicious cycle. You feel bad because you're fat and then you overeat to numb the pain of how bad you feel.

There might be an even bigger problem waiting. The fat issues are familiar; they feel comfortable. We all know how to handle fat — we complain about it! If it were to disappear, there might be an even bigger problem waiting in the wings. Keep the fat around, and you get to keep the other problems at bay forever.

What would you do with yourself? What would you talk about, worry about, read about, plot about? How would you occupy your time, if weight and food were no longer the big issues of your life? What would the new purpose/obsession of your life be?

There would be no more excuses. If you lost the weight, you would have to confront relationships, success, and all those things on your "after I lose weight" list. Now you can blame the fat for not having those things. Listen, you can blame almost anything on fat. It covers a multitude of sins, and who wants to blow a great excuse?

Soul-Searching Exercises

1. Make a list in your journal of any other reasons that we haven't listed that have prevented you from losing weight in the past. Please list them in detail.

2. Now list the obstacles you've come up against in the past when you have tried to have the body you wanted.

3. These are all the fears I can think of that might be stopping me from losing weight:

4. This is what I think it would take for me to break through these reasons and fears:

5. What is the first step I would have to take to break through these fears?

6. What is the next step?

What do all these reasons for not losing weight have in common? They all work! They keep you from losing weight on a subconscious level. No matter how motivated you think you are, none of your reasons for losing weight will work for you if the subconscious reasons for keeping the weight are stronger.

If you have failed in the past, you're going to have to make a complete and dramatic shift in your attitude and point of view about your emotional weight. In order to make this shift, you'll have to give up every notion you've ever had about losing weight; give up your ideas about what works and what doesn't work; and forget everything that's happened in the past. The past does not equal the future.

You are on a new journey now with a different set of beliefs. Sometimes you need to ask yourself a better set of questions. In this next chapter we are going to look at some of the emotional triggers and feelings that may be operating beneath the surface.

*I have never seen a person grow or change
in a constructive direction when motivated
by guilt, shame, and/or hate.*
– William Goldberg

*Honesty is the first chapter in the book of
wisdom.*
– Thomas Jefferson

CHAPTER 2

■ ■ ■ ■ ■ ■ ■ ■ ■

Oh...The Games We Play!

I just wish I had the courage to get it over with,
and get really FAT!

– Kathy Bates, from the movie *Fried Green Tomatoes*

We are going to look at some of the behaviors you may have developed with your relationship to food and some of the ways you have kept yourself fat. You are probably already familiar (way too familiar in fact) with some of the reasons you eat, that have nothing to do with giving your body the fuel and nutrition it needs. In this chapter you may even discover more reasons.

This book is a tool designed to transform your relationship with food so that you can metabolize fat; it is not a book to beat yourself up with for having a fat body. You need to get your body, mind, and spirit in harmony to reach your goal of a healthier you. Before you can repair your relationship with your body you must understand how it works on all levels, emotionally and physically.

Remember, our purpose here is not to make you a wise fat person or a negative fat person; our purpose is to end weight as a problem in your life forever. Being negative is part of the diet mentality and only encourages the kind of negative attitude that gives rise to the cycles of weight loss and weight gain that we are trying to avoid. Some people are merciless on themselves with negative self-talk, if they "cheat on their diet" or eat something they believe they are not supposed to. It can seem that no matter how fast or far you go, it's never fast or far enough. You can devote your whole life to looking at the glass as half empty instead of half full.

If you have a weight problem and you begin to examine your emotional issues, you may have a tendency to beat yourself up over past dieting failures. You have the courage (congratulations to you) to examine unhealthy behaviors and tell the truth about them. Most importantly you can finally tell the truth about yourself. After recognizing these unproductive behaviors, you can work to change them.

When you are gentle with yourself and love yourself, the positive and creative aspects just bubble to the surface without any effort. It's like watering the flowers instead of the weeds. The attractive and thin person inside you will come forth when he or she knows that it's safe. A loving, accepting, nurturing environment will draw the thin person out much faster than a negative environment.

So let's look at some of the ways that you may have used food for the wrong reasons.

USING FOOD FOR THE WRONG REASONS

> *He that but looketh on a plate of ham and eggs*
> *to lust after it, hath already committed breakfast*
> *with it in his heart.*
>
> – C.S. Lewis

The warm fuzzies. Sometimes there's nothing in the world as comforting as eating. Food doesn't talk back to you. It doesn't withdraw its love. If something upsetting happens at the office, if you have a problem with your relationship, if your kids are making you nuts, or if you just feel depressed for any reason, eating will soften the pain. Ah! Emotional bliss at last.

Falling in or out of love. Whether you're falling in or out of it, love can lead to eating. It's easy to see why you'd eat if you were falling out of love, or if someone were falling out of love with you. It's the end of a relationship. You're depressed, upset, anxious, confused, and hurt. Did we mention crying a lot? Yes, you are also crying a lot. You yearn for the comfort and temporary sedative effect that food can give you. All you want to do is go unconscious. Besides, now that it is over, who cares whether you're a hottie or not?

It is not so obvious why people eat when they're falling in love. But falling in love is an exhilarating time. It brings new feelings, including its own set of anxieties. Even though you've longed to have these feelings, they can be unfamiliar, unsettling, and just downright scary. One surefire way to numb out uncomfortable feelings is by eating.

The quest for wholeness eating. You just are not getting what you want from your life or your relationship. You are looking for something to make you feel better, but you just don't know what it is. Maybe some fudge brownies will help clarify things for you. Every day you stand at the refrigerator and stare, hoping to find the answers to life's problems between the pizza and the box of Krispy Kreme donuts. You can find life's answers, but I will give you a hint: they are not in the refrigerator!

Guilt eating. You just screamed at the kids, or your spouse, or maybe your co-worker. You are really on edge. Now you feel guilty. So how do you deal with the guilt and numb out the feelings? Just eat. Since you have blown your diet, now you can feel guilty about eating on top of everything else. So you might as well just keep on eating.

"I am really angry/upset" eating. You are upset. The quickest sedative to calm that anxious feeling is to eat. You are really angry or frustrated, you are going through a personal crisis, a

divorce, a personal loss—you name it. Instead of experiencing the emotions you stuff them down with food. However, this is just a stall tactic. These feelings will come back sooner or later, usually toward someone else who does not deserve them. This syndrome is also known as "I am so angry with you! But I can't tell you to your face, so I will eat a whole chocolate cake instead." For many years this was my personal favorite!

"I'll start my diet on Monday" eating. Monday morning is doomsday. You are going to succeed this time by losing the weight, or die trying. It is Sunday night and the clock is ticking. This is it! Your last supper. Anything that you feel that you might want to eat in the next two years . . . you had better eat now, because as of tomorrow morning you are officially on a *diet.* It doesn't matter how much you eat today because you will lose it on your diet or you will be dead, in which case it won't matter anyway.

It is now six days into your diet and you have spent the whole week picking at grapefruits and eating hard-boiled eggs, and now the thought of either of them makes you want to vomit. Besides, you have been good all week and you will never go back to eating the way you used to. So why not have just a few cookies for a reward?

"I'm grown up now" eating. When you were a kid, your parents and other adults could tell you how, when, and what to eat. Now you can eat anything you want. If you want to eat raw cookie dough, no one can tell you not to. We've all heard the starving children in China stories. Personally, starving children stories never made me like liver or brussels sprouts any better. You may have unconsciously taken the viewpoint that when you grow up and have your own money you can and will eat whatever you want and no one is going to tell you what to do.

Creative eating. You love to cook, and you're good at it. It's one of the ways you express yourself. Or you are into exploring new foods. It is part of your adventurous spirit, your zest for living, for discovering the finer things in life. You certainly can't be expected to give that up. And once you've cooked a glorious gourmet dinner, you can't be expected to toss it down the disposal, either. Someone has to eat it, right? It might as well be you.

Holiday eating. From Thanksgiving through New Year's, it is a nonstop eat-a-thon. You don't want to be a wet blanket at parties and family gatherings. Besides, you will keep your New Year's resolution to lose the weight anyway.

Ritual eating. You are conditioned to eat certain things at certain times of the day; if you can't do that you are very uncomfortable. There are certain times, places, and situations in which you just eat as if part of you were an automatic eating machine. If you go to a movie you just have to have popcorn with tons of butter and a giant Coke, no matter what. You go unconscious and the next thing you know your hand is in a bunch of oily popcorn seeds.

Maybe you meet the guys to watch the game, and the next thing you know you have inhaled a bowl full of peanuts and a gallon of beer, because everyone else is doing it. Or if the eating ritual is going across the street on your afternoon break for junk food, you'll do it even if it is hailing golf balls outside.

Secret/closet eating. You go out with friends and eat nothing but a salad. You're on a diet after all, and all your friends are watching you watch your weight. They admire you and praise you for having such willpower. If your spouse is wanting you to lose weight, the heat is really on. He may be watching your every move. Well, when no one is around, look out . . . drawers, closets, any place you can hide food may be your sacred sanctuary. Also, eating in the car is a way of eating where no one can really see you. You can go to the grocery store and eat your forbidden morsels before you return home from shopping.

Don't forget to throw away the grocery receipt before your well-meaning spouse checks for indiscretions. I actually know a woman who would have her husband blow his breath into her face to check and see if he had been eating Snickers candy bars.

Premenstrual syndrome munchies. There is the ten-day pre-menstrual cycle hunger during which even the wallpaper looks pretty appetizing. You feel cranky and unlovable. You feel so emotional that even a hardened criminal would think twice about tangling with you. You feel tired, and you're a bloated blimp. So what are a few more pounds? Who cares anyway? You'll get back on track as soon as your period is over—better yet, the *Monday* after your period is over!

Procrastination. You really don't feel like washing the dishes, doing that work project, balancing the checkbook, or . . . (you fill in the blank). Before you know it you are standing in front of the refrigerator, procrastinating, hoping your project will just disappear into thin air.

The reward. You were so good today on your diet you deserve a reward, right? It is 10:00 P.M.: it is dark, it's quiet, the kids are in bed, your spouse is sawing logs on the couch again. It's just you, David Letterman, and the refrigerator. Besides, the day has been so hectic and stressful that a few cookies, or at the very least a few Twinkies, wouldn't hurt. Anyway, if no one sees you eat them they don't count, right?

The free meal. Someone else is paying for this, so why not have the dinner, drinks, and the dessert? You don't get taken out to dinner every day, so you should get as much out of it as you can. As long as it is free, why not? Free samples at the supermarket, the buffet table at a party, or even free meals on an airplane. Now that is a stretch! Is a bag of peanuts considered a meal? How can you overeat on airplane food?

The grazer. You just love the taste of any food. If it is there, it is meant to be eaten. You are always on the hunt. Just

> **Ask yourself, "Am I furious because I am fat?
> or am I fat because I am furious?"**

a few bites won't hurt. This may be your last chance. What if you die tomorrow?

Grazing reminds me of Oprah on her popular television show reciting the experience of pulling out a frozen hot dog bun and pouring maple syrup over it before eating it. It is just that oral fixation to have something in your mouth, just grazing through your day!

BEATING YOURSELF UP WITH LIMITING BELIEFS

If there is to be any peace it will come through being, not having.

– Henry Miller

There are many more reasons that people overeat. You probably know some I haven't mentioned here. You know the games you play with yourself? But this gives you a sampling, so you can start to identify your own. It really shows you how much you can rationalize overeating with other events in your life.

Exercises

Now take out your journal and complete these exercises.

1. These are the reasons I overeat. (To obtain answers, keep asking yourself, Why do I overeat?)

2. These are the specific circumstances in which I'm likely to overeat.

3. These are the payoffs or benefits I get from eating for these reasons. (Example: "I always overeat when I am at my parents' house because I want to avoid a fight.")

If you had trouble completing these exercises, observe yourself for a few days. Keep asking yourself these questions and write down your answers as they come to you.

These exercises will make you more aware of your behaviors on a conscious level. When you realize that you may be eating for emotional and not for physical reasons (hunger, energy, etc.), you will see that a diet program is never going to succeed because it does not address your emotional responses and needs. Examining these reasons will show you the contrast between having a diet mentality and working with your body in a non-diet context, so that you can see how out of touch with your body you probably are right now. Furthermore, by examining these reasons, you'll come to see that there are even deeper reasons, an unconscious agenda that underlies them.

It is my belief that until these unconscious reasons come to light, there is no way to gain mastery over them. These unconscious reasons come from our experience, some event or events in our life that have caused us to make a decision about ourselves, about how to operate in life, how to succeed, or how to survive. These unconscious agendas had their purpose when we adopted them, but when they stay unconscious and start operating automatically, we are prisoners to them long after they have served a useful function.

Many of the most powerful unconscious agendas are often misguided because they were made when you were too young to have an accurate picture of who you are or of what the world is actually like. In the case of eating, as long as you try to motivate yourself with all kinds of very good reasons for losing weight, but don't stop to really examine the underlying unconscious agendas that are keeping you fat, you will always be in the heat of the battle.

Ask yourself what limiting beliefs you might have created that would cause you to act the way you do. Just stay aware, keep asking yourself these questions, and eventually the unconscious agenda will become clearer to you. Many of you still operate on beliefs that served you when you were a child but no longer serve you as an adult.

If you have a belief, for example, that being overweight runs in your family, then you will produce results that support that belief. If you become aware of your conscious and unconscious beliefs then you can reevaluate them and decide how to make choices that better serve you. Once you discover what motivates you to overeat, you can choose to do something about it to produce a different result. All of these reasons may not become clear to you at once: this is a process. In that case these exercises will function like a time-release capsule; their effect will be realized gradually, as you go along.

Additional Exercises

Take your time. It may take days or even weeks to come up with all these answers.

1. What were the circumstances in your life when you first began to gain weight? Provide as much detail as possible. How old were you? What was your family of origin like? What were your relationships like? What was your financial situation? How successful were you in school or in your career? Was there some trauma, crisis, or pressure in your life? Provide as much detail as possible.

2. Under what circumstances do you overeat today? Describe your circumstances in detail, as in the previous exercise.

3. When you attempt to imagine yourself being thin, what objections come to mind? What is your belief system that is running riot with your desire to be thin? Some examples:

- Good mothers aren't thin and sexy.

- People might expect more from me.

- My friends or family will not like it if I change.

- Men/women will come on to me and make sexual advances.

Now look back over your answers to the previous questions and see if you can discover the unconscious agenda that motivates you to overeat and keep you fat. What is it?

Look at your unconscious agenda closely. Are these limiting beliefs still true? Are they limiting your life in a way that you have not been aware of? Do they reflect an accurate picture of your life, as you now know it?

4. These are the different emotional hungers I try to satisfy with food: _____

When I feel _____ I want to overeat.

These are the specific foods I use to try to satisfy those hungers: _____

To keep your emotional equilibrium my suggestion is that you journal every day. You will be amazed what you what you learn about yourself.

Dieters live a life of "if only":

- If only I could stop eating.
- If only I could lose ten pounds.
- If only I were thin.

There are problems, however, when dieters say "if only." The first is that "if only I were thin" is really another way of saying, "I hate myself the way I am." The second is that "if only" is a wish for magical transformation, not a realistic approach to change.

People rarely know how to say "I want to be different from the way I am" without putting themselves down at the same time. When you put yourself down in an effort to change yourself, the healthier part of you refuses to budge. When you say, "I am disgusting, I have to lose weight," that healthier part of you heads for the fridge. I understand that you want to be different from the way you are. I also know that, ironically, accepting yourself as you are is a prerequisite for change. Giving up the "if only" syndrome makes it possible for you to begin to resolve your rigid dieting behavior and to begin to lose weight.

Louise Hay, in her book *You Can Heal Your Life*, explains her viewpoint about overweight:

> *Overweight* is another good example of how we can waste a lot of energy trying to correct a problem that is not the real problem. People often spend years and years fighting fat and are still overweight. They blame all their problems on being overweight. The excess weight is only an outer effect of a deep inner problem. To me, it is always fear and a need for protection. When we feel frightened or insecure or "not good enough," many of us will put on extra weight for protection.

> To spend our time berating ourselves for being too heavy, to feel guilty about every bite of food we eat, to do all the numbers we do on ourselves when we gain weight, are just a waste of time. Twenty years later we can still be in the same situation because we have not even begun to deal with the real problem. All we have done is make ourselves more frightened and insecure, and then we need more weight for protection.

> So I refuse to focus on excess weight or on diets. Diets do not work. The only diet that does work is a mental diet; dieting from negative thoughts. I say to

clients, "Let us just put that issue to one side for the time being while we work on a few other things first."

They often tell me they can't love themselves because they are so fat, or as one girl put it, "too round at the edges." I explain that they are fat because they don't love themselves. When we begin to love and approve of ourselves, it's amazing how weight just disappears from our bodies.

◆　◆　◆

> **You must accept and treat yourself the way you've always wished others would. You can start living with yourself in a new way. As you do so, you will feel better and be encouraged to move forward.**

Remember that your self-hatred is the factor most responsible for keeping you at a miserable standstill. Self-contempt makes you feel bad, and when you feel bad you become immobilized. Each critical remark you make to yourself puts you at risk for out-of-control eating. I encourage you to stop every time you make an unloving remark to yourself. If you think about it, you would never make such hurtful remarks to someone you love, such as your spouse or your child. Why then would you make those critical remarks to yourself? Your body hears and believes everything you say. The rebel within you will not bow down to your abuse. When you accuse yourself, that rebel will take you directly to the fridge in an attempt to feel better.

I am advocating being kind, positive, and gentle with yourself. Being overweight is not a crime. The person inside your body—the real you—is a capable, worthy individual and a beautiful being. I invite you to put self-recrimination behind you and start now to be loving toward yourself.

CHAPTER 3

■ ■ ■ ■ ■ ■ ■ ■ ■

Feelings Buried Alive Never Die

*It is what we all wanted when we were children—
to be loved and accepted exactly as we were then,
not when we got taller or thinner or prettier . . .
And we still want it but we aren't going to get it
from other people until we can get it from ourselves.*

– Louise Hay

I really want you to peel off your emotional onion layers with this book. If your inclination is to skip to the end of the book and get to the "what do I do?" or "what exercises would I use to lose weight?" section, stay right here. Be willing to experience discomfort in order to grow and move to a new level of understanding. Be willing to step out of your comfort zone—that is where the growth takes place.

This is your exercise right here and now. It is an exercise in humility, raw humanness, and going backwards to where these issues may have started, in the beginning of your life. The theme of this book is about your body's resistance to weight loss and yes, it may very well be metabolic, but it also may be emotional resistance, or both.

Like myself, you may have started out with emotional issues as a child that were the precursor for metabolic issues later in life. Right here and now, it is time to get honest and get real with issues in your emotional closet. This is where the real journey begins.

HEALING THE CHILD WITHIN

I believe that many of your health and weight problems could have their foundation in unresolved emotional conflict. I began to learn about this theory of emotions being related to unhealthy eating behaviors from a recovering alcoholic named John Bradshaw in the late 1980s. John Bradshaw catapulted to national fame with a PBS show, *The Family*, discussing dysfunctional behaviors and unhealthy family systems.

John Bradshaw describes emotions as "energy in motion." When this energy is blocked or does not find its proper natural expression (i.e., anger, rage, sadness, grief, etc.), then it stagnates inside the body. It becomes an emotional "toxin." I have also heard it said that every pound is an unshed tear.

I believe these hidden emotions manifest themselves in physically destructive and unnatural ways — namely disease (dis*ease* of the body). These buried feelings can manifest themselves through physical illness or obesity. Just as the physical toxins or poisons must be cleansed from the body for healing to occur, unresolved emotional issues must also be cleansed from the whole body system for healing to occur.

This comes from my viewpoint as a holistic health educator, but more importantly, from my heart as a human being. I feel that you need to accept, acknowledge, and love that part of yourself that is ultimately alive, energetic, creative, and spontaneous — your child within or your authentic self. As someone who admittedly has struggled with my own inner conflicts and unresolved emotions, it was quite healing to discover a beautiful, precious blonde girl, deep within my heart. Coming to know, love, and accept her has truly changed my life. Though she can be very outrageous at times I can now accept that part of myself without judgment.

Most of us have been taught from our life experiences going back to childhood to stifle or deny our inner child or our real self. As a result we have developed a false or public self. Our false self is a cover-up—a mask, if you will. It is inhibited and fearful (will people love me if they know who I really am?). It is envious, critical, idealized, blaming, shaming, and perfectionistic. Alienated from our real self (the child within), the false self focuses on what it thinks others want us to be; it is overconforming. It gives love conditionally, rather than unconditionally. It covers up, hides, or denies feelings. It is what John Bradshaw describes as a "human doing" instead of a human being.

Inner child work is not about judging or condemning your parents. It's about learning how to nurture and protect yourself in each stage of developmental need, without using food and overeating as a coping mechanism. It is about a beautiful transformation from people-pleasing to self-actualization.

DENYING FEELINGS

The possibility of denying your true feelings and your truth is a common problem for children who lived in troubled homes. To grow in self-worth, you must give up the fantasy of your memories and the convenience of your past as all good or bad.

– Sharon Wegscheider Cruse, *Learning to Love Yourself*

If you ignore your inner experience (that which you feel), you disown part of your truth. Your reality therefore can become distorted and you may not be able to see your situation clearly.

As a child, teenager, or adult, when you experience a loss or a trauma, whether real or threatened, you most likely respond to that experience with fear and hurt. However, when feelings can't be expressed, you might feel as though you caused the loss or trauma and you feel guilt. Guilt can come from inappropriate responsibility to something you can't control. Teaching experiences can come in some very painful lessons.

When I was a teenager I had the traumatic experience of seeing my dad pack his belongings and drive away as I stood sobbing at the window. My parents were divorcing after 19 years of marriage. As a teenager I took this all on with fear, guilt, and hurt, as if I had some control over the situation. The truth is my parents' divorce was not about me, it was about their life unraveling. I was just caught in the circumstances.

Believe me, I did not have this all figured out at the time. When my dad was leaving, I was coming apart at the seams watching him drive away. If you can imagine being alive and breathing, but feeling like you are going to die at the same time, that is how I felt. It wasn't until many years later (I will go into detail later in this chapter) in counseling, when all these repressed feelings were oozing out in every other aspect of my life, that I was willing to really take a look at this. With some profound teachers I was able to revisit these feelings.

Somewhere you may have gotten the message that your feelings were wrong or unacceptable. Let me assure you, there is no right or wrong to feelings; they just *are*. John Bradshaw talks about kids being told to be robots where they are not allowed to show emotions, especially anger. The old tape plays in your head, "If you don't have anything nice to say, don't say anything at all. Nice girls don't get mad." So you may feel even more angry and hurt, and if you were to express that, you are squelched again. I will tell you what nice girls get, and that is "fat and furious." With each bite of food you are stuffing down the real anger and rage, bite by bite.

REPRESSING FEELINGS

With repeated stuffing or repressing of such feelings your child within is left feeling confused, sad, shameful, and empty. As these painful feelings build up and accumulate, they begin to become intolerable. With nowhere to ventilate them your only choice may seem to be to block them all out as best you can, to become numb, to deny that anything is really wrong (even though you are feeling depressed), or to hold them in until they become unbearable. Unable to let your feelings out, the body will step in and speak its mind by gaining weight or getting sick.

Sometimes your body can say loud and clear what your words cannot. Gaining 50 or 100 pounds really gets everyone's attention. It says very loudly, "Hey everybody. Look at me, I'm furious." Or you may want to blow up and explode, what I call *losing it!* The other side to this is, you may not blow up at all. You may just shut down and become numb and depressed.

You can also blot out your pain by becoming obsessive/compulsive with food, alcohol, drugs, sex, shopping, etc. You can numb and repress feelings, or you can express the pain and work through it with safe and supportive people. Although the last option seems the most logical, it involves moving out of denial, taking risks, becoming vulnerable, becoming real with yourself and others. Usually most people move through the aforementioned unhealthy behavior until they surrender to facing their own reality and making new healthy choices.

Then there are those of you who may resist taking emotional risks at all costs and may need a crisis to reach your surrender point. You may have a critical health crisis because of your weight, or a family member may be in your face because they can very clearly see your unhealthy food behavior. You may be trying to protect your comfort zone like a grizzly bear protecting her cubs. You may be the last to acknowledge your behavior because you are so emotionally checked out and repressed.

On your journey of self-discovery the toughest part will be looking for the truth of your growing-up years and finding your own sense of reality. Why look back? Why dredge up situations and feelings that are old and forgotten? Why reopen wounds?

The most important reason to look back and examine your early years is this: While the situations and the feelings might be old and forgotten, your attitudes, thoughts, and feelings affect your day-to-day current relationships and choices. Feelings are linear, and they stay alive in our unconscious as if the event happened yesterday. Unless you access your buried emotions and heal them, they will come up when a situation triggers them. If we do not recover, we repeat. John Bradshaw states, "What we don't work out we will act out."

GOING INTO THE DARK

My life script with my parents for the first 16 years of my life was very volatile. My father was a raging alcoholic and my mother was stuck in severe codependency. When I say volatile, I mean severe, bordering on life-threatening—an environment of trauma, physical abuse, and verbal abuse.

One of the most significant events that was frozen in time in my memory was the night my father physically beat my mother so badly I thought he was going to kill her. My father, in a drunken rage, was kneeling over my mother, slamming her head into the floor with blood going everywhere. My sister and I ran to her aid, pulled my father off of her, called the police, and had him removed from the house, guns and all. My father was a big man, six feet tall and weighing over 200 pounds. For two young girls to take him on, in absolute fear and terror, had to be an adrenaline protective reaction. My sister and I were terrified of my father and rightly so; he physically abused us as well. Being hit, slapped, or kicked was as normal in our house as taking out the garbage.

When I was 16 years old my mother was diagnosed with breast cancer. In the midst of her trying to save her own life, she finally put an end to a miserable marriage and proceeded with a divorce. As I shared with you earlier, my father left, my mother was fighting for her life, and I was in so much emotional pain that I didn't know what to do with myself. I couldn't cry, I couldn't express my emotions. I was frozen inside like a Popsicle, but on the outside I looked as if I had it all together. I was outgoing, well liked at school, dating the captain of the football team, and performing well in speech and drama (my favorite subjects). Watching me you would have thought I came from a functional, sane household.

When I was 18 my mother lost her battle and died of breast cancer. I was devastated. I used food as a way of numbing out the feelings that I was too scared to feel. Everyone said how mature I was and how well I handled such a horrible event, still managing to go on with my life. Are you surprised that was my MO (method of operation)? Just bite the bullet, take it in the gut, don't cry. Show the world you have it all together.

Four years later when my infant son, Brandon, was just two months old, I was dealt another tragic blow that would change my life forever. I was told that my 64-year-old grandma Tina had been found raped and brutally murdered. My grand-mother and I were very close. I cannot begin to describe the pain you feel when you lose someone in such a violent way. The shock is so devastating that it shakes you to the very core of your being. What followed was a murder investigation, an arrest, and finally a trial of the man who committed this heinous crime. The trial left me in a nauseous emotional state; my emotions were just black and numb. Nothing in the court system can make you feel vindicated, because you can't have your loved one back. You go on wondering how your heart will heal from this tragedy.

When an event is as shocking to you (especially as a child) as some of these personal events I have shared with you, your brain actually cuts the memory cord so it can block out the event. For example, your eyes may have seen the event but the actual feeling around it is frozen. If these traumatic events are not dealt with and healed, they will operate at a very deep unconscious level. You think as an adult you have forgotten the event, gotten over it or dealt with it, but your body in its infinite wisdom has stored the actual pain in your tissues. Until you actually *feel that pain* it cannot be released from the body.

What I did when all these traumas occurred was what many of you have done without even knowing it: blocked them out, detached from my feelings, froze these events and suspended them in a timeless warp to be dealt with later. I went to counseling and learned a great deal, but when I talked about these events I had no emotion attached to them. I could not get deep enough into the original pain of it.

It took me 12 years of struggling with these frozen feelings to finally get the courage to experience what I call *going into the dark*. I had to go deeper. I had to jump off into the abyss and feel the pain that was never felt originally. As John Bradshaw said so eloquently, "The only way to the other side of the pain is through."

Buckle your seat belts because what I am about to share with you is not for the faint of heart. I am emotionally naked with you, describing the original pain work that I experienced over 13 years ago at the John Bradshaw Center to help heal these events that I have just shared openly with you. Original pain work is about understanding and accepting pain and loss from an earlier time in our life. It is about *feeling* the pain, sadness, and grief which was not allowed to be felt during the actual event.

If I had not had this amazing, incredible experience with my own body, I would not have believed it! When I say that feelings buried alive never die, this is the most profound example I can share with you. These painful secrets were held in the vault of my memories and my body tissues, until they were healed in a safe place with loving support.

After participating in a weekend workshop with John Brad-shaw, I decided I had some original pain issues that I needed to attend to, but I will admit I was scared. It was predictable for me to try to stay in denial, go about my daily life, ignore my increasing internal uneasiness, or resist stretching myself out of my comfort zone. I decided to go into John Bradshaw's 30-day codependency inpatient program. That's right: locked up for 30 days. I know myself and I can be a hard nut to crack. I am overly responsible. If I stayed busy and distracted (as I had learned to do my whole life) I would not let myself fall apart and get to my emotional wounds. I made all the arrange-ments, said goodbye to my husband and two young sons, and left to take care of myself and do some much needed healing.

The first day I went to the group therapy session I could not breathe because of fear. I saw group members doing what they call original pain work, which is much like role-playing and acting out scenes from painful events in their lives. People were becoming hysterical, screaming, crying from their guts, and uttering sounds that seemed inhuman. Sounds that you would only hear out in the wild, from animals. This was reality like I had never experienced before.

I saw one woman actually vomit on the floor during group therapy. She had a memory of an uncle forcing her to perform oral sex when she was a child; her body memory in the group showed her physical reaction to that event by gagging and vomiting. Before coming to the center she did not have a conscious memory of any sexual abuse having taken place. Another woman reacted physically to the body memories of being raped by a family member with a broom handle. It was heart wrenching, brutal, shocking, and downright unbelievable. I am telling you the truth: if I had not seen it with my own eyes I would not have believed it. Your body records everything that happens to you, whether you are conscious of it or not.

Silly me, I thought we would just sit around in a group,

talk about our feelings, and get to the deeper issues. I am telling you, reality television could not hold a candle to this drama. I never saw anything like this in my drama classes in high school. The first few days of group therapy I spent literally curled up in a ball, in the corner of the room (they won't allow you to leave), crying my eyes out because I was in such terror and in emotional reaction.

The way original pain work is facilitated is by putting you "into a scene" with issues that the therapists know are deeply traumatic for you. Your body, fueled by the feelings and memories, takes over and goes into the original pain that you did not feel at the actual event. One of the reasons that I described my father beating my mother was so I could explain how this original pain work healed this issue for me.

I was asked to pick players (group therapy participants) in the room who might resemble my parents. There was a man, Bill, in our group, whose masculine, overpowering energy scared me, so I picked him to be my father. I then picked another woman for my mother, and someone to play myself and my sister to act out this horrendous scenario. In this scene the therapists wanted me to observe the traumatic event from outside myself.

Bill, my role-playing father, came in and violently slammed the door and the scene was off and running with fighting, yelling, mock physical violence, and abuse. When I saw myself and my sister as young girls (by the actors) pulling my father off my mother, seeing her terror and fear (as if for the first time), my visceral reaction was nothing short of a cellular catharsis. Now it was my turn to make sounds that would come out of a wounded animal, only they were screeching out of my own throat. My whole being was crying. It was so intense and deep that my body convulsed as if I was vomiting with my tears. I was humped in a ball on the floor, in the middle of the room, sobbing, grieving for my inner child that had to witness such a violent act upon another human being, the mother I dearly loved. I laid on the floor for hours (the group has to stay in the room and wait it out), convulsing and crying out all the pain that my body had hidden in the dark for all those years.

My skin became pale and gray that day, and it took about three days for this pain to finally move all the way through. I was physically nauseated for all three days, unable to eat while my body was healing and grieving. My husband came down for Family Week and was shocked when he saw me, because I was so visibly affected by this work.

That was only the beginning. After that experience there was no going back. I did this work for a whole month, day after day. My two emotional closets were of course the loss of my mother and the murder of my grandmother. I knew there was more pain buried in my soul in those deep and dark places, and so did my therapists.

This work enabled me to see how I had hidden anger about my mother not leaving my father, and putting all of us in this violent and dangerous situation. I chose a woman named Phyllis (who physically reminded me of my mother) to play my mother in all my scenes. It felt very real to me. I was able to hold Phyllis as my mother and get closure on the loss of her. I was finally able to tell my mother all about her two beautiful grandsons, Brandon and Christopher. I was able to tell her how much I had missed her in my life. You have to realize that this was not a logical adult play-acting, this was a wounded, abandoned child who wanted her mother.

When it came to the issue of my grandmother I had no idea what the therapists were going to come up with for that scenario. They handed me a foam bat (which we all used a lot for anger work) to face my grandmother's murderer. I was very resistant to go there in my fear. As a logical adult I knew that I was in a group facilitated by therapists, in a safe room, and that there could be no danger to me. Here again, my inner child and unprotected adult went into panic, facing a perceived danger where my grandmother was raped and murdered and I was powerless to stop it.

The therapists goaded me (damn, they're good) into tapping into the rage I felt for the atrocity that was inflicted on such a powerless, fragile, sweet, kind-hearted, loving woman. I had gone to the trial of this man, and I could remember his physical features. So when I finally gave myself permission to bring him into the room (figuratively speaking), and let the rage fly it was scary. I scared myself. I never knew I had so much rage inside of me. I was beating walls and chairs, screaming like the wild animal I had become. I was physically exhausted for days after that anger/rage catharsis.

Then came the healing and grieving piece of that scene where I also got to physically hold and say goodbye to my sweet grandmother. I still really miss her contribution to my life as a mentor and a teacher.

In his book, *Homecoming*, Bradshaw says, "Until we reclaim and champion that child, he/she will continue to act out and contaminate our adult lives. That child will be expecting someone else or something else [such as food, for the context of this book] to make him/her feel good and will be constantly frustrated as a result." Now you have a better set of questions to ask. "What do I need right now instead of food to nurture myself and my inner child? How can I give that to myself? Am I really hungry, or am I angry, lonely, or just tired?"

I am so grateful that I valued myself enough to give myself these healing experiences. My hope is that you will give yourself the courage to go into the dark places of your own soul and move towards healing. If you go backwards, sometimes it will actually lead you forward. Moving towards being your authentic self, who you are meant to be, can be so freeing.

Healing your inner emotional wounds to become the complete essence of your true self is a journey back home to yourself. Welcome home.

◆ ◆ ◆

The following is excerpted from *Healing the Child Within* by Charles L. Whitfield, MD.

Please hear what I am not saying
Don't be fooled by me.
Don't be fooled by the face I wear.
For I wear a mask, a thousand masks,
Masks that I'm afraid to take off, and none of them is me.
Pretending is an art that's second nature with me,
But don't be fooled.
So I play my game, my desperate pretending game,
With a façade of assurance without
And a trembling child within.
So begins the glittering but empty parade of masks,
And my life becomes a front.
I idly chatter to you in the suave tones of surface talk.
I tell you everything that's really nothing,
And nothing of what's everything,
Of what's crying within me.
So when I'm going through my routine,
Do not be fooled by what I'm saying.
Please listen carefully and try to hear what I'm not saying,
What I'd like to be able to say,
What for survival I need to say,
But what I can't say.
Who am I? may you wonder.
I am someone you know very well.
For I am every man you meet
And I am every woman you meet.

CHAPTER 4

■ ■ ■ ■ ■ ■ ■ ■ ■

The Feelings Behind the Fork

I address my inner child to make sure that I keep in touch with my emotional needs each day. I notice that doing this allows me to take care of myself on a regular basis. I feel positive about this self-nurturing. Food is not a choice for this nurturing. I choose other and more effective ways to soothe my body. One example of meeting my needs is speaking up for myself rather than remaining passive. I am aware of the pattern of remaining passive and then needing to binge. I utilize my newfound ability to speak for myself to refuse food when others encourage me to eat. I also reach out to others who will listen to me rather than attempt to find misguided comfort in food.

— Susan Ward, MA, MSW, *Beyond Feast or Famine*

Food was designed to give us nourishment, to create and maintain healthy, functional bodies. Food was not designed to nourish our wounded souls and mend our broken wings. Every food we take into our body has an emotional and biochemical component, either positive or negative.

Just as environmental toxins can invade your body, negative thoughts, emotions, and stress can increase biochemical toxicity. Mental clarity and emotional consciousness are critical factors in your healing process. Detoxifying your body, mind, and spirit of negative thought patterns and emotions that are stuck is imperative for the weight to leave your body.

With her book, *Heal Your Body,* Louise Hay has been instrumental in the lives of thousands by showing the connection of health conditions and the probable emotional underlying cause. The following is excerpted from her book.

> *Overweight.* Probable cause: Fear, need for protection. Running away from feelings. Insecurity, self-rejection. Seeking fulfillment. *New thought patterns: I am at peace with my own feelings. I am safe where I am. I create my own security. I love and approve of myself.*

> – Louise Hay, *Heal Your Body*

FOOD RESPONSIBILITY

> *Life is the sum of all your choices.*
>
> – Albert Camus

Take full responsibility for everything you choose to eat, and eat foods in the spirit of moderation and healing consciousness. My gift to you is positive affirmations to set the stage for conscious choices.

Strive to:

- Know when enough is enough.

- Know when not to eat.

- Develop a healthy emotional relationship with your food and eating habits.

- Take full responsibility for everything you choose to eat.

- Commit yourself to eating nutritionally superior, nontoxic food.

- Appreciate the food you eat and relax before you eat each meal.

- Eat in the healing consciousness with patience, calmness, control, and composure.

- Chew your food slowly, one bite at a time.

- Engage in good conversation and laughter to aid in your digestion and assimilation.

- Enjoy your food and be creative. Take time to enjoy preparing and eating your meals.

And avoid:

- Overeating. You are "eating to live" by nourishing your body, not "living to eat."

- Becoming emotionally attached to your food.

- Eating when emotionally upset, anxious, uptight, or depressed.

- Constantly snacking, nibbling, tasting, raiding, or the ol' famous grazing.

- Consuming foods containing toxic chemicals, diet sodas, or other harmful pollutants.

- Eating food that is lifeless (devitalized) and/or over-cooked.

- Overindulging in refined carbohydrates such as refined table sugars and syrups (chocolate, candy, ice cream, rich desserts, cake, donuts, white sugar, white rice, and white bread).

- Trans-fats and hydrogenated oils.

And *especially avoid* large amounts of these foods in a short amount of time, also known as a *binge*.

You are the only one who may truly know in your heart of hearts if you are engaging in an unhealthy relationship with food. You may have had it brought to your attention by a close friend or family member. If you are not sure, consider therapy or Overeaters Anonymous. The old sayings are true: "It takes one to know one," and "Don't try to kid a kidder." In a group setting or with a therapist, where there is an understanding of unhealthy eating behaviors and patterns, your behavior will be exposed from the cloud of denial. You may even be relieved to finally have your secret *out in the open*. It takes a lot of energy to hide.

You may try to white-knuckle it while saying to yourself, "I just won't eat anymore when I am upset." This may sound well and good but your experience may prove otherwise. Your unconscious mind may have another agenda. You may have issues that are buried so far below the surface, you are not even aware that they are still running your ship. As I have previously shared with you, my experience at the John Bradshaw Center should be a real case in point.

If just giving you a list of foods to avoid would have done the trick for you, why would you have needed this book? You would have just followed all the other diet advice in the numerous other books that you bought and then donated to charity or sold at your last garage sale for a quarter. You are depending on me to deliver the goods, to give you the weight loss answers that you could not find previously, and I will. I just want you to know that you are a puzzle just like I am. All the components of this book will give you the puzzle pieces, but you will have to fit them all together. You will have to do the work to make your puzzle pieces fit, creating the beautiful being that you truly are.

Personally it took a conscious effort, group support, journaling, and therapy for me to not want to *stuff my body* with food when I was angry. I used to joke and say that if I was not supposed to eat when I was angry, then I would not have eaten the whole 21 years I was married!

But seriously, it is a pattern I developed as a child to avoid painful feelings. When I became conscious of this as an adult I would really watch myself wanting to go unconscious and run to the refrigerator to numb out with food when I was feeling uncomfortable. I remember one instance when I was going to therapy and I became acutely aware of my unhealthy patterns of using food when I was upset. One night—I can't remember the issue at hand—I caught myself walking into the kitchen about ten times (I am not exaggerating), opening the refrigerator door, and just staring. Then I would catch myself, close the door, and leave the room.

After about the tenth time my former husband said to me, "Loree, are you having a problem? Why do you keep going into the kitchen, repeatedly opening the refrigerator, looking in, and then coming back in here to watch TV? You have been up and down like a yo-yo all night. What's up with you?" I was annoying him and finally had to cop to the fact that I was also annoying myself. But I was anxious and frustrated, and had wanted so badly *to just eat! Damn it!* Was I hungry? Hell no! I just wanted emotional solace in the leftover whatevers in the refrigerator. I had to learn that the leftover whatevers were not going to solve my problems.

The emotional aspect aside, overindulging in all of these "avoid foods," especially junk foods, will throw your body chemistry and hormones into severe imbalance, which will lead to weight gain. I am not just talking about the obvious *excess calorie theory*. You are probably thinking that struggling with your jeans the next day is the only consequence of going on a binge, but it is the chemical consequence that is also physically damaging. Staying in balance emotionally and physically is the whole key to winning your weight game.

CHAPTER 5

■ ■ ■ ■ ■ ■ ■ ■ ■

The Shame Game

Guilt is I MADE a mistake.
Shame is I AM a mistake.

– John Bradshaw, author of *Healing the Shame That Binds You*

I will never forget the emotional impact John Bradshaw's words had on me the first time I heard them in a recovery workshop. Just sit for a moment and let his words sink in.

Is that *shame* you feel gnawing at your guts? Do you feel that *you* are a mistake? Are you using food to cover up your uncomfortable feelings, and then feeling ashamed because you could not control your eating? Do you feel ashamed for feeling inadequate? Ask yourself, is the shame you feel really about *you*? Or was it given to you by significant others in your life and you *took it on* as your own?

> **Codependent thought for the day:**
> **Toxic shame is like toxic waste —**
> **nobody wants to own it.**[1]

---

[1] From *Codependent for Sure! An Original Jokebook,* by Jann Mitchell.

Several years ago when I was a radio show host in the San Francisco Bay Area, Deirdra Price, Ph.D., was a fabulous guest on my show. In promoting her book, *Healing the Hungry Self: The Diet-Free Solution to Lifelong Weight Management,* we talked about the very same emotional issues I am covering here and now in *Fat and Furious.* Her book is nothing short of phenomenal as a guide to opening your awareness of your existing patterns with food and emotional hunger.

In her book, Dr. Price expounds on this issue of shame. The following section is excerpted with permission from *Healing the Hungry Self: The Diet-Free Solution to Lifelong Weight Management* (Plume 1996).

◆ ◆ ◆

Shame is one of the major emotions a child feels when wounded.[2] Appropriate amounts of shame help a child to learn right from wrong, to feel remorse, to grow, and to change. However, when an adult uses extreme amounts of shame on a child, it becomes debilitating and destructive to the child for a number of reasons:

1. The child learns to feel guilty about every error or mistake made.

2. The child develops little, if any, trust in her or his ability to make decisions based on feelings, instinct, or gut reactions.

3. Self-esteem is low due to near-constant critical internal dialogue.

4. Self-worth is minimal.

---

2   Much of the information on shame comes from the "Ending Shame" tape series by Lazarus (Part I: Infancy; Part II: Psychic Contracts of Pain Childhood; Part III: Those Adolescent Years; and Part IV: Adult Shame). © 1990 concept: Synergy. Used by permission.

Shame is passed from one person to another. When adults shame a child, they're passing on the shame they received as a child. But children don't realize they're taking on someone else's shame, fueled by that person's internalized belief system. Rather, children begin to believe there is something wrong with them, and that they're being told about it. The child has no idea that negative beliefs are being passed on through the act of shaming. Statements adults make to a child during the wounding process build the foundation for negative beliefs and the critical internal dialogue that stems from the beliefs. Statements that form negative beliefs sound like:

- "Stop eating that cake, or you're going to get fat."

- "No one will ever love you if you act like that."

- "Don't you cry!"

- "I'm putting you on this diet for your own good."

- "Once you lose weight, you'll look pretty."

- "We'll go clothes shopping when you lose five pounds."

- "You can't have cake like your sister can—she's thin."

- "Either you get an A on your math test or you're grounded."

- "You look fat in that outfit."

- "Don't talk back to your mother like that."

> **Shame is easier to feel than pain.**

This is when children begin to reject the parts of them seen as undesirable. If the adults around them think aspects of the children are not acceptable, the child will think the same. The flaws are the very things the critics criticize.

Underneath the shame is the actual pain felt during the wounding experience. Shame is much easier to feel than pain. The pain gets buried, and shame is readily felt throughout life. As these children grow into adulthood, they're likely to pass on their unresolved shame to their children, partners, other family members, friends, coworkers, and acquaintances, by creating similar wounding experiences for these people.

THE CRITIC

This part of the self enforces internal rules based on the belief system developed during childhood and adolescence. The dialogue many people hear in their heads is a barrage of critical comments that ensure that feelings, thoughts, and behavior (decisions) stay in line with the negative beliefs. These self-statements are automatic and conditioned. Your critic knows no other belief system, only the one taught by the adults who had an impact on you while you were growing up. The critic's reinforcement of beliefs serves many purposes. Ultimately, the critic offers protection. It makes sure you don't fully trust other people, which guards you against being hurt or betrayed. To guarantee you'll get approval from others, the critic pushes you to engage in efficient, helpful, people-pleasing behaviors. The downside to having a critic is that it doesn't allow the development of self-trust or self-esteem.

> **If you listen to what your critic says, it sounds similar to what you heard while growing up.**

◆ ◆ ◆

This inner critic can also be referred to as *the committee!* You know what committee I am talking about. The one that won't *shut up in your head!* The committee likes to play the shame game. Shame is taking on perceived negative beliefs about yourself, and then beating the hell out of yourself with those beliefs.

If no one else is shaming you and telling you, "You're a pig!" "You're fat and ugly," "You're stupid," "You're unlovable," "Who would want to love you until you lose weight?" then you learn to do it to *yourself.* No one can even *begin* to beat you up better than yourself. Does this sound like anyone you know intimately? Maybe someone you see in the mirror every day?

I implore you. *Stop right here and now!* You *are* going to turn these internal verbal assaults and negative beliefs around. You *are* going to learn a new set of beliefs. Stay tuned!

When I embarked on the *Fat and Furious* journey I asked Dr. Price for her expertise and for a contribution to my message. She has graciously contributed the following section.

◆ ◆ ◆

NEGATIVE BELIEFS AND FOOD ABUSE
by Deirdra Price, Ph.D.

You are the person you believe you are. If you hold positive beliefs about yourself, you're more likely to interpret experiences as pleasant and maintain high self-esteem when difficult situations occur. In general, you'll accept, appreciate, and feel good about the person you are. Conversely, if you hold negative beliefs, you're more likely to interpret life's experiences as painful, frustrating, or unsatisfying. You'll dislike and blame yourself for any perceived failures, which will produce depressed moods and anxious moments. The way you see yourself is how you see others and assume they see you, affecting how you react to people and events in your life.

Everyone has a set of beliefs they developed during childhood and adolescence. You received spoken and unspoken messages from people who were and maybe still are important:

parents, grandparents, extended family members, teachers, coaches, friends, and bullies. These messages told you about your personality, appearance, performance, abilities, and talents.

Harsh criticism during the early years makes it difficult for a person to develop a healthy self-image. A sense of not being "good enough" emerges. Being unattractive, inadequate, unlovable, or lacking worth may also arise. It all depends on things that happened to you and the messages that were conveyed about these events.

Most people are "wounded" while growing up. It's an inevitable part of the human experience. When you're being wounded, you receive negative information about yourself in the form of shame. Statements such as "You're fat," "You screwed up," and "How could you have done that?" make you think less of yourself. The shame leads to pain and hurt. You learn that there are aspects of yourself that are flawed, and you reject them just as others have done. You see them as unacceptable, and so you put yourself down in your own head. At the same time you also strive for perfection with the hopes of pleasing others and liking yourself. It never works because perfection doesn't exist. Eventually, you'll make a mistake and remind yourself how bad you really are.

This is how our beliefs create our reality. These ingrained beliefs shape how you feel about yourself, what you think and therefore tell yourself, and ultimately the decisions you make. People who struggle with food, weight, and body image often hold less than flattering self-views. You resort to starving, bingeing, purging, or grazing to change either your appearance or emotions. You incessantly try to lose weight to make your body more appealing or turn to food to numb out. These attempts don't stop the unpleasant emotions and judgmental thoughts for long. How can they? You're trying to alter your external presentation to eliminate internal suffering. Instead, you create a secondary layer of emotions such as self-disgust, distress, and guilt for engaging in behaviors that ultimately leave you feeling out of control.

Now that you're an adult, it's your responsibility to heal unresolved issues stemming from the past. To do this, you work in these four areas: beliefs, feelings, thoughts, and choices. Start with addressing your feelings and choices. You need to sit with whatever comes up and not turn to harmful behaviors. It's easier said than done. However, you do build up the capacity to cope by facing emotions instead of avoiding them. It actually becomes less difficult over time with practice. You also need to change how you eat and exercise, being moderate with both.

If you eat three balanced meals a day, letting yourself become full and satisfied, then the reasons for consuming additional food right after a meal are either emotion-based or a bad habit. If you're eating for emotional reasons, identify what you're feeling and use alternative coping strategies. Try writing, talking with a confidant, or doing something else that is soothing to dissipate the intensity of the experience. If you're breaking a habit, it takes 21 days of doing a new behavior every day to create change, and six weeks for the new habit to become fully ingrained.

To alter beliefs, you must start working with compassionate self-statements to counteract the critical ones. Come up with phrases such as, "My body is fine the way it is today," "I did the best I could," and "I don't want to be mean to myself anymore." Daily repetition for months will start to chip away at the old beliefs. It is important to make a conscious effort to not beat up on yourself. Then you can add other sentences like:

- "I release my body hatred."
- "I let go of my unworthiness."
- "I can be me and still be okay."

Efforts in the four areas (beliefs, feelings, thoughts, and

choices) will eventually erode your negative beliefs so you can let them go. Then a new space opens up for a more encouraging and realistic perspective of yourself."

◆ ◆ ◆

USING SHAME AS LEVERAGE

Loree, you're fat! Do something about it!

– My grandma Gladys, 1995

Shaming someone into losing weight, or trying to make changes in his or her behavior to match your agenda, is cruel and abusive. I know from experience, because all my life from childhood to adolescence and through a failed marriage I put a lot of wasted energy into trying to change others. (Of course, this was before I got my self-righteous, codependent ass kicked in therapy). I speak from experience when I say that it is easy to take someone else's inventory and give suggestions on how *his or her* life could be so much better with *your* blueprint. I feel a codependent country-western song coming on . . . *Stand by your man,* or take your pick of numerous whiney *I'll fix your life* songs. I am going to come out punching on this issue because shaming is such an abusive travesty. I have three words for you, if you are attempting to shame someone else into losing weight with your well-meaning "but if you would just listen to my advice" codependent behavior. No disrespect intended, but . . . *back off, Bucko!*

If someone you love has an unhealthy addictive relationship with food, alcohol, drugs, or compulsive toenail painting . . . guess what? This may come as a shock to you, but, it is *his or her* issue not *yours*. It is very arrogant and self-righteous to subscribe to the theory that you can fix *his or her* problem. This is a harsh reality, but here it is, straight to the point, from me to you. The truth is, the only person's behavior that you are responsible for, can change, or even control, is *your own!*

> **Codependents are the only people who go to a marriage counselor by themselves.**[3]

For the purpose of this book we are going to discuss shaming only as it relates to a food addict. You want to see a food addict gain 20 pounds in ten minutes? Tell them they're fat and they need to lose weight. They'll eat everything that is not nailed down, plus more. The shortest distance between a food addict's fork and a ransacked kitchen pantry is overt shaming. The truth is, all your harsh judgments about them (even though your belief is that it is well-meaning and in their best interest) will result in weight gain, the quickest nonverbal way for an addict to give you a "middle-finger salute"!

> **Q: What does a codependent have in common with God?**
>
> **A: They both have a plan for your life!**[4]

Remember what you just read earlier in this chapter about taking on shame that is given to you from critical adults in your life? If your shame issues are alive and well in your consciousness, and your pattern is to use food to cope, guess where you're going to sprint when someone is attempting to shame you into losing weight? Lock up the refrigerator, here you come! It is a vicious cycle and guess what? No one wins this shame game! This becomes a power struggle of the largest magnitude. Both sides lose trust, dignity, and respect.

I will refer to the receiver of the shaming abuse as "the shamee" and the imposer of the shaming abuse "the shamer." The overweight person, the shamee, feels a double whammy—

[3, 4] From *Codependent for Sure! An Original Jokebook,* by Jann Mitchell.

first victimized by critical adults, then possibly taunted by other children dispensing shame in schools full of peer cruelty. Victimized as an impressionable child and then by a codependent as an adult, you have a perfect set-up for deep-seated resentment and major passive-aggressive behavior and more overeating behavior.

The shamer feels even more self-righteous, angry, and confused about why this overweight person just doesn't "get it" and go on a diet and lose weight. "What is your problem?" he laments. "Don't you [spouse, family member, child, or friend] realize that you are fat? Don't you realize the harm that you are doing to yourself? Don't you see that I can really help you?" Without intervention, therapy, or behavior modification on both sides, this can and will rip relationships apart.

Let me share with you a personal experience involving my own self-righteous behavior. The universe has a way of humbling you when you need it. My former husband was a periodic alcoholic (also known as a binge drinker), and I was very self-righteous about his drinking behavior, because I do not drink. I always had the finger pointing to shame him about his irresponsible drinking behavior. How could he drink and compromise our family life? How could he do that?

I had such a deep-seated issue with alcoholism because my father, grandmother, and uncle were alcoholics. I finally sought counseling and group therapy. In one of my first counseling sessions I began with, "If my husband would just stop drinking and (blah, blah, blah), then our marriage would be fine." Who in the hell did I think I was? How arrogant, really! I had my own sugar addiction going on, but I was always focusing on his shortcomings and issues. I was a codependent walking around with a giant "C" on my chest like Wonder Woman.

My husband acted out his addiction with alcohol like I did with sugar. Was I any stronger than he was? No! Was I being self-righteous and arrogant? Yes! So he drank alcohol when he couldn't deal with his anger and his feelings, and I ate Oreos and a half of a chocolate cake. What is the difference?

As I started to unravel my own codependency issues, I became very aware of the struggles of all addicts, whether they are getting buzzed on beer or mainlining Oreos. An addict is an addict. I have learned finally to have compassion for others and myself.

True, you can't get arrested for having an open bag of Oreos in the back seat of your car. You won't be asked to walk a straight line and get a breathalyzer test for suspicious weaving while driving back from the bakery with a dozen donuts. It is socially acceptable to be a sugar addict (actually encouraged from a young age), but if you are guzzling sugar, you just have a different drug of choice.

If you have an unhealthy relationship with food and realize that you could be a food addict, then *you* are responsible for dealing with these issues. You are *not* absolved of responsibility. Step up and face the music! Let your recovery begin!

If you also see yourself in this picture as a shamer, let go of the *drama you crave* by trying to impose your will on others. I hope you learn what I did ... *get over yourself*. If you are going to take a searching and fearless moral inventory of someone's character defects ... *take your own*.

BEWARE OF FINGER-POINTERS IN WHITE LAB COATS

Doctor: "You're fat and you need to go on a diet."
Patient: "But doctor, I want a second opinion."
Doctor: "Okay, you're ugly too!"

– Rodney Dangerfield

The doctor walks into his examination room, where an overweight female patient waits. "Still fat," he says, shaking his head.

The woman lets out a nervous chuckle, hoping for a punchline to ease the shame. But the doctor says nothing more, and she is too humiliated to bring it up again.

Within one year, the woman finds a new doctor — a nutrition specialist who deals sensitively but directly with her obesity—and drops more than 75 pounds. "The doctor shook her up, but in the wrong way," said her new doctor, researcher Pamela Peeke. "He ended up losing her as a patient."

There is yet another dimension to this issue. If you, the overweight person, are *not* a food addict but have an underlying and undiagnosed metabolic issue, there is all the more reason for the shamer or finger-pointer to watch his/her step.

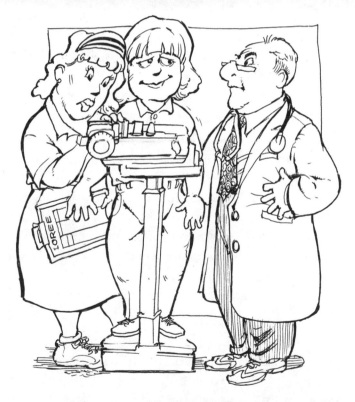

**"I can't believe you haven't lost any weight.
You must be cheating."**

Your shamer could even be a medical professional who shames their patients with statistics and accusatory weigh-ins. In this type of explosive situation, the "cannoli" can really hit the fan!

There is nothing more humiliating than your doctor or family member accusing you of lying because if you did "A" (diet and exercise), the result would be "Y" (lost weight). Somehow your metabolic dysfunction has left the equation: doing "A" leaves you stuck at "H" (hormonal hell!) with no weight loss in sight.

If an overweight person is putting all the essentials in place to lose weight, such as eating a healthy food plan, exercising, and taking supplements, and the weight is not budging ... shamers should look out. Any shamee in that situation would be absolutely out of his or her mind with frustration. You may get more than you bargained for if you go aggressively shaming and finger-pointing. Better yet, all shamers should wear a bullet-proof vest and helmet at all times!

I use the example of a man who is well on his way to becoming "follicly challenged." Would walking up to this man and giving him attitude or shaming him about his hair falling out change anything? Would it prevent his hair from continuing to fall out? Of course not! That is a ridiculous statement. Yet others feel compelled to give obese people major attitude about their weight and shame them, as if they didn't notice that they are fat or just don't care. Trust me ... *they care!* Sometimes there is a legitimate hormonal problem the overweight person is struggling with and unaware of. Shaming and finger-pointing are not going to correct someone's metabolism! Not to mention that shaming is nothing less than abusive.

To all shamers wanting to play the shame game ... unless you have a medical degree or a Ph.D. and are qualified to diagnose metabolic dysfunction or eating disorders *at a glance*, exercise humility, compassion, and tenderness of heart in dealing with other people's weight issues.

My grandmother Gladys, bless her heart, was very shaming in attributing my weight issue to lack of moral character on my part. Several years ago, she asked me to come into her bedroom and sit on her bed, and she gave me her well-meaning pep talk: "Loree, you're fat. Do something about it!" I was stunned at her insensitivity and obvious judgment of me. I realized that these were the only tools my grandmother had to get her point across; however, she was being abusive to me.

I stood up (without judgment), looked her straight in the eye, and stated firmly (but kindly), that my weight issue should not be of concern to her, it had nothing to do with her, and to respect me by never speaking to me in that manner again. She wasn't pleased, but she knew by my words and body language that she had stepped over the line with me. She knew that I meant every word I said.

> *Kiddo, you have gained weight. You need to go on a diet!*
>
> – Bob, my dad, on his deathbed, 2002

This last year, I was given the news that my dad, Bob, had just a few months to live. He was dying of colon cancer. My father had lived in Florida, and even though we kept in contact, we had not seen each other for several years. My sister and I flew him to Oregon to live out his last days in a beautiful hospice home environment.

When I walked into his room, it was very emotional to see him. He was dying. It was visibly obvious, and it devastated me. When I looked into his big brown eyes, they looked expressionless but so sad at the same time. He knew his life was ending. It was all I could do to not drop onto the floor in a sobbing heaping mess.

He asked me to pull up my chair to the side of his hospital bed and he looked at me with complete seriousness. I thought he was going to say something about his condition or ask for the nurse because he was in pain, or something like that. I moved the chair and sat down next to him. He looked me directly in the eyes and said, "Kiddo, you have gained weight. You need to go on a diet!"

What? Was he kidding? I was screaming to myself! I was screaming so loud inside my head I thought for sure the whole state of Oregon (and a few neighboring ones) could hear me. God help me, this was neither the time nor the circumstance to make a federal case out of this issue. I was in utter shock!

Geeeez, I can't take this any more! Just a month before I had gotten my metabolic panel from a new physician, Dr. Dommisse (you will hear all about this later in the book), confirming that my hypothyroid condition was a contributing factor to my inability to lose weight.

Come on Dad, I was screaming to myself. *What is wrong with this family? First my grandmother's shaming, and now you, on your deathbed, no less. I am a successful mother, author, and health professional, but everything comes back to what I weigh? I am not valuable unless I lose weight, is that what you're telling me, Dad?*

I got control of my voice and said, "Dad, we have only a few weeks to get closure on our 47 years together, say our goodbyes, and your concern is that you want me to go on a diet?"

"I just want to know you're doing something about it," my dad said.

"I'm seeing a physician for a thyroid and metabolic imbalance, Dad, and I hope to get it under control soon. I am *doing the best I can.*"

"Okay honey," he said. "As long as you are doing something."

After my initial internal temper tantrum, I let it go, and Dad and I moved on to getting closure.

My saving grace in all these circumstances is Lori Jean (my birth name). She is the beautiful, funny, silly-nilly, outrageous little girl that lives in my heart and soul always.

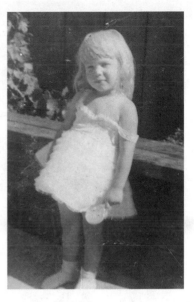

Here is a daily affirmation that can help you stay in touch with your inner child.

I am becoming my own nurturing parent to my beautiful inner child. It is okay to be vulnerable and listen to my innermost thoughts. I will learn to answer the depth of my own needs without judgment or fear. My life will get easier as I channel my resources within myself. I begin each day with gratitude by checking in with myself as I wake up. I love myself.

My suggestion is that you find a picture of yourself as a child that you really connect with and carry it with you at all times. Stay rooted in yourself on a deep level. Your inner child always has *you* for protection. Realize that you are a valuable, loving human being—regardless of what the scale says.

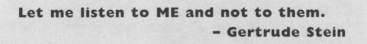

Let me listen to ME and not to them.
– Gertrude Stein

CHAPTER 6

■ ■ ■ ■ ■ ■ ■ ■ ■

Recovery of Your Self-Esteem

No one can make you feel inferior without your consent.

– Eleanor Roosevelt

I am renewed by my strengthening sense of self-worth. I respect myself in a different way now. I acknowledge the value of my feeling and my personal expression. I allow my inner worth to grow in strength as I assure myself of its presence. My actions reflect this belief. I respect myself and ask for respect from others through my new sense of self.

– Susan Ward, MA, MSW, author of *Beyond Feast or Famine*

Woman are especially vulnerable to feeling inadequate and depending on the approval of others for their self-esteem. You may have been taught at a young age to be a "good girl," do as you are told, keep your voice down, be willing to help out, and always mind your manners. Codependency, another common problem with women, also involves getting your sense of self-worth from the approval of others, rather than generating it from within yourself. It is therefore not surprising that so many of us have limited or fragile self-esteem. If this is your problem, you need to learn to value yourself for who you truly are.

Many women cannot self-nurture because they have been brought up to think that they should always be a giver and not a taker. Society teaches women that giving is good, and that taking care of yourself is selfish. You may have been taught to take care of everyone else first (e.g., buy all the kids' clothes first, or never go to the beauty salon so you can save money for the family) and leave yourself at the end of the line. You're taught to fulfill all your responsibilities before you're allowed to give to yourself.

I believe that this is exactly the mindset that can lead many of you to overeat or participate in other compulsive behavior as a last-ditch effort to nurture yourself. If you are not giving yourself the respect you deserve, food can become an emotional crutch. Then you feel guilty, lose respect for yourself, and start the self-critical cycle all over again.

This self-punishment doesn't work, and in fact even backfires, thereby lowering your self-esteem even more and making you feel hopeless. The only solution you often come up with is to criticize yourself. This self-perpetuating cycle, where self-perceived failure leads to self-belittlement, further decreases self-esteem. Low self-esteem produces feelings of hopelessness and despondency, which sap your energy and faith needed to strive and achieve, thus producing more failure. Does this sound familiar to you? Do you think whatever you do is just not good enough? Do you *awfulize* and hold yourself to a seemingly impossible standard?

You may use your achievements as a way to value yourself. This can be a set-up, because sometimes no matter how much you achieve, you may feel that it is never enough. Often, despite receiving the respect and admiration of others, you may feel like an imposter inside—afraid to expose your real deficiency. You look at each achievement as something that only increases others' expectations of you, and that sets you up for a harder fall when your unworthiness is revealed. You may long to feel content and pleased with yourself, but self-contentment is the one thing you cannot achieve.

Self-esteem is an inside job. It can come only from the inside, from inner acceptance and approval. If this self-approval is not there, then the effects of outside commendation and rewards last only as long as the compliments keep coming in. When they cease, you may suffer a dramatic drop in self-esteem, and you may become depressed. To be truly anchored in feelings of self-worth, you need to approve of yourself for who you are.

SELF-ESTEEM TOOLS

Somehow we learn who we really are and then live with that decision.

— Eleanor Roosevelt

Here are some nurturing acts and attitudes that will help you grow and flourish.

Compassion

Compassion, when it is genuine, creates a healing energy that goes directly to where you're hurting, warming and sustaining you. Reach into your heart and think of how it felt when someone was truly caring and compassionate to you. Compassion does not make the problem go away, but you have a much stronger outlook when sharing your concerns and being treated compassionately.

If you were to see a child crying and upset, would you not be compassionate to that child? You would not berate that child when he or she was hurting. Then why would you be any less compassionate to yourself?

Circumstances may not always provide a friendly confidant when problems arise. In that case you can learn to give compassion to yourself. You can learn how to develop an inner voice that is caring and loving, ready to encourage you and give you the courage to go on.

Acceptance

Your friend is the man who knows all about you, and still likes you.

– Elbert Hubbard, *The Notebook*, 1927

Compassion goes hand in hand with acceptance. If you respond to yourself with compassion rather than beating yourself up with disappointment, you are accepting yourself as the imperfect human being that you are. Sometimes things in our lives just don't go well or as planned. As the saying goes, *sh*t happens!* It may have nothing to do with you. If your self-esteem depends on external circumstances, then *anything* and *everything* will bowl you over with self-doubt.

You need to learn to accept yourself as you are and *to be there* for yourself. We all have problems and failings, and things we could have handled better, but that does not make us undeserving of caring, empathy, and assistance. How many times have you said to yourself, "I should have done that, I could have done that"? It is the "shoulda, woulda, coulda" syndrome. On the contrary, you need to accept and appreciate yourself as you are, even as you are attempting to improve yourself and your life.

Facing yourself and accepting in a non-judgmental, nurturing way the things you previously denied or hated about yourself helps you to change these "character defects" into positives. *Not* accepting yourself keeps you stuck.

Learning to accept yourself is something that happens one baby step at a time. As you move forward, there are bound to be old habits and patterns that cause you to step backward at times. Therefore, one of the first things you have to accept is that you are not going to change overnight. Change takes place slowly, and at each step along the way you need to give yourself credit for what you *are* doing, rather than focusing on what you are *not* doing.

> **When you accept yourself, you start to be close to yourself and to fill yourself up. In doing so, you also become more able to accept what others have to offer. The more you are able to genuinely receive from yourself and others, the more you have to give.**

Respect

As I become more honest with and respectful towards myself, I can be more honest and respectful towards other people. My inner light is guiding me, and my self-respect is no longer based on the approval of others. I can accept their approval as support; however, my own standards are what I am learning to live by. I am receptive to compliments, because I am worthy of my own respect and approval. I am not perfect, and therefore I do not expect others to be perfect either.

— Susan Ward, MA, MSW, author of *Beyond Feast or Famine*

A very popular singer, Aretha Franklin, is famous for belting out the song, "R-E-S-P-E-C-T"! If you are always feeling taken for granted, unappreciated, or devalued by others, then it may be time to look at how you are disrespecting yourself by staying in relationships with them. When others in their own unconscious way do not treat you with respect, you need to learn to give it to yourself. People treat you the way you *allow* them to!

Can you remember a time when you were feeling really low, and then someone let you know that he or she really appreciated something about you? Do you remember how that made you feel? You can feel that glow of self-respect warming inside of you. You can feel the positive energy that it gives you. Self-respect may take some time to rebuild, especially if you have been criticized or verbally abused about your weight.

I know you may have grabbed this book off the shelf and thought it would be another diet and exercise plan to lose weight. All this introspective work is more than you bargained for. Rebuilding yourself is an inside job and it is a foundation of what appears on the outside. You must be *willing* to do the work!

I will tell you my personal gauge of how much I have learned to respect myself. After my divorce and going out into the dating world, I felt like a Christian thrown in the Coliseum by the ancient Romans. My previous lack of self-respect had me turning into a contortionist trying to please someone or trying unsuccessfully to be the apple of his eye.

I have now learned to respect myself in many situations where *men behaved badly* toward me. *Now it is, "NEXT!"* No hesitation. I actually had a date stand me up (first date) and then beg and plead to give him another chance. He had a very lame excuse. My criteria is unless you are in the hospital on life support, severely bleeding, or in the morgue with a tag on your toe you had better *call* if you can't make it. If you just don't respect me or my time to primp for a date (yes, there is a lot of primping) and forgot how to dial a phone, it's *goodbye!*

I could not do that before. My lack of self-esteem and self-respect kept me in situations that were not healthy or to my emotional benefit. Before, I would have given this guy another chance (or many chances) to disrespect me or blow off *another* date. Okay, just to recap. I respect myself. If you don't respect me

(I don't care who you are), then it's *"NEXT!"* Sing it, Aretha: *R-E-S-P-E-C-T!*

Encouragement

> *If you think you can't . . . you must!*
>
> – Anthony Robbins

We all need encouragement to stretch ourselves to behavior that at first seems uncomfortable. If you were teaching a young child how to ride a new bike, you would be patient when the child didn't get it on the first try. You can count on it, it will take many attempts for a child to fully learn how to ride a bike. You would encourage that child and say, "Come on, you can do it!"

It's the same with you: you're learning behaviors that are different. You may feel emotionally wobbly (like the child on a bike) as you get your emotional balance. You may need encouragement from others to help you realize you *can do it.* This may come in the form of a support group that deals with your specific issues. If you are a compulsive eater or binger, then a support group such as Overeaters Anonymous may give you the encouragement you need. There are also many groups with therapists that may be helpful.

There is tremendous healing in knowing that you are not alone in your issues. Knowing others are struggling with the same feelings and issues that you are helps you realize that you are human just like they are. Support groups can give you tools to encourage yourself and help you with acceptance.

Have you ever felt so bad that you just wanted to pull the covers over your head and stay in bed and hide from the world for a day, a few weeks, or months? Inside you feel discouraged, hanging out with your two best friends, *whiney* and *poor me?*

You long for a shoulder to cry on, someone to love and support you (sniffle, sniffle), someone to give you the encouragement to go on.

We all long for this kind of support, for the knowledge that you have a loving, caring, nurturing parent behind you, encouraging you, telling you, *"You can do it!"* When you support yourself, you are being this kind of loving parent to yourself, assuring yourself that no matter what happens, you always come home loved. Encouraging yourself is letting yourself know that no matter how bad things get, no matter what losses or disappointments you may suffer, you always have yourself in your corner for encouragement and support.

I will leave you with this final thought: *Forgive yourself.* Just as you would forgive another if they made a mistake that hurt you, *forgive yourself.* Don't you deserve the graciousness of forgiveness for yourself that you extend to others? You need to look at your mistakes, learn from them, forgive, forget, and move on. You cannot go through life with a gunnysack of guilt draped on your back. Forgive . . . forget . . . move on.

I am my own heroine.
— Marie Bashkirtsell

In the middle of difficulty lies wisdom.
— Albert Einstein

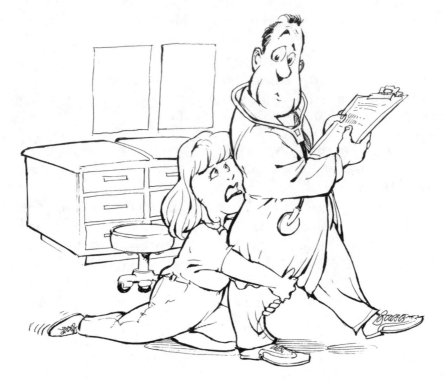

"Doctor, doctor . . . give me the news."

Metabolic Mayhem

*My doctor is wonderful. Once,
when I couldn't afford an operation,
he touched up the X-rays.*

— Joey Bishop

Either the human being must suffer and struggle as the price of a more searching vision, or his gaze must be shallow and without intellectual revelation.

– Thomas de Quincey

CHAPTER 7

■ ■ ■ ■ ■ ■ ■ ■ ■ ■

My Day of Reckoning

*I had no intention of giving her my vital statistics.
"Let me put it this way," I said. "According to my
girth, I should be a ninety-foot redwood."*

— Erma Bombeck, *If Life is a Bowl of Cherries,
What am I Doing in the Pits?* 1978

There I was, sitting in the doctor's treatment room, coming down from the high of my celebration of the release of my first book the night before. I had also written and produced a theater production surrounding my book, and I was still feeling the adrenaline rush of this magical night. Even with these feelings of success and excitement, I was angry as hell—angry because the night before, I had to do the best acting job of my career. I say acting because I came out on stage as if I owned it and the world was mine! But inside I felt like the biggest failure in history—because I was at my heaviest weight. The shame I felt was overwhelming.

As I was waiting for the doctor to come in, I was reflecting on the spectacular night before. I wanted to come out on that stage feeling thin and beautiful. Instead I had been scrambling for weeks trying to figure out what I was going to wear, so that I could present myself in the best possible light. (I thought about my bathrobe—no, that wouldn't work.) I talked with my friend Ned, who was to be my master of ceremonies, a few weeks before the event. I was sharing with him how absolutely out of my mind with frustration I was that I had lost no weight from the intense running and marathon training program I was participating in. Although I wanted to run the marathon, another one of my motives was to lose weight to shine at my own event.

Ned and I had been to many Tony Robbins events together, and he had seen me jump 50 feet off a pole into midair, for Pete's sake. He knew that when I committed to an outcome, I busted my butt to get there. I was telling him I was following a low-carbohydrate food plan and running my ass off, but the weight was hanging onto my body for dear life. My legs were so strong and solid from the running that my acupuncturist could not put a needle in my lower leg without bending the needle! But I was still fat! Ned, being the adoring and supportive friend that he is, just listened to my fears about coming onto the stage in my "obese condition." But what was I going to do? As they say in show business, the show must go on, regardless of what the scale says.

The doctor came in and sat on his stool, peering over his bifocals to read my chart. I was sitting on the exam table trying to contain my tears. I just wanted to explode into a crying tantrum. If I could have gotten away with it, I would have hurled myself onto the floor, kicking and screaming like a two-year-old. That's how *furious* I was! As tears started to roll down my cheeks I began to explain to the doctor how the only way the scale would register a weight loss for me would be if I cut off a limb! I told him that I had been eating a low-carbohydrate diet, running for six months, until I thought I would absolutely drop dead on the track, and *I was frustrated.* I had legs as solid as tree trunks, but I was still fat! *Still fat!* I wanted to scream at him! He asked me why I was so angry. Me, angry? No reason— I was just living in an alien body that had a mind of its own, and I was sick of it. I hated my body because it had betrayed me. Why would the doctor ask if I was angry?

Again he peered over his glasses, making eye contact and trying to be patient with me, but I would say he was conde-

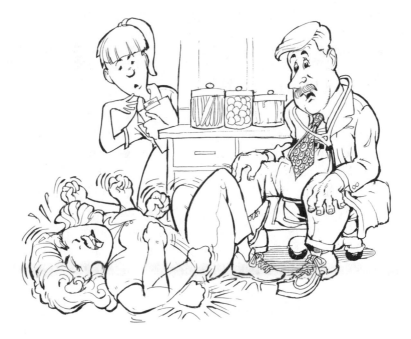

scending (I do not see him any longer as a patient—more about that later). I got the feeling he thought I was lying to him or just being a drama queen. I will admit that I had major attitude, but geeeeez, let's figure this out already. My life was ticking away. I was in fat prison serving a life sentence with no possibility of parole. I wanted out! Keep in mind that at that point I had been struggling for 14 years, in vain, to be thin.

The doctor said, "By looking at your weight distribution [heavy in the abdomen area and upper hips] I suspect that you have a serious problem of insulin resistance and Syndrome X."

"Syndrome what?" I asked.

"A severe form of insulin resistance," he explained, "where the insulin stays in the blood, can't get into the cells, so your body can't burn fat, and you become a fat-making machine." A fat-making machine—that was me, all right. "We will schedule you for blood work to determine your fasting insulin levels." I would have agreed to donate a kidney at that point if it was necessary to get to the bottom of my weight issue.

Below is an excerpt of the doctor's report for that office visit, dictated to his office staff:

> The patient is in the office with multiple complaints, over an hour discussion. She has a weight problem with serious insulin resistance, Syndrome X. She has tried every diet on the market and she is frustrated. She has tried a high-carbohydrate diet and then a low-carbohydrate diet. She has tried high protein, low fat, etc. She has run as much as 13 miles a day. I demonstrated the trochais of water [live water], exercise, and diet, all working as one. I talked about the concept that 3,500 calories equals one pound anywhere. She wants to get into a relationship and hates her body. There is depression clearly evident.

> The patient has insulin resistance. She had many questions about this and wants to learn as much as possible, maybe to write another book. She has impaired glucose tolerance associated with aging, which is correlated with her weight gain. The obesity is visceral/abdominal for this patient, which is a textbook, classic symptom. She was told that when she returns to a normal weight, the glucose levels will normalize.

My blood work confirmed that my insulin was indeed high: 114 points. You should be around the 80 to 90 mark. My doctor discussed with me prescribing glucophage. Although I am very anti-prescription, I listened to what he had to say. The glucophage, he said, would bring down the insulin so it could go into the cells and be burned as fat. I asked about the possibility of just taking it for a few weeks because of my holistic "let's-take-a-supplement-or-an-herb instead" beliefs. I really struggled with this, because it went against everything I believe in (holistic nutrition), but I was becoming such a frustrated raving maniac I was willing to consider anything.

I agreed that I would take the glucophage for only six to eight weeks to jump-start my body, but then I would search for a natural alternative instead. (I have since found a natural alternative, which we will discuss later in the book.) This gave me time to research, read, and strategize a holistic approach.

In six weeks, without changing my diet or exercise regimen, 25 pounds just fell off my body. I am not kidding you. Without any effort whatsoever—and without having to lose a limb— the weight just dropped off. It became evident that the insulin's inability to get into the cells and burn fat was the immediate issue at hand. I am telling you I just don't drop 25 pounds. The only time this had happened before was water loss three days after my first son was born.

Well, I wish I could tell you this was the end of the weight problem, but that would be too easy, and there would be no book! After I experienced this tremendous drop in weight, my weight stabilized, and again I stopped losing. I stopped the glucophage after about eight weeks, and the weight loss stopped as well. I had also started having serious conflicts with this doctor and his staff. The first conflict was due to the condescending tone this doctor used when speaking with me. He was God, and knew everything; I was not to question him. The second conflict was that, as I was reading and learning more about Syndrome X, I was starting to question advice given to me by this doctor and his staff. The biggest issue was their wanting me to use their products, which contained fructose. Even though fructose is considered "safe sugar," because it does not raise glucose levels, it actually promotes insulin resistance.

I also asked—begged was more like it—that this doctor have all my hormone levels tested, because my low energy indicated that I was entering into menopause and had a possible low thyroid. In his own words (from a medical dictation that is too lengthy and too medical to put in this book) he states, "Excess insulin in overweight people can lead to other problems, water retention, sleep disorder, LDL, increase in the liver enzymes, interference with thyroid, aggravating low metabolism, etc." The irony of this whole situation was that I had seen this doctor in my early twenties and he had given me a prescription for low thyroid then. But since my records were sealed in the tomb of archived patient charts he could not verify it. This doctor flatly refused to test my thyroid, saying that it was unnecessary. I loudly disagreed with him, and he did not like it. Let the power struggle begin! Now it was a matter of preserving

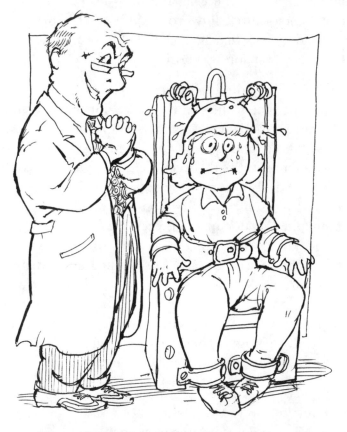

"I am God! You have disobeyed me!"

his need to be right and an ego that could barely fit through his office door! Maybe he should have gone back and read his own report!

I had a handle on the insulin issue. It was now at normal levels, but something else was going on. I could feel it, I knew it! and I wanted to get to the bottom of it. All I was getting from him were the accusatory eyes peering at me over the bifocals again, when my weight loss stopped. The way he looked at me you would think I was sitting there in his office eating a chocolate glazed donut!

Okay, enough of this holier-than-thou doctor. It was over! It was time to move on. Next! It took me more than a year to find Dr. Dommisse, who would consult with me and take my concerns seriously. Before I met this new doctor, I had lost no weight. I was in the same place. Time was standing still—just spinning my wheels, bursting out of the seams in my pants, but what are you going to do? I had to drive all the way from California to Arizona to see this new doctor, but that was a small price to pay for sanity.

In my first consultation with Dr. Dommisse I began to explain my saga of the failure to return to my goal weight. I tried to stay calm and state the facts, but my irritation was obviously evident by the subsequent medical report I received from him. He told me that there were thousands of people in the United States with thyroid problems that are undiagnosed. Many medical doctors are not taking their patients' complaints seriously and are not checking for thyroid dysfunction. I told him that I had taken my underarm basal temperature, and it did in fact indicate a possibility of low thyroid. At least he validated the possibility of a metabolic issue with me and did not suggest that I was running around town stuffing my face with pizza and then whining because I was fat.

Below is an excerpt of Dr. Dommisse's metabolic evaluation, after meeting with me.

Ms. Jordan is referred by the *Alternative Medicine Weight Loss* book in which some of my case histories apparently are chronicled. She has been very fatigued since 1988 but has still managed to write a book, *Detox for Life,* and is working on a second one. She also has significant brain fog, memory loss, concentration difficulties, low functioning. She has perimenopausal symptoms. She has low libido, moderate depression, and a huge weight gain of 85 pounds in the last 14 years, despite being on the Syndrome X diet and lots of exercise. A TSH was 1.55 back in 1998, which I would have treated because a T4 level was low–normal at that time already. She had an insulin level of 121 back then as well, and I would have put her on the high-protein, low-carbohydrate diet then if she wasn't on it already. She is now on this diet. Ms. Jordan is very frustrated, angry, and emotional about what she sees as the ineffectiveness of the medical profession to address all these significant symptoms and problems.

Her diet is low carbohydrate, high protein, but ineffective at this time and she's even talked to the author of the *Syndrome X* book, Jack Challem. She is not diabetic. I suspect primary hypothyroidism and will test adequately and sensitively for that.

After the initial consultation and subsequent medical testing, it was determined that indeed my thyroid was low functioning, and my perimenopause state was the root of my low energy level. At one point Dr. Dommisse asked me how I had written a book and kept the schedule that I did with such low energy. I am a very determined person, that is all I can say.

I began taking Dr. Dommisse's recommended protocol with supplementation to support my hormones and activate my thyroid function. I was also contributing my own knowledge to healing with natural supplements and herbs.

Right on the heels of my consultation with Dr. Dommisse, my father was diagnosed with terminal cancer and given just a few months to live. It was hard to assess my energy and metabolic improvement on the new regimen because I was emotionally upset and in grief. My father subsequently passed away and my energy was low for quite some time due to grieving.

The weight started to come off, not dramatically, as in dropping 25 pounds in a few weeks, but slowly. For the first time in 14 years, I began to feel hopeful and confident that my body was slowly working its way into hormonal balance.

I began training with a personal trainer three times a week for muscle definition to reshape my body. He wanted me to come in and perform cardiovascular training twice a day to inprove my metabolism. I felt that this physical exertion would also help me work through my grief. This worked well for about eight months after the hypothyroid diagnosis from Dr. Dommisse. Then came the metabolic crash.

The easiest way I can describe it is like a flashlight battery that has been left on and the light is growing dimmer and dimmer. Every workout left me increasingly drained and weary. My recovery time between workouts became longer and longer. My enthusiasm to get to the gym became lower and lower. My trainer's lack of knowledge about low thyroid and metabolic issues became apparent, and he kept pushing me beyond what I thought I could comfortably bear. His theory was to push me harder so I would speed up my metabolism. I did the workout and then went home and dropped dead!

I bluntly told him I was frustrated. I felt that he was not fully understanding my issues when I told him I felt so tired I could hardly train. I was not trying to wimp out. I was just beginning to realize that I was doing too much training too soon. My hormonal system was improved, but still struggling for balance under seemingly adverse conditions.

During all the research for this book and talking with all the metabolic specialists, I realized (and it was validated by all of them) that I had used up my reservoir of energy in my metabolic bank account. I was on a fast track speeding to metabolic bankruptcy if I didn't repair and build up my reserves again.

I opted to discontinue training with a personal trainer and work out on my own. I now have more control over my energy output and stamina. My dogs are in heaven because they get walked more than usual!

I decided to consult with a medical doctor located near my home rather than being treated out of state. I am now working with Richard Shames, MD, and Karilee Shames, RN. In my initial consultation, Dr. Shames kept revisiting my Epstein Barr diagnosis in 1988 with extreme interest. This was the beginning of my hormonal hell. My body has never returned to my thin pre–Epstein Barr weight. His belief is that this was the catalyst that blew out my thyroid and adrenal glands.

As you can see, metabolic situations can be detailed, complicated, and time-consuming. Not to mention the absolute crazy insanity you feel trying to figure it all out! It is not as simple as taking a few supplements for one issue and then you have boundless energy. The metabolism takes time to heal, sometimes a year or more, and *all* the hormones must be taken into consideration and balanced. Getting to the core metabolic issue can be challenging at best. You have to find a physician who is willing to do the detective work to get to the beginning of the ball of yarn!

I am also engaging in acupuncture with Richard Nuesteder, OMD (doctor of oriental medicine), to assist my metabolic system in the healing process and to increase my energy.

I am not at my goal weight today, but I will be. I am working with my health care team and improving one day at a time. I am striving for progress, not perfection—as you should be.

Later in this book I will present a laundry list of criteria you can take to your doctor or health professional to assist you if you see yourself in this picture. You have lived with yourself the longest; you know your body better than anyone. If you have a gut feeling about health concerns, you owe it to yourself to find a health professional or doctor who will assist you. Take care of yourself by preserving your self-respect and dignity. Do not allow any doctor or health professional to belittle your concerns or opinion. There is only *one God,* and trust me, he is not working in a lab coat. Have a cooperative spirit and be open to all the possibilities of where this journey will take you.

Nothing ever becomes real until it is experienced.
Even a proverb is no proverb to you until your
life has illustrated it.

– John Keats

CHAPTER 8

■ ■ ■ ■ ■ ■ ■ ■ ■

If Your Diet Doesn't Fit You, How Can Your Clothes?

Written by Robban A. Sica, MD

WHAT TYPES OF DIETS HAVE YOU TRIED?

Most diets are based on calorie restriction, fat restriction, fasting, and restricting foods to certain limited (not to mention boring!) food choices. You can maintain the diet, if you are highly motivated, for a period of time. But sooner or later, something will make you go off the diet: feeling deprived, celebrating a special occasion, etc. Then you are back on the weight roller-coaster, often gaining back whatever weight you've been successful in losing and usually a few pounds more.

Why do we believe that there is a "right diet" that everyone will lose weight with? Or that people gain weight only because they eat excessively?

Why diets don't work:

♦ The wrong diet for a person's unique type.

♦ Boredom, severe restrictions, regimentation, lack of variety.

♦ Calorie restriction actually causes the body to hold onto fat! When you consume an insufficient amount of calories, your body goes into "starvation mode." In other words, your body thinks it is being starved, so it tries to store whatever food it gets for future use. The body does this by converting calories into fat stores that can be broken down at a later time to produce energy.

◆ Dieting slows down the functioning of the thyroid gland. The thyroid gland controls the rate of metabolism and thus the rate at which calories are burned by the body. Severe dieting slows down your body's metabolic rate, which slows down weight loss and predisposes you to gain weight more easily once you go off the diet.

◆ Most rapid weight loss achieved on calorie-restrictive diets results from water loss and muscle wasting. This type of weight loss is not lasting. Losing muscle mass decreases your lean-muscle-mass-to-body-fat ratio, which causes your metabolic rate to slow down even further. This means that this type of dieting predisposes you to gain weight more readily.

◆ Quick weight loss—through starvation, calorie restriction, laxative use, vomiting, and other diet methods—causes nutritional deficiencies and imbalances in the body which can lead to serious and long-term health problems, especially cravings that lead to binging.

◆ Crash dieting is a stress on the body that can lead to the production of toxins and free radicals, which increases the rate of aging and degenerative diseases.

◆ Toxins are usually stored in fat tissue. When the body is overloaded by toxins, it increases fat stores in an effort to sequester these toxins and protect the rest of the tissues.

◆ Besides obesity, prolonged or cyclic (yo-yo) dieting predisposes you to many chronic illnesses such as:

Hypoglycemia
Fatigue
Insulin resistance
Diabetes
Thyroid disorders
Menstrual and hormonal disorders

What you really need, instead, is an eating plan or "dining style" that you can maintain day in and day out for the rest of your life to maintain your optimal weight and health!

AN EFFECTIVE DIET HAS NOTHING TO DO WITH STARVATION OR DEPRIVATION!

Each person—body/mind/spirit—is unique. Beliefs, goals, feelings, reasons for eating, physique, health status, biochemistry, metabolism, blood type, allergies, etc. are all individual. Every human is as unique biochemically as they are physically. Thus, biochemical and nutritional needs vary considerably among the population. Variability in nutritional requirements has been linked to genetic makeup, blood types, lifestyle factors, insulin response to carbohydrate intake, environmental pollution, food processing techniques, hormonal balance, and health conditions. These combined factors indicate that all people should not have the same diet. Therefore, their diet, exercise plan, and lifestyle choices must be unique too! One size truly does not fit all.

The most significant individual variables that affect weight issues and diet include:

◆ Carbohydrate sensitivity and insulin resistance

◆ Adequacy of trace minerals

◆ Optimal thyroid function, which controls metabolic rate

◆ Hormone balance, including estrogen and progesterone, cortisol and DHEA, growth hormone, testosterone

- Toxicity
- Food allergy
- Optimal digestion and absorption
- Metabolic type
- Blood type
- Body type
- Exercise tolerance and ability
- Age
- Emotional issues
- Belief systems about weight
- Lifestyle habits
- Stress levels
- Genetics
- Other medical conditions

BIOCHEMICAL INDIVIDUALITY

Individuals are as unique in their biochemistry as they are in physical appearance. Thus, biochemical and physiologic needs vary considerably among the population. While many bestselling books have touted the latest, supposedly best diet for everyone, they are destined to fail if they ignore the truth: One diet does not fit all!

In helping a person to find the keys to his or her unique situation, I think of myself as a detective, seeking the keys to unlock that individual's particular needs. Over many years of practice, I have realized that honoring the uniqueness of each person is the way to guide them on the path to their optimal wellness. When these individual variables are addressed, we arrive at the answer: an integrated and truly individualized approach to weight loss.

CARBOHYDRATE SENSITIVITY AND INSULIN RESISTANCE

Warning: What you are about to read may totally contradict much of the advice given by doctors, dieticians, and diet authors. "Fat phobia" that has been generated in our society arises from a total misunderstanding of how food is handled physiologically in the body, along with the simplistic thinking that "fat makes you fat." Contrary to the "low-fat" advocates, fat (in and of itself) does *not* make you fat! Nor does it raise your cholesterol! The body is much more complex than that, as you will see.

I've found that the single most important factor in how you will fare on a given diet is your body's reaction to carbohydrates. Virtually any carbohydrate intake causes the body to produce increased levels of insulin in order to metabolize these sugars that *all* carbohydrates break down to eventually. Every dieter knows that some carbohydrates are "better" than others. However, for some, understanding the reason why often unlocks the mystery of dieting. Among other benefits, some fruits and veggies have a lower glycemic index versus high-glycemic carbohydrates such as sugars, grains, and flour-based products. The higher the glycemic response, the more insulin has to be produced to handle the sugars. Insulin is a storage hormone: It tells your body to take everything you have just eaten and store it basically as fat. You simply cannot lose weight with that higher insulin level telling your body to go into storage mode!

This applies to everyone. Higher insulin levels take their toll many ways: weight gain, poor concentration, fatigue, impaired performance, generalized inflammation, hypertension, elevated cholesterol and triglycerides, decreased HDL, insulin resistance, adult onset diabetes, and cardiovascular disease. *Food acts as a drug.* What we eat profoundly affects insulin production. Insulin is the most powerful mediator of the short-term chemical messengers called eicosanoids or prostaglandins, which mediate inflammation in the body (for example, arthritis), and affect serum lipids and blood pressure. High insulin decreases the sensitivity of hormone receptor sites, causing hormonal imbalances and aging.

SO WHAT'S WRONG WITH THE FOOD PYRAMID?

◆ According to the food guide pyramid that we all had to learn in school, you need to consume 20 to 30% of your calories as fat, 15 to 20% as protein, and 50 to 65% as carbohydrates. Unfortunately, this emphasizes large amounts of carbohydrates, which is inappropriate for many, and worsens weight problems. Also, the food pyramid makes little distinction in food quality. It tells you to minimize the intake of fats without discriminating between necessary fats and harmful ones.

◆ Many Americans do not eat a balanced diet, even those who feel they eat well. Almost 40% of the calories in the average American diet comes from highly processed convenience and snack foods that are high in unhealthy fats and refined sugar, and depleted of valuable vitamins, minerals, and essential fatty acids needed for health. If you are eating processed "low-fat" and "no-fat" foods, you're still not helping yourself. These foods are extremely high in sugar (they have to get them to taste good somehow!). Sugar, which comes in many different varieties, has the strongest effect on the release of insulin. The higher the amount of circulating insulin in our blood, the more likely we are to store our calories as fat.

How much insulin is produced depends not only on the type of carbohydrates but also on the carbohydrate tolerance of the person who ate them! Some people produce increased amounts of insulin in response to carbohydrates. This hyperinsulinemic state is also called Syndrome X, insulin resistance, and, eventually, carbohydrate intolerance, also known as adult-onset diabetes. People with this tendency are much more prone to health problems induced by insulin.

Not uncommonly, I see patients like Adam, who, at 48, had already had bypass surgery several years before and was having chest pain again. His cardiologists were recommending a second surgery. His cholesterol was 281 with a low HDL (good cholesterol) of 18, and triglycerides of over 800! And his weight and blood pressure were climbing. His conventional doctors wanted him on a very low-fat diet and statin drugs immediately, but he didn't want the side effects. Since this lipid pattern is classic for hyperinsulinemia, I immediately explained to him why he needed to lower his carbohydrate intake. After only ten days on a very low-carbohydrate, moderate fat and protein diet, Adam lost ten pounds and lowered his blood pressure significantly. His cholesterol fell to 230, HDL went up to 31, and triglycerides fell to 90! All without cholesterol-lowering medications. Best of all, his energy level went up dramatically and his chest pain stopped, probably because high triglycerides make the blood thick and harder for the heart to pump, among other factors. The standard low-fat recommendations were literally killing him!

When someone tries to follow a low-fat diet, they generally replace protein and fat with carbohydrates, causing them to overeat carbohydrates. Low-fat diets cause another problem: since they are less calorie-dense, people will generally lose weight initially due to the calorie restriction. As the effects of the elevated insulin levels and the resultant insulin resistance take their toll, gradual steady weight gain occurs and often exceeds the amount lost. Blood pressure, lipids, and blood sugar often rise as well. The resulting frustration is considerable!

This illustrates another misperception about diet: that all fat is bad! There are many benefits of fat in the diet, including slowing down metabolism of carbohydrate and lowering the glycemic index, which in turn slows down production of insulin. Fat signals the satiety center in the brain, telling you that you've had enough to eat. This satiety center is only stimulated by cholecystokinin, which is produced in response to fat in the diet. Unfortunately, carbohydrate does not trigger the satiety mechanism that tells us to stop eating! Low-fat diets, therefore, actually *cause* overeating because of the absence of this signal. Only adequate fat content will produce a satiety response.

Think about the portion sizes at typical Italian restaurants. Often, pasta is served in an enormous bowl. This gives the impression of generous portion size, but actually pasta is relatively inexpensive, as is bread. In addition, large portions have affected what people view as a normal portion size. Now think about someone trying to eat a large serving of prime rib. Halfway through, they will usually push the plate away, exclaiming that they can't eat another bite! This is due to the higher fat content. Not so with the person who ordered the pasta dish. Most likely, they will continue nibbling until they've finished most of it.

Another example is the difference in fat content in types of ice cream and frozen yogurt. The expensive gourmet ice creams have higher fat content, but notice the package size is usually smaller than the low-fat frozen yogurt. Most people will consume a small serving of the gourmet ice cream and savor it but will overeat on the low-fat varieties, trying to gain the same level of satisfaction. (I often tell my patients that, if they are going to "cheat," at least get the good stuff and enjoy it!)

All fats, however, are *not* created equal! Essential fats such as omega-3 fatty acids—found in fatty fish such as salmon, mackerel, cod liver oil, and flax seed oil—decrease appetite, lower inflammation by building of good eicosanoids, and give many other health benefits. Unfortunately, eating too much large fish (like tuna or swordfish) can expose you to high levels of mercury, pesticides, PCBs, and other fat-soluble poisons. So I recommend taking supplements of flax seed oil or omega-3 fish oils, purified to remove these toxins, to aid in weight loss. Arachidonic acid, found in fatty red meats, egg yolks, dairy, and organ meats, increases inflammation in the body, so those on higher protein diets need to choose from a variety of protein sources. Also, excessive amounts of omega-6 fatty acids found in sunflower oil, safflower oil, and soybean oil can increase arachidonic acid. Mono-unsaturated fats are hormonally neutral, so foods such as olives, olive oil, avocado, and nuts are good for snacking as they are satisfying with minimal effect on insulin.

The good news: A diet composed of the proper balance of protein, fat, and carbohydrate reduces insulin levels and results in normalization of blood sugar, blood pressure, cholesterol, triglycerides, HDL, LDL, and energy levels. In my opinion, anyone's diet should contain no more than 40% carbohydrates (preferably fruits and vegetables), and approximately 30% each of protein and fat. However, the optimal balance of macro-nutrients is *very* individual, according to the person's tolerance for carbohydrates. People with diabetes, hypoglycemia, ex-tremely high triglyceride levels, polycystic ovarian syndrome, or fatigue after eating carbs are very carbohydrate-intolerant and need to reduce the percentage of carbohydrates in their diet accordingly. From what I've observed in my patients, this explains the mystery of why some people do fine on the food pyramid diet, while others lose weight only on an extremely low-carbohydrate diet, and still others need something in between. Balancing these macronutrients and moderating por-tion size to maintain this balance are the keys to losing weight and feeling great consistently.

Far too often, I am frustrated and angered when I hear from a new patient a horror story of going to doctor after doctor, seeking out nutritionists and personal trainers and diet pro-grams, carefully following all the recommendations and not losing weight. To add insult to injury, these unfortunate people are told that they must not be following the diet, that it is somehow their fault! I hope that you have never had that experience, but I know that too many people have!

Fortunately, certain blood tests can allow your doctor to monitor your progress and determine how strict you need to be with carbohydrates. These tests include lipid profile, glucose, hemoglobin A1C, fructosamine, and fasting insulin levels. With these tools, you have the power to individualize your carb intake to ensure you are successful with your weight goals.

THYROID FUNCTION AND METABOLIC RATE

Ever wonder why some people have "slow metabolism"? Thyroid hormones control metabolic rate, which of course affects your ability to lose weight. The metabolic rate, which is the rate at which your body turns food into energy, affects the health of every cell in the body, so many health problems have their roots in hypothyroidism, or low thyroid function. I could easily write a whole book on this subject, but the most frustrating effects of a sluggish thyroid are fatigue and weight gain. Many overweight people suspect that their metabolism is not what it should be, yet they find little help or support in solving this mystery. Often they are blamed for their inability to lose weight, yet I often see patients who are eating 1,000 calories or less per day and still not losing weight! Sometimes they exercise two to three hours a day and still can't lose.

I recently saw a 23-year-old girl who gained a large amount of weight during puberty and at 15 became anorexic in her frustration to be thin. She did lose the weight, but at a tremendous price. At our first meeting, Maryann was pale, with puffy dark circles under her eyes. She suffered from dry skin, severe constipation, depression, and fatigue that only improved when she exercised to extreme—all signs of hypothyroidism. Her temperature was very low and she frequently felt cold, which is an indicator of metabolic rate. While she was very wary of any dietary intervention and fearful of eating more than 800 calories, as we cautiously corrected her underlying thyroid problem with natural thyroid replacement, she became free of the torture it took to maintain her weight. Her skin improved and the sallow color disappeared. Maryann now has plenty of energy and is no longer depressed. Best of all, she is able to eat more normally, although she did maintain a lower carbohydrate intake. (Most hypothyroid patients have a hyperinsulinemic tendency.)

Unfortunately, her conventional endocrinologist did not recognize or treat her thyroid problem, because her blood tests for thyroid function were within the laboratory's reference ranges, although on the lower side. These ranges are usually misconstrued to mean "normal" range but really only represent a statistical average of the last 800 tests run by that particular lab! In no way do they represent optimal function for a given individual. There are at least a dozen reasons that I know of that thyroid blood tests can miss the diagnosis of hypothyroidism. Various authors have estimated the percentage of low thyroid people in the population from 30 to a whopping 80% (could this account, in part, for the epidemic of obesity?) and the percent of those missed by blood test from 30 to 50%! That is why I prefer to use a clinical method of diagnosing and treating hypothyroidism: looking for clinical symptoms and signs like those Maryann was suffering from. While thyroid hormone is *not* a magic weight loss pill, and other factors still must be addressed, many of my patients have benefited from this approach and are living happier, healthier lives as a result.

THE DELICATE HORMONE BALANCE

Besides thyroid, the balance of other hormones such as cortisol, DHEA, estrogen, progesterone, growth hormone, and testosterone affect weight gain as well as percent body fat and distribution of fat. As we age, many of our hormone levels decline, causing imbalances and deficiencies. This affects our overall well-being and many aspects of our health, not the least of which is the tendency to gain fat and lose muscle mass. It is essential to identify individual imbalances and correct them.

BALANCING ADRENAL FUNCTION

Our adrenal glands help in several ways to maintain normal function under a variety of stressors. Cortisol is an adrenal hormone that stabilizes blood sugar. A low cortisol level can result in low blood sugar and the need to eat frequently. This type of adrenal deficiency can lead to fatigue after exercise, a real obstacle to losing weight and getting in shape. Cortisol is also essential for utilization of thyroid hormone, leading to the problems associated with low thyroid. Small, physiologic doses of cortisol can be helpful and actually improve thyroid function and weight loss.

High cortisol levels, a common side effect of too much stress, can also be problematic. Cortisol is catabolic, meaning it breaks down tissue. This can cause loss of muscle mass and excessive fat gain, especially around the middle! Worse yet, high cortisol suppresses the production of DHEA, an adrenal hormone that is anabolic, meaning it builds and repairs muscle and other tissues. Stress management and DHEA are the keys to reversing this imbalance.

WHAT ABOUT FEMALE HORMONES?

Estrogen and progesterone balance each other in a delicate dance. When a woman has too much estrogen relative to progesterone, she tends to gain weight, have fluid retention, and have other premenstrual symptoms, including chocolate or sweet cravings. Improving this balance with magnesium, vitamin B6, the herb vitex, or natural progesterone restores the natural balance and helps to smooth out the month.

After menopause, women who take hormone replacement therapy (HRT) very often gain weight. But do naturally occurring hormones cause weight gain? Or is something else going on? The most commonly prescribed HRT is made from horse urine. These conjugated waste estrogens are strong enough for a thousand-pound animal! Hence, they lead to estrogen dominance, including increased risk of weight gain, blood clots, and breast cancer. These problems are compounded when combined with the synthetic progesterone derivative, which has side effects of severe water retention, bloating, and breast tenderness. No wonder so many women resist the idea of HRT. Fortunately, when natural hormones that are bio-identical to human hormones are used in a balanced fashion, a woman can realize the benefits of HRT—including the prevention of osteoporosis, diabetes, and cardiovascular diseases—without the risks and the weight gain. I use estriol predominately, the estrogen highest during pregnancy. This hormone actually seems to provide some protection from breast cancer, and, since it is far weaker than estradiol, has far less tendency to cause weight gain, etc. Estrogen dominance can be prevented by pairing estriol with bio-identical progesterone. Natural progesterone actually opposes the negative effects of estrogen and has some positive anabolic effect.

Sarah came to my office at age 55, on Prempro that her gynecologist had prescribed to treat her severe hot flashes. She got rid of the flashes only to suffer significant fluid retention and a weight gain of 18 pounds. The resultant mood swings caused food cravings and binge eating, compounding the problem. She felt stressed and out of control, afraid to stop the HRT and have the hot flashes return, but equally afraid of continuing to gain weight. I helped her get out of this vicious cycle by switching her HRT to an estriol and progesterone combination and adding DHEA (in the 7-Keto form to prevent conversion to estrogen) to balance the stress-induced cortisol. First she noticed feeling calmer and sleeping better. As she gained control of the stress, she was able to make the necessary adjustments to her eating habits and begin exercising regularly. Her weight loss was gradual but steady, until she returned to her original weight six months later.

WHAT ABOUT MALE HORMONES?

Testosterone and DHEA are androgens, or anabolic steroid hormones, that start to decline sometime after the age of 45. We don't talk much about male "andropause" but it happens all the same. Although attention is often focused on diminishing sexual prowess and libido, low testosterone levels can affect cardiovascular health, carbohydrate metabolism, memory, cognitive function, bone density, and sense of well-being. As these androgens decrease, muscle mass starts to turn to flab, and it's harder to build muscle from those endless workouts! Weight gain around the waistline increases conversion of testosterone to estrogen by up-regulating the aromatase enzyme, causing increasing weight gain and gynecomastia (enlarged breasts).

Steve, at 50, was already feeling the effects of a falling testosterone level, with weight gain, diminishing muscle mass, and decreased libido. He felt like something was missing in life, like he was "not himself." His testosterone levels were in the low–normal range; not unusual, since the laboratory reference ranges are broad, encompassing the range for 20- to 80-year-old men. After starting natural testosterone replacement therapy, he initially felt some increase in fluid retention with chest and abdominal swelling. After checking his estrogen level, we realized he was converting all his testosterone to estrogen. By using aromatase blockers, we were able to prevent this. His testosterone levels came up to normal, along with the disappearance of his symptoms. He felt like himself again! He was able to return to his individualized diet and exercise program with vigor and, in time, his physique returned as well.

The metabolites of testosterone are as important as the

hormone itself in terms of libido, arousal, and optimal sexual function. Not just for men, women need testosterone too—especially menopausal women and those whose high cortisol/stress levels are suppressing testosterone. Improved libido helps with weight loss. Feeling sexy helps self-esteem, and sex itself is a much better stress reducer than maladaptive eating. And sex burns calories instead of adding them. Testosterone builds exercise tolerance and ability, aiding weight loss and fitness efforts.

Steroid hormones have gotten a bad rap, and none worse than testosterone. A steroid hormone is, by definition, a hormone built on a cholesterol frame. Steroid hormones include testosterone, DHEA, cortisol, estrogen, and progesterone. All affect every cell in your body and are absolutely essential to feel great, look great, and prevent disease and the effects of aging. Testosterone, particularly in synthetic form, has been abused by athletes, causing excess levels and a variety of horrific side effects. However, when testosterone is properly supplemented with bio-identical hormones, the benefits can be wonderful!

ADEQUACY OF TRACE MINERALS

Too often, cyclical starvation diets are devoid of nutrients, leaving the dieter in a nutrient-depleted state. To complicate matters, the myth that multivitamins cause weight gain continues to raise its ugly head. Deficiencies of vitamins and minerals cause craving and binging on certain foods. For instance, chocolate is rich in magnesium (among other things), so when you're deficient, your body craves chocolate. Premenstrually, the demand for magnesium and vitamin B6 increases sharply, as do chocolate cravings and weight gain. Chromium and vanadium are trace minerals, often ignored, that are necessary for normal carbohydrate and insulin metabolism. Deficiencies create cravings for sweets and carbohydrates, as well as blood sugar swings, high insulin, and hypoglycemia. It a vicious cycle that is so easily prevented. Since over 60% of the population is deficient in one or more nutrients, I believe that our food supply is significantly depleted in essential nutrients, made far worse by restrictive low-calorie weight loss diets. I recommend a high-quality, balanced multivitamin to all my patients, especially those interested in losing weight. And I often look for nutrient deficiencies with specific testing, allowing me to correct imbalances unique to a given person.

DIGESTION AND ABSORPTION

Food cravings and overeating may also result from an inability to digest and absorb nutrients. Malabsorption leads to subsequent deficiency of essential nutrients. Sandra was a typical patient who complained of indigestion and fullness after eating, but overate because she always felt hungry. Comprehensive digestive testing revealed that she did not produce the enzymes to break down proteins. Starved for amino acids, she overate to get the protein she craved. Once we corrected her digestive enzyme deficiency, the bloating ceased and she felt satisfied with a reasonable portion size. Unable to lose weight before without "starving," she found she could easily follow a diet individualized for her and start to achieve her long sought-after "ideal weight."

TOXICITY

One of the overlooked issues of weight loss is that fat is often a protective mechanism. Toxins are sequestered in fatty tissues to protect the other tissues from damage. The body then holds onto the fat stores to prevent release of these substances, including pesticide residues, heavy metals (mercury, lead, etc.), and other fat-soluble toxins. Detoxification is essential to allow the release of this excess weight.

The story of Jason, the body builder, illustrates what can go wrong when you don't listen to the body's wisdom. Jason's job while in the Navy was to sandblast old paint from the inside of his ship's metal hull. Since he didn't wear adequate protection, residues of lead, cadmium, and mercury seeped into his system through his skin, lungs, and gastrointestinal tract. Being a young and otherwise healthy young man, he ignored this exposure. That is, until he couldn't. Jason decided to sign up for a body building competition that meant he had to drastically reduce his percent body fat to be competitive. He put in hours at the gym and did whatever it took to get to 10% or less body fat. He looked fantastic but didn't feel that way. In fact, he received a medical discharge from the Navy.

I met Jason four years later; he was completely disabled with chronic fatigue syndrome. He still looked the picture of health, so doctors ignored his complaints and told him it was in his head. They thought he was malingering. After hearing his story, I checked and found astronomical levels of the heavy metals he was exposed to back on the ship. As he lost the protective fat, the heavy metals flooded his system, poisoning his cells. Using chelation therapy, we were able to remove those toxic metals and restore Jason to health. I shudder to think what his life would have been like if we had not found out he was toxic. Most people don't drive to win a competition like that so, fortunately, they don't go through the same agony. But many feel the anguish as Jason did of pushing against an unseen barrier to weight loss that is caused by the resistance of losing that protective fat.

FOOD ALLERGY

Food allergies are often overlooked because they don't cause classic allergy symptoms: stuffy nose and itchy eyes. In fact, allergies to foods are most often delayed IgG reactions that can manifest in a variety of symptoms. Sometimes, the only symptom is difficulty losing weight. You see, there is an allergy-addiction cycle with foods that we're allergic to. The more allergic, the more we crave them because we get some relief, like a high, when we eat them. You can be allergic to almost any food, even "healthy" foods. Studies have demonstrated the food allergy/weight gain phenomenon. If your weight loss is stuck on a plateau, consider food allergy testing.

Linda had been a patient of mine over ten years before but had long since forgotten my recommendations because she was "feeling well." Gradually over time, lack of attention to her health caught up with her. She gained over 100 pounds and felt terrible. She was exhausted, depressed, and her allergies were getting worse. She had a sinus infection at least once a month and was taking antibiotics almost continuously. Her cholesterol and triglycerides were edging skywards and her primary care physician was harping on her to lose weight. But he couldn't give any effective advice, and she was at her wit's end. Then she remembered that she had seen me years before, and things seemed better then. When she returned to my office, I barely recognized the young girl I had once known.

After hearing her story, I started her back on thyroid medication that she had taken previously, and her immune system improved significantly. But her allergy symptoms were still severe. Using antifungal medication and probiotics, we were able to stop the yeast overgrowth that was causing a great deal of discomfort and fluid retention. But she still didn't feel well, and her weight was sticking with her. Since antibiotic-induced yeast infections often cause yeast infection and damage in the gut, I suggested we test for food allergies that result in these situations. Sure enough, she had many significant allergies, including corn, dairy, tomatoes, wheat, and yeast, among others. While it was difficult for her to cut out all of them, she knew she needed to. Her determination paid off immediately: her allergy symptoms diminished and she dropped ten pounds in two weeks. We supported her immune system with allergy desensitization drops, and she rapidly improved with this combined approach. She lost an additional 25 pounds in the next two months and felt so much energy returning that she started a rigorous walking program five days a week. When she came back a month later, I barely recognized her in a new dress she had bought. All the puffiness was gone from her face. But she was very upset. She had been to see her primary care physician, who had insisted she lose weight when she was at 240 pounds, only to be told now that she was anorexic, and she should stop what she was doing! Since she felt fantastic, she decided to ignore that advice and continue to follow the allergy elimination diet (which, by the way, did *not* restrict calories!). She has gradually continued returning to her optimal weight. A year later, she has lost over 100 pounds, but more importantly, Linda has regained her self-esteem and her health.

METABOLIC TYPE AND BLOOD TYPE

Dr. William Kelly and his best known protegé, Nicholas Gonzalez, MD, have long studied human variability in metabolic type. Individual differences of the autonomic nervous system (ANS) and digestive integrity affect which diet a person will thrive on and which diet will contribute to disease, particularly specific cancer types related to the metabolic type. While Kelly's original system included over 12 types, the most common are sympathetic-dominant and parasympathetic-dominant, depending on which half of the ANS is strongest. Sympathetic-dominants have weaker digestion, and tend to be healthier on a lower animal protein diet, higher in grains and vegetables. Parasympathetics, with stronger digestion, need to eat more protein and avoid excessive grains. While metabolic type has been studied mostly in reference to cancer, not weight loss, it is a good illustration of how many factors contribute to individualization of your diet.

Probably the clearest evidence that individual genetic variation affects what foods we should eat to lose weight and be healthy comes from blood type. This work was pioneered by two naturopathic doctors, Drs. James and Peter D'Adamo. Years of observation and study of any reference in the literature to blood type led the doctors to the conclusion that the lectins (sticky cell membrane proteins that differentiate the four blood types) interact differently with foods. These lectins occur not just on blood cells but on many cells in the body. I tend to de-emphasize blood type because I've seen patients get fixated on the concept. On the other hand, while the D'Adamos' theories are far from conclusive fact and much research still needs to be done, I have also observed dramatic differences when blood type is taken into account.

I'll make some fairly sweeping generalizations to make a complex subject simpler. Blood type O, the most common type, stems from humanity's "hunter-gatherer" phase, so the best diet for a person with this blood type is a higher protein (from hunting and fishing) with vegetables, nuts, and fruits (from gathering). The O types tends to have stronger digestion, resulting in more stomach acid problems and intestinal reactions when eating the wrong foods. Grains, the product of farming, weren't available in the hunter-gatherer days and the O is poorly adapted to these foods. Often, an O individual complains of indigestion after eating even the smallest amount of wheat. O types do much better avoiding grains, and with this restriction, many digestive problems disappear. They also produce more insulin to store nutrients to get them through long periods when food isn't available, causing increased risk of hyperinsulinemia and diabetes. Wheat and corn, in particular, contain lectins that block insulin receptors on the O type cells, worsening insulin resistance. This can prevent the O type from losing weight and getting blood sugar under control. It may take up to six months of avoiding these foods for the insulin problems to resolve and weight loss to accelerate.

A person with blood type A, on the other hand, is much more adapted to a grain-based diet, later in evolutionary development. Weaker in digestion, they find animal proteins harder to digest and suffer from lectin interactions. A types often feel better eating more vegetarian diets and do poorly with excessive dairy and animal products. Nevertheless, some A types are still insulin resistant and need to limit dense carbohydrates. The other two types, B and AB, are the rarer types with their own unique dietary needs. I won't go into details, but I think you get the point.

Kim, in her mid-fifties, had been slowly gaining a pound or two per year over the last ten years. She was also beginning to experience some nagging health problems, worsening allergies, skin problems, and arthritis. She stuck rigidly to an extremely low-carbohydrate diet, the only way she could lose any weight at all. If she ate even one slice of bread or a dessert, the scale would jump up five pounds or more, and it would take two weeks for her to lose it again. Frustrated by weight gain, she traveled from Florida to Connecticut to my office. We assessed and treated her hypothyroid condition, put her on natural hormones, and tested for food allergies. Weight loss was easier but the extreme carbohydrate intolerance remained. I suggested we check blood type and was shocked to find that she was an A type. With trepidation, I sent her the diet recommendations, largely carbohydrates. Two months later, I received a distressed call that she had gained over 20 pounds. She had been so relieved that she had really enjoyed herself, but it took its toll. We explored her food choices and decided to try a lower carbohydrate diet but using A type food choices with more vegetarian protein choices, such as soy products, eggs, protein powder, and beans. She continued to eat poultry and fish. Another three months went by. Kim called me, ecstatic. Not only had she achieved her premenopause weight, but her arthritis, allergies, and skin problems virtually disappeared! Interestingly, after all those years of struggling with dieting, Kim told me that this diet was effortless for her and she was enjoying eating for the first time in years!

I experienced the relevance of individual metabolic and blood types in a very personal manner. Over 15 years ago, I was vegetarian, having been convinced that this was the healthiest way for everyone to eat. Only I felt less and less well. My cholesterol level dropped too low and affected steroid metabolism, and all my hormone levels were scrambled. I felt hypoglycemic most of the time and often felt shaking chills, almost feverish. I had no idea what was wrong until a nutritionist friend of mine who had studied with Dr. Kelly suggested that my metabolic type was parasympathetic-dominant and I should be eating meat. That day I went out and had a steak and immediately started improving. Several years later I met Dr. D'Adamo and realized that, as an O blood type, I was much better suited to a lower carbohydrate, even higher protein diet. And I felt the difference immediately!

THE BODY-MIND CONNECTION

While I've left this until last, the profound connection between our mind and what happens in our bodies is critical in achieving our weight and health goals. Our individuality is most evident in how we think and feel and what choices we make to create our unique lives.

Many emotional issues affect our ability to stick to a diet. Feeling nervous, bored, frustrated, or depressed can lead to binge eating as a reward. Individual lifestyle issues like ingrained eating habits, dining out often, eating alone, eating in fast food restaurants to save time, traveling on business, high stress levels from work or family obligations, feeding children, or hating to cook, also create the need for unique solutions to these diet problems. Doctors can't just expect that everyone can follow through with diet recommendations. By identifying which situations are most difficult for you, we can discover creative ways of adapting the diet to your lifestyle, not forcing you to adapt your life to a diet!

Most powerfully, entrenched belief systems affect every aspect of our lives and often limit our possibilities. What we've heard and learned in the past causes us to make assumptions that allow for only that possibility. "I'll always be fat." "Losing weight is hard." "I hate dieting." "I love desserts." "I'm a chocolate addict." Our body hears those beliefs and our subconscious mind sets out to make sure they happen. The resulting internal conflict produces increased stress, low self-esteem, and self-sabotaging behavior. Our beliefs determine what we allow or don't allow in our lives. We cannot change our experience without first changing our beliefs. The difficulty often arises from the fact that many of our beliefs are unconscious. We may have picked them up as children or in response to some negative event that happened to us. It may have made us decide, "Not me, I never can have what I want." If you've tried to lose weight several times before and were unsuccessful or regained the weight, you probably have some strong beliefs that losing weight is difficult, hard work, or even impossible for you. These beliefs must be released in order to make room for new beliefs that allow you to create what you want.

Rosalyn, a 35-year-old woman who was divorced and had two children, had been overweight to varying degrees most of her life. She knew and had tried many diets successfully but always gained back the weight. She was referred to me for thyroid evaluation, but even correcting her sluggish metabolism didn't do the trick for long. It became evident to me that she had some pretty strong beliefs about weight, so powerful that no amount of dieting could overcome them. Her belief that she would always be fat clashed with her belief that, unless she was thin, she would not be sexy and no one would ever love her. This profound conflict led to depression and self-sabotaging behaviors like binging on cookies at night, fulfilling her prophecy. I convinced her to forget the diet for awhile and concentrate on finding some new thoughts about herself. As she worked on just accepting herself, she started to feel happier than she had in years. Then she met a new boyfriend whom she thoroughly loved and enjoyed. That convinced her that the second belief was false and opened the door for her to change many other limiting beliefs. Now she is free to diet or not, can lose weight when she chooses to, and is making different choices. No longer obsessed with her weight and diet at every moment, Rosalyn is now living to enjoy her life.

Your body is unique. No one is just like you. Your body also has the innate wisdom to know what is right for you, what is consistent with your health and happiness and what is not. You have a flawless inner guidance system. Most people have been taught by society to suppress their intuition, their feelings, and most signals from their body. You can learn to access and listen to the body's wisdom. The body can communicate only through feelings and sensations, which often are ignored. These are often far more subtle and quiet than the negative beliefs we have picked up from others or from society. You just need to "tune in" to this extremely useful inner wisdom.

There are only two steps to creating a new reality about weight, health, or virtually anything, in your life:

- ◆ First, intend it.
- ◆ Second, allow it.

Intending means creating in your thoughts the outcome that you desire. This sets the creation into motion. The stronger your positive feelings, the more you enjoy your visualization, the faster and more completely your goal will manifest in your life. Allowing means expecting you will receive what you want and believing that you can and will have what you desire. It is just a matter of time. Shift your picture of yourself in your mind from that of an overweight person to that of a fit and healthy person who just happens to temporarily be in a costume, acting the part of an overweight person. All that you are and want to be is already there, just temporarily hidden underneath.

Once you've pictured your result, don't allow negative thoughts like "That can't happen, I'm still fat" undo your creation. Intend to feel joy in each moment, and you'll connect with that allowing state. Then you'll find the right keys to unlock the secrets of achieving your dreams.

Patience and diligence, like faith, move mountains.

– William Penn

Trust yourself. You know more than you think.

– Benjamin Spock

CHAPTER 9

■ ■ ■ ■ ■ ■ ■ ■ ■ ■

Medical Doctors Speak Out About Metabolic Imbalance

I feel blessed! Blessed because these doctors have contributed to *Fat and Furious* and to your life in ways that you have only just begun to understand. These doctors are just as frustrated as you are at the misdiagnosis and mistreatment of patients trying to lose weight and uncover their metabolic imbalances.

They all have my undying gratitude. I want you to know that I did not know any of these doctors prior to writing and researching this book. They are not just doing me *a favor* by contributing to my book, or for publicity. Just as you are, they are caught in a medical system of ignorance. Regrettably, patients like you and me have paid the price. They want to lend their knowledge and voices to make a positive change.

In my conversations with them during the writing of this book they are *all* without a doubt humanitarian caregivers and loving healers. They are giving *you* a priceless gift, my friend.

METABOLIC REHAB IS NECESSARY FOR MANY TO OVERCOME AN IMPAIRED METABOLISM

by Gina Honeyman-Lowe, DC

I have often had patients who for years exercised faithfully, watched their diet (sometimes to the extreme!), taken nutritional supplements, and didn't lose weight or shape up as they had hoped to. Their doctors, friends, and family told them that they just needed to work harder and watch their diet. I'm not saying this to let anyone off the hook for failing to adopt a wholesome diet, take nutritional supplements, and exercise. These are essential for anyone to achieve optimal health, and they are included in our metabolic treatment protocol. If you haven't honestly cleaned up your diet, aren't taking nutritional supplements, and aren't exercising to tolerance, then you know what you need to do next. However, if you're already doing these health practices and you're still not losing weight, undiagnosed or undertreated thyroid disease may be your problem.

To appreciate how thyroid disease can keep you from losing weight despite a healthy lifestyle, it's important to understand some basic information about thyroidology—the study of the thyroid gland and the thyroid hormones it produces. It is a complex topic so I'll mention a few of the most important ideas. Thyroid disease, including primary or central hypothyroidism, and thyroid hormone resistance can cause sluggish metabolism, which we call hypometabolism. In hypometabolism, the person's thyroid gland doesn't produce enough thyroid hormone. In thyroid hormone resistance, the person's tissues don't use thyroid hormone efficiently, and they have the same signs and symptoms as people with hypothyroidism. In a person with resistance, the thyroid gland can be functioning properly, and thyroid-related blood tests can be within the laboratory reference ranges.

The thyroid gland makes two types of thyroid hormone. It makes mostly thyroxine (T4) and just a little bit of tri-iodothyronine (T3). The T4 *has* to be converted to T3 to drive metabolism. If it is not, it has no ability to affect metabolism. If people do not convert T4 to T3 properly, or if the T3 doesn't bind properly to thyroid hormone receptors, the thyroid hormone in the bloodstream doesn't effectively stimulate metabolism. Hormones and their receptors in cells must bind properly for the hormone to do its job. If a receptor's shape changes, the hormone can't bind to it and affect the target tissue.

As you see, there are many processes involved in the pro-duction and use of thyroid hormone by the body. Disruptions can occur in one or more of the processes, and when they do, metabolism becomes impaired, and the person develops health problems and impaired function. Since nearly all tissues in the body demand adequate thyroid hormone stimulation to func-tion properly, a myriad of symptoms can occur if tissues aren't properly stimulated.

Some common signs or symptoms of impaired metabolism are fatigue, pain, muscle stiffness, depression, anxiety, poor memory, constipation and/or diarrhea, abnormal coldness, poor sleep, low sex drive, menstrual difficulties, infertility, urinary frequency, and hair loss. And, of course, the inability to lose weight is a common symptom of hypothyroidism and thyroid hormone resistance. You may have only a few of these signs or you may have many.

It's important to get an evaluation for thyroid disease if you suspect hypothyroidism or thyroid hormone resistance is an obstacle to your goals of improving your health and fitness. But getting an adequate evaluation for thyroid disease can be quite a challenge. This is due to the current standard of care that has been established by the endocrinology specialty. To diagnose hypothyroidism, many doctors rely solely on a person's blood level of TSH, the pituitary hormone that stimulates the thyroid gland and thyroid hormones. Some doctors look at the thyroid hormone levels, as well. A person's clinical symptoms and signs of thyroid disease are usually ignored. Often these classic symptoms and signs of hypothyroidism are considered to be "mysterious illnesses," because blood levels of TSH and thyroid hormones are not grossly out of the reference ranges. Many times people are told, "It's all in your head!" because their lab tests are inconclusive. This leaves many people untreated or undertreated for thyroid disease. It also leaves people angry, frustrated, and disillusioned with the medical community, and rightfully so. After reading this far, you already know more about thyroidology than many of your doctors.

In a well-meaning but misguided attempt to help, many doctors prescribe a different medication for each symptom of poor metabolism. People then have such a "chemical soup" in their body that it gets difficult to sort out which of their symptoms are due to thyroid disease and which are adverse effects of medications. Be aware that medications such as antidepressants, painkillers, and beta-blockers used to treat high blood pressure can also impair metabolism. Subjecting patients to these metabolism-impairing medications is a dismal standard of care, and results in diminished quality of life for many people and even premature deaths for some people.

Misdiagnosis and mistreatment of people with thyroid disease is a serious public health problem worldwide. My husband, Dr. John C. Lowe, and I consult with people in many countries, and we hear the same stories of poor diagnosis and management skills of their local doctors. Many doctors aren't even aware of the possibility of thyroid hormone resistance or what to do about it. When they do prescribe thyroid hormone for a person, it's usually a product with T4 in it, such as Synthroid, and this is woefully inadequate for most people. In one study, we found that 44% of patients with symptoms of hypometabolism had completely normal thyroid test values, even though they had symptoms of hypothyroidism. Most finally recovered by using enough thyroid hormone, along with other health-inducing activities.

One treatment protocol, called metabolic rehab, is a comprehensive treatment protocol which includes wholesome diet, nutritional supplements, exercise to tolerance, physical treatment as needed, and the right kind and amount of thyroid hormone. There are some over-the-counter thyroid medications, but most of our patients require a prescription written by a co-treating doctor. Patients fill out pencil and paper forms so we can objectively monitor changes in their symptoms. We score the forms and post the scores to line graphs that show us precisely which of the patients' symptoms are changing and to what degree. This method of data collection provides essential information we need to give our patients intelligent recommendations. While the treatment protocol has set components, it is tailored to the needs of the individual.

This management style, which uses objective feedback in making decisions, has proven highly effective. Our latest statistics show that 85% of our patients have either fully recovered or significantly improved. We don't recommend the usual management style of medical doctors, which is to recheck blood levels of TSH and/or thyroid hormones. That method keeps most people ill and dysfunctional.

Many people lose weight when they are engaging in metabolic rehab. One reason is that thyroid hormone powerfully regulates the lipolytic enzymes that are responsible for breaking down fats. When they find an effective dosage of thyroid hormone, these enzymes become more active and reduce the amount of their body fat. Other reasons for the weight loss include adopting a wholesome diet, using nutritional supplements, and exercising. As an example, Darlene, a 56-year-old elementary school music teacher, started metabolic rehab in February 2003. She was not eating a wholesome diet or exercising, but she was taking some nutritional supplements. Breakfast was coffee, toast, and juice, lunch was a canned diet drink, and her dinner was a balanced meal. She didn't have the stamina to exercise and had cut calories to an unhealthy level. Darlene was determined to recover her health and has diligently participated in her metabolic rehab. Over the past five months she has lost 25 pounds by improving her diet, adding a few nutritional supplements, walking for exercise, and using the right kind and amount of thyroid hormone. The weight loss is gradual for most people, and they maintain the loss over time. Darlene's experience is typical of the majority of our patients who need to lose weight.

Exercise to tolerance is one area where most hypometabolic people need some guidance. It's true that to increase fitness one must push beyond the usual activity level. But for some people, pushing just a little past their current capabilities causes debilitating aches, pain, stiffness, and fatigue that can last for days or weeks. Taking weeks off from exercise while the symptoms subside can, of course, allow fat to accumulate again. When people have impaired metabolism, they usually can't tolerate the same duration or intensity of exercise as people with normal metabolism. I know people who have been humiliated, cursed at, and generally abused by personal trainers because they weren't able to maintain the intensity of the workouts that the trainers demanded. You have to trust your own perceptions of your body and abilities, and set boundaries with your personal trainers or workout partners. If they won't respect your boundaries, find new trainers or partners. I also hear stories of sensitive, compassionate trainers who understand that baby steps are necessary for some people to reach their health and fitness goals.

Trust your intuition and your intelligence. Most of my patients tell me that they have known that their problems are thyroid-related, but their other doctors won't listen to them. You don't have to put up with bullying or intimidation by anyone, regardless of his or her diplomas and degrees. Find a practitioner to help you with your health and fitness goals, one who will listen to you, respect your intelligence, and collaborate with you.

Dr. Gina Honeyman-Lowe and her husband, Dr. John C. Lowe, practice in Boulder, Colorado. They are the authors of YOUR GUIDE TO METABOLIC HEALTH, *which provides step-by-*

step instructions in the proper method to help you with your own metabolic rehabilitation. If you feel that you have some of the symptoms of an impaired metabolism you can find additional information on their website listed in the resource guide at the end of this book.

IT'S ALL ABOUT BALANCE
by C. Richard Mabray, MD

Balance! Balance! It's all about balance. Nature does not like for us to be too hot or too cold, too wet or too dry, too thin or too fat. So, as we think about fat and thin, let's look at some of the balances that are necessary.

We'll come back to diet later, but one of the obvious areas where balance is important is the food we eat. Thousands of years ago God told our ancestor, Noah, and his sons to eat a diet of balanced protein and vegetables. The key concept is that simple. When we eat a pound of meat, fish, or fowl, and balance that with a pound of vegetables, it is most difficult to not be healthy and have reasonable fat and protein distribution and fitness.

But before we get into the nuts and bolts of the diet, let's look at some issues that affect Loree and a huge number of us who struggle with excess body fat. That area is hormone activity and status.

Pituitary-Controlled Hormones

One of the most powerful and active systems to keep us in balance is the trio of thyroid, adrenal, and gonads (sex organs) controlled by the pituitary gland. Abnormal, defective, or sluggish function in any one or all three of these results in producing symptoms and struggles affecting our whole body and sense of well-being.

Sex Hormones

Consider that one of the most powerful realities for each of us is our gender. Loree is obviously female. That means that in the best of times, her hormones are on a constant roller coaster ride. These ups and downs of estrogen, progesterone, testosterone, DHEA, and other hormones make getting to steady state most difficult. Even past the onset of menopause and/or with hormone administration, steady state may be most difficult.

One of the obvious gender differences is that most of us men have a much easier time of weight loss with equal expenditure of energy and good food choices. It simply is easier for most men than for most women.

A major reason for this is the balance we mentioned before. Nature does not like too much or too little of any hormone. One of the ways this is manifested is that women who have estrogen excess or deficiency — either one — have a marked increase in the resistance of cells to properly utilize insulin and therefore glucose (blood sugar). So, as cellular resistance to insulin rises, there is a tendency for the body to enter a vicious cycle of sugar craving, leading to excess consumption of carbohydrate foods, leading to weight and fat gain. Now, this cycle becomes a cruel joke in that body fat tends to convert certain pro-hormones into active hormones. So, the fatter the woman becomes, the more estrogen-dominant her hormone pattern becomes, and this leads to yet more sugar cravings and weight gain.

Many of the hormone regimens used over the last couple of decades have not been realistically in balance. There are excellent laboratory tests available to help document hormonal balance. But remember that most of the time our bodies do try to keep us informed. We just need to listen to symptoms of imbalance such as fatigue, mood change, poor libido, weight gain, headaches, and breast tenderness. So, work with your health practitioner and listen to your body to get into balance with those sex hormones.

Thyroid

This little butterfly-shaped gland located low in the anterior neck is a major player in determining metabolic competence. Along with insulin it facilitates getting energy into cells throughout the body. When it is in balance and working well, the body functions the way it is supposed to.

When thyroid function is not in balance, the symptoms can affect any organ or system in the body. Common symptoms of dysfunction are fatigue, abnormal menstrual bleeding, vascular headaches, and mood disorders such as depression, dry skin, and heat or cold intolerance. An often-overlooked association is that benign and cancerous breast disease occurs with both over- and underproduction and utilization of thyroid hormone.

A major problem here is that we doctors have been taught that just as with hand grenades and horseshoes, getting close is good enough. So, if one's thyroid stimulating hormone (TSH) is anywhere near normal range, we have been taught that all must be well with thyroid function. Unfortunately, someone forgot to convince our bodies of this. For example, the "normal" range for TSH is usually listed as somewhere between 0.35 and 6.5. However, there is a significant amount of information in the medical literature that says when the TSH is over 1.9, there is a tendency to have elevation of cholesterol, which can be corrected by even low-dose thyroid hormone supplementation. In fact, the TSH is not even a thyroid test. It is a test of pituitary gland function and can be fooled in several important ways.

And then there is the problem that even when they prescribe thyroid supplements, most doctors still give the synthetic form of pure pro-hormone in a T4 product such as synthyroid or levoxyl. These are good products; however, studies strongly suggest that most folks feel and perform better when the active hormone, T3, is given at the same time. This may be done by either adding the T3 to the T4 preparation or by going to the natural hormone (e.g., Armour thyroid).

Adrenal Gland

These little powerhouses sit atop the kidneys. They provide front line defense against the myriad occurrences and consequences of stress in our lives. When your medical condition is not responding the way it should, trying to identify and handle stress well can make all the difference.

Stress is not just having a bully for a boss. Stress is also about sleeping well, not taking ourselves too seriously, minimizing chemical exposures, avoiding high carbohydrate intake, balancing hormones, and getting exercise. God tells us that "a merry heart doeth good like a medicine."

As the body senses itself to be stressed, it begins to shift gears toward increasing cortisol production, which increases insulin resistance, which makes us form and store fat in anticipation that even more harmful events are in the offing. Work with your health practitioner to get and keep adrenal hormone balance.

Diet

Here we are back to balance again.

There have now been shown to be "essential" amino acids, fatty acids, and carbohydrates. Essential amino acids are protein building blocks that our body can't make. Therefore, we have to eat them in the form of protein. Adequate protein intake is therefore mandatory. For most of us not given to running marathons, three servings per day about the size of the palm of your hand should be sufficient for minimal requirements. The foods that are either all or mostly protein are meat, fish, fowl, cheese, eggs, and tofu.

Essential fatty acids are those lipid or fat-building blocks our bodies must have as dietary intake in order to make our hormones, cell membranes, and more. Look for healthy sources such as extra virgin olive oil, and pressed oils such as sunflower, safflower, and flax seed. Much can be said for the anti-inflammatory and health benefits of the omega-3 oils found in deep-sea, cold-water fish such as sardines, cod, orange roughy, and salmon. These are indeed very beneficial, but their biggest drawback is their tendency to be contaminated with mercury and other heavy metals. This makes pharmaceutical-grade fish oil a wise choice for supplementation. It is important to avoid the damaged and toxic highly processed fats such as deep fried anything, trans-fatty acids, and hydrogenated fats.

Until a few years ago, it was not recognized that there are essential carbohydrates. But we now recognize that some of the simple sugars are not present in the typical diet and can't be made in the body to a meaningful extent. Therefore, we must do our best to eat the highest quality we can find of less processed and organically grown vegetables and even green supplements. Let me emphasize that these essential sugars are not the highly processed sugars that are sweet to taste, so don't use this as an excuse to eat candy, white bread, and potatoes.

So, what really is important?

1. Work with your body and your health practitioner to get and keep a balance of hormones.

2. Balance good healthy protein with healthy fats and vegetable intake.

3. Drink plenty of the cleanest water you can find and afford.

4. Keep your body active and physically working.

5. Set goals and make meeting them enjoyable.

6. Laugh and have fun. Life is short.

7. Don't get sidetracked by fads. God gave us our dietary formula in Genesis 9 a long time ago.

C. Richard Mabray, MD, is the author of LOSE WEIGHT, NOT YOUR HEALTH. He currently practices in Victoria, Texas.

PURSUE YOUR BLISS AND STRIVE FOR EMOTIONAL BALANCE

by David Parrish, MD

In our current society we have reached a new high water mark in the number of stressors we face. The individual, when facing a stressor, should ask him- or herself, "Am I in immediate danger?" If not, the person should choose a more purposeful and peaceful attitude. There are no saber-toothed tigers lurking behind nearby trees. The rapidly advancing technological age with its flood of information has a strong tendency to overwhelm us with details, most of which are not relevant to our daily existence. This is extremely distracting and harmful to our physiological balance. One of the biggest secrets of the universe is that under all circumstances, we can choose how we want to feel: either happy or fearful.

Our inability to peacefully handle red lights, stop signs, slow traffic, and starting times for soccer matches has resulted in a level of stress that blows a major circuit breaker in the midbrain, the hypothalamus. This region regulates body functions, such as blood pressure, heart rate, respiratory rate, temperature, and sleep. This impairment causes hypothalamic-pituitary axis dysfunction, further causing a cascading effect, that trips other circuit breakers in the thyroid gland, adrenals, pancreas, ovaries, and testes. This process can be viewed as protective, but certainly not adaptive. The resulting aggregate of impairments can become extremely chronic, severely impairing energy and adaptability. One of the results of this kind of impairment is a reduced metabolic rate due to thyroid hypofunction and insulin resistance. The resulting lethargy leads away from physical activity, as well as a reduction in the efficiency of the body to burn calories. Another associated aspect of unbuffered stress is the motivation to handle anxieties and disappointments via food and to eat to a point beyond satiation, where frightening emotions become dulled.

My approach to these problems involves (1) having patients recapture eight to eight and one-half hours of uninterrupted, restorative sleep, (2) restoration of hormone balance, (3) addressing nutritional requirements and habits, and correcting digestive enzyme deficiencies, (4) diagnosis and treatment of chronic infections often occurring in the gums, sinuses, or lower intestinal tract due to overgrowth of pathogenic bacteria or yeast, and (5) having patients devote a portion of the day to stress management, the choice to be happy rather than right, and meditation, where we can listen for guidance. This approach can be very useful in treating the problem of obesity by a process that uses a holographic view rather than a single-dimensional view.

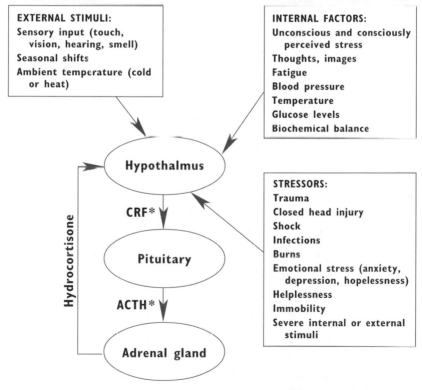

EXTERNAL STIMULI:
Sensory input (touch, vision, hearing, smell)
Seasonal shifts
Ambient temperature (cold or heat)

INTERNAL FACTORS:
Unconscious and consciously perceived stress
Thoughts, images
Fatigue
Blood pressure
Temperature
Glucose levels
Biochemical balance

Hypothalmus

CRF*

Pituitary

ACTH*

Adrenal gland

Hydrocortisone

STRESSORS:
Trauma
Closed head injury
Shock
Infections
Burns
Emotional stress (anxiety, depression, hopelessness)
Helplessness
Immobility
Severe internal or external stimuli

* **CRF** – corticotropin releasing factor
* **ACTH** – adrenalcorticotrophic hormone

Used with permission by David Parrish, MD

Remember that, in the course of life, you will never finish what you are doing. At any time you are precisely where you want and should be, and wherever possible you should pursue your bliss. In a word, staying in the present is the best way to cultivate preferences rather than requirements. A burgeoning list of requirements almost always ends in emotional imbalance, an excessive need to eat, and an attendant inability to utilize calories.

David Parris, MD, is board-certified and practices in Scottsdale, Arizona. A multi-specialty physician, he specializes in neuro-endocrinology, endocrine modulation, and psychopharmacology.

HORMONE HAVOC IS PREVALENT
by David Overton, PA-C

Ever wonder why so many people have hormone problems? There must be reasons why so many people suffer from stress hormone imbalances, thyroid problems, PMS, menopause, and impotence, especially since drug treatments often fail to alleviate the symptoms or correct the problem.

First, it helps to understand there is a sequence of events that happens over time to cause unbalanced hormones. For example, the thyroid does not become underactive or "hypo" overnight. It takes a series of events over time for any hormone system to become unbalanced.

The first problem in the sequence is with what I call the foundations of good health. This includes diet, stress handling, organ system functioning (digestion, liver, kidneys, etc.), nutritional factors (minerals, fatty acids, vitamin deficiencies), and toxin accumulation. For example, we make our hormones from the foods we consume. The typical high-carbohydrate diet often causes blood sugar problems (either high or low blood sugar), which in turn will imbalance the adrenal hormones. Adrenal imbalances lead to thyroid and sex hormone problems. The best way to find out if you have these problems is to do a simple four-hour glucose tolerance test. Standard blood glucose testing will miss the vast majority of blood sugar handling problems, until a disease like diabetes has set in. But glucose tolerance testing *will* detect low blood sugar and high blood sugar (before the need for diabetic drugs), and both conditions are treatable with diet, lifestyle changes, and natural medicine approaches. Restoring blood sugar helps hormone balance.

Hormone imbalances can be checked with blood tests, but just as with blood sugars, they may not detect problems until a disease develops. And blood levels of hormones check only the levels carried around in the bloodstream. What you really want to know is the hormone level available to the cells and tissues. More accurate tests include "free" or available hormones and saliva free hormones. These tests provide more accurate information of the hormone levels (adrenal, thyroid, sex hormones, etc.) actually available to the cells for metabolic activity.

Many people have mild or subclinical hormone imbalances. This is particularly true of the thyroid. I see people all the time who just know they have a thyroid problem, but their past blood tests are "normal."

If your digestion is poor, you don't assimilate the nutritional building block to make hormones. Digestive problems can be determined by symptoms, exams, and testing. We also live in a toxic environment with exposure to thousands of potential toxins (metals and chemicals). The thyroid and sex hormones are commonly unbalanced by toxins.

Minerals act to stimulate hormone production. Most Americans have mineral deficiencies and don't know that most calcium supplements contain lead. Simple tests performed in the doctor's office can determine the best minerals for you. Your physician or health care professional can recommend supplements free of toxins. Stress depletes B vitamins, which the body needs to support the adrenals and thyroid. The thyroid needs phosphorylated B vitamins, which are not sold at most health food stores. Hormones are made from fatty acids like cholesterol, so if you lower your cholesterol too much in an attempt to prevent heart disease, you'll be fatty acid deficient, which contributes to hormone imbalances.

A final note—it's best to work the entire sequence of hormonal balance or you may not make the progress you seek. For example, just taking a thyroid or female supplement rarely get results; working the sequence does.

David Overton, PA-C, is the author of FUNCTIONAL & NUTRITIONAL BLOOD CHEMISTRY: WHAT THE NUMBERS REALLY MEAN. *He practices at Natural Medicines & Family Practice in Tumwater, Washington. He presents an extensive case study in the next chapter to illustrate exactly how hormonal imbalances are uncovered.*

OBESITY IS A COMMON COMPLAINT
by Ron Manazero, MD

Obesity is one of the most serious epidemics facing our nation today. It is a complex subject that is confusing to the lay public and poorly understood by the medical profession. In my medical practice, obesity is a chief complaint. At least 90% of my patients—who are mostly female—are overweight, fatigued, stressed, and eating fast foods.

Is diet the only problem? Not at all. Though I am educated in family medicine, much of my practice evolves around endocrine-based problems. I have found it useful to rule out potential concurrent problems: hypothyroidism, insulin resistance, and anabolic/catabolic imbalances. There are certainly other matters to evaluate, but I usually start with these three issues.

Regarding hypothyroidism, if you are highly symptomatic, don't be satisfied if your doctor says your tests are "normal."

The main blood tests for hypothyroidism are the TSH (thyroid stimulating hormone) test, free T4 (the main hormone made by the thyroid gland), and free T3 (the active form of thyroid hormone the body uses). The standard TSH range is 0.3 to 5.1. Many doctors use only the TSH test and, if your TSH level falls within this range, they will dismiss your symptoms and conclude that you are "normal." But in my experience, if you are tired and have brain fog, depression, cold intolerance, dry skin, brittle nails, low body temperature, constipation, weight gain, and muscle aches, you are probably hypothyroid, regardless of the TSH range! Recent studies have confirmed that the average TSH in healthy individuals is around 1.0 to 1.5. Optimally, the T4 and T3 ranges need to be evaluated as well. A standardized combination of T4 and T3, Armour thyroid, has proven effective for many people.

After checking the thyroid status, the next thing I look for is insulin resistance. This can be a precursor to Type 2 diabetes and is a common cause of obesity. Some clues are a family history of diabetes, a diet high in refined carbohydrates, and obesity in the lower abdomen. I confirm the diagnosis with the following tests: hemoglobin A1C (tests the three-month average blood glucose level), fasting insulin, and a fasting lipid/cholesterol profile. These tests also need to be viewed from the perspective of "what is optimal?" An optimal hemoglobin A1C test will be less than 5.1 despite the "normal" range of 4.0 to 6.0. So if your A1C is greater than 5.1, and your triglycerides are greater than 100, you could have insulin resistance syndrome.

Insulin resistance is triggered mainly by consumption of refined carbohydrates and lack of exercise. Did our ancestors have white bread, toaster tarts, and soft drinks? No, they generally had to chase their foods or pick them from the ground or from trees. Their diet consisted of primarily low-fat proteins like buffalo, deer, turkey, fish, and whatever nuts, eggs, green veggies, and fruits they could find. Notice that "hunter-gatherer" foods tend to be low fat and low glycemic.

The final aspect of my evaluation involves looking at the anabolic/catabolic balance, or forces of "wear and tear" on an individual. As teenagers, our bodies are in high "build and repair," or anabolic, gear; but as we age and add emotional and dietary stresses to our bodies, our "wear and tear" metabolism, or catabolism, increases. (This anabolic/catabolic seesaw has been described in detail by Stephen Cherniske, M.Sc., author of *The Metabolic Plan.*) Increased catabolism exacerbates the symptoms of aging and can result in low muscle mass and obesity.

To understand catabolic metabolism, look at hydrocortisone that is made by our adrenal glands as a stress response hormone. Without it we couldn't live and survive stress, but with excess cortisone we begin to break down, and DHEA declines. Decreasing DHEA levels have been correlated with aging effects like obesity, insulin resistance, osteoporosis, and cognitive decline. Cherniske has shown that by signaling the brain with small doses of DHEA and its metabolite, 7-Keto DHEA, along with proper diet, exercise, and lifestyle, we can shift our metabolism back towards an anabolic balance and reduce obesity. I have outlined a treatment protocol to help regain a more youthful, anabolic metabolism.

In summary, my prescription for correcting obesity involves ruling out or correcting suboptimal thyroid functioning with full-spectrum T4/T3 hormone, ruling out or correcting insulin resistance, and helping the metabolism to become more anabolic. There is hope, and people are finding that they can lose weight and regain their youthful vitality.

Ron Manzanero, MD, practices in Austin, Texas.

MANY DOCTORS WILL BRUSH OFF PATIENTS WITH "NORMAL" LABORATORY TESTS
by Neal Rouzier, MD

Let me first introduce the concept of "normal" and discuss laboratory tests. Normal laboratory levels are determined by measuring levels of an average population. Young people will have high normal levels and older people will have low–normal levels. Eighty-year-olds will have normal levels for their age, but certainly not what they had when they were 20. If a 20-year-old had the levels of an 80-year-old, he would feel lousy and we would say he needs replacement to feel better. When an 80-year-old has the levels of an 80-year-old and feels lousy, we accept that as normal. However, it is not appropriate to settle for a "normal" value when improvement of this value can improve health and quality of life. The concept of normal covers a wide range of values, but normal does not imply that which is the most beneficial. The thyroid level is like a dimmer switch: the higher it is, the stronger the effect; the lower the level, the less the effect. It is not an on-or-off phenomenon; rather, the more you have, the better off you are.

The other factor that begs understanding is receptor site sensitivity. This is easily understood by looking at diabetes. As we age, the insulin receptor site becomes less sensitive to stimulation, thereby requiring a higher insulin level to effect a change. This is known as insulin resistance. The same occurs with other hormones, including thyroid. In spite of normal levels of hormone, receptor site insensitivity results in low thyroid symptoms due to lack of adequate stimulation of the receptor site. The only way to increase receptor activity is to increase thyroid hormone to higher or more optimal levels. This is exactly why people have low thyroid symptoms in spite of "normal" thyroid levels: poor receptor site stimulation. And the reason we see improvement of symptoms with treatment is due to better receptor site activation. Therefore, having normal lab values in no way guarantees adequate thyroid function. Frequently I see reversal of thyroid symptoms and weight gain only with high, optimal thyroid levels obtainable only with adequate thyroid hormone replacement.

Finally, in order to understand which treatment works best, one has to understand the lab tests. Historically we monitor thyroid stimulating hormone (TSH) levels. This is an indirect measurement of thyroid hormone. The thyroid hormone produced by the thyroid gland is called T4 and is not active. This T4 hormone must be converted in the body to a hormone called T3 in order to become active. It is the T3, not the T4, that is the main metabolic hormone responsible for all the metabolic activity. Unfortunately, the enzyme that makes this conversion of T4 to T3 becomes less effective as we age. Often we produce plenty of T4 but little T3, thereby resulting in low metabolism. The main reason our metabolism falls as we age is because of the ineffective conversion of T4 to T3. It is not possible to correct this enzyme deficiency. Therefore the best way to assure adequate thyroid replacement is to use a preparation containing T3. In my experience, this is best replaced by a medicine that is a combination of T4 and T3 called "natural thyroid." Armour thyroid is the most common name, although there are multiple other names for this natural thyroid.

Once we understand the above mechanism, then we can understand why the thyroid medication that most physicians prescribe is ineffective. The thyroid insufficiency that most people encounter is not inadequate thyroid T4 production from the thyroid gland, but rather inadequate conversion of the T4 hormone to the active T3 hormone. Therefore, even if we replace T4 (thyroxine) the problem still exists, because our bodies do not adequately convert T4 to the active T3. Most physicians prescribe only T4 as Synthyroid (synthetic thyroid), Levoxyl, or generic L-thyroxine. The body poorly converts this synthetic T4 to T3. Thus synthetic T4 replacement is largely ineffective and for most people is not a worthwhile therapy. Low thyroid symptoms and low metabolism prevail in spite of this customary treatment.

A landmark study appeared in the *New England Journal of Medicine* (Feb. 11, 1999; 340(6): 424–429) that demonstrated the efficacy of natural thyroid hormone (T4 and T3) over the synthetic T4 by itself. Those patients treated with the combination thyroid containing T3 all felt better, had more energy, less fatigue, better memory, and improved well-being. These same results were not seen with any patients treated with just T4. Nevertheless most physicians continue to prescribe only the synthetic T4 medicines. Drug company marketing and prejudice against the natural thyroid continues to influence physicians' approach to treatment. Other studies continue to show improvement with the natural thyroid due to the increase in T3 levels. Because of the poor conversion of synthetic T4 to T3, we do not see the same increase in T3 levels when using T4 preparations. This can easily be measured with laboratory tests. In my clinical practice, I routinely find improvement of symptoms and laboratory tests with natural thyroid. The key is replacing the correct hormone to optimal levels to obtain optimal metabolism. Optimal levels occur only at the upper end of normal ranges. The levels that we had when we were young are necessary for maximum metabolism. This can only be accomplished by natural thyroid and T3 hormone replacement.

Most patients will find that their hormone levels are low–normal. Doctors frequently will brush them off as "normal" and ignore their symptoms and metabolic disturbances. It is therefore of utmost importance to seek out a physician who is familiar with prescribing, monitoring, and adjusting thyroid to optimal levels. Thyroid is vital to any cell, organ, and function in the body. The body can suffer from elevated cholesterol, poor memory, weight gain, or low energy. The symptomatic spectrum is vast, and includes depression and mood disorders that are frequently not improved with antidepressants. People often get depressed because they feel lousy, not from being psychologically depressed. Thyroid makes them feel better, thereby alleviating their depression. Diet and exercise can be frustrating and unsuccessful if one has low–normal levels of thyroid. Our thyroid works to ensure an efficient utilization of energy, and maximal levels are therefore preferred. It may be up to you, the patient, to become aware of this, because most physicians are not.

Thyroid hormone affects every cell in the body. It regulates temperature, metabolism, and cerebral function. The low energy, fatigue, and weight gain seen with aging is partially due to insufficient thyroid function. This hormone is indispensable to better health and well-being. Replacing thyroid to the optimal levels that we had as a young adult alleviates many symptoms and allows our body to function more effectively and efficiently.

Laurie, a friend and fellow physician, was always freezing. Cold hands and feet were a way of life for her. I had suggested that she try thyroid to just warm her up a bit. Convinced that it would not work because her labs were perfectly normal, she was surprisingly pleased when it did work. She was amazed that it was so simple and yet overlooked by herself and other physicians. Not only was she now warm, the normal metabolism resulted in shedding the few pounds that were impossible before. She is not only a believer but she also now preaches about how well it works for her. She encouraged her support nursing staff to be treated with thyroid to improve body temperature and fight the fatigue they once encountered working 12-hour shifts. They no longer wear sweaters to work and their work is more productive as energy improves. After six months they noticed positive changes in skin, hair, and nails.

Laurie was like a typical physician and ordered only the typical thyroid blood tests, which don't usually include free T3 levels. And even if she had, she still would have failed to realize the significance of a low T3 level. She also did not appreciate how optimal levels of the hormone result in symptom improvement due to better stimulation of thyroid receptor sites. Doctors rely solely on a few lab tests and miss the diagnosis. This might become the most difficult task: locating a physician who understands all this and prescribes accordingly. Fortunately, there is a national network of physicians who are knowledgeable in thyroid matters.

Neal Rouzier, MD, specializes in the treatment of hormonal and nutritional deficiencies. He practices in Palm Springs and is the author of Natural Hormone Replacement for Men and Women: How to Achieve Healthy Aging.

HYPROTHYROIDISM: AN UNDERTREATED ILLNESS
by Ralph J. Luciani, DO

Hypothyroidism is usually described as a condition caused by an underfunction of the thyroid gland. However, I prefer to describe it as a condition whereby the body is deprived of the influence of an active thyroid hormone. I prefer this definition because there are several conditions wherein the thyroid gland may be functional, but either the quality of the active hormone is inadequate, or toxic substances in the body curtail transport of the hormone across cell membranes, thereby depriving the cell of adequate amounts of hormone. It is also possible that the thyroid gland itself may be dysfunctional, unable to produce adequate amounts of thyroid hormone or, as we age, active thyroid hormone is produced less in the body.

Symptoms of low thyroid function are fatigue, sleep disturbance, weakness, depression, weight gain, dry skin, falling hair, cloudy thinking, or abnormal hormone function. Many patients have these classic signs but are never diagnosed with this problem because their thyroid tests are normal.

As with all glands in the body, the pituitary gland exerts primary control. Thyroid stimulating hormone (TSH) is produced in the pituitary and stimulates the thyroid gland to produce thyroxin T_4, liothyronine (T_3), and triiodotyrosine. T_4 is not metabolically active but must be converted to T_3 to be effective. T_3 is the most active hormone, which stimulates normal metabolic function within each cell. A normal amount of T3 and T4 in the blood feeds back to the pituitary to curtail production of TSH.

Therefore, if a poorly functioning thyroid gland does not produce enough T3 or T4, the pituitary produces more TSH in an attempt to stimulate the thyroid gland to produce more hormone. So a high TSH level in the blood would indicate an abnormally low T3 and T4 production, which in turn means low metabolic function. A very low TSH level, on the other hand, means a greater production of T3 and T4, since the pituitary does not have to prime the thyroid gland quite as much.

Most physicians rely solely on the TSH level to determine whether the thyroid gland is producing enough T3 and T4. This test can be exceedingly misleading if someone is taking thyroid hormone as therapy for low thyroid function, or if the quality of the T3 produced by the thyroid gland is not normal. A person with a normal T3, T4, and TSH can be hypothyroid if the thyroid gland produces reverse T3 instead of normal T3. Reverse T3 is not metabolically as active as normal T3; therefore, despite normal blood tests, a person can be suffering from a lack of normal thyroid hormone in cells. This condition is known as Wilson's Syndrome. It is also a medical fact that as one ages, the de-iodinase enzyme which converts T4 to T3 becomes less efficient in its activity. Therefore, despite a normal TSH level, actual influence of thyroid hormone on the system can deteriorate.

Toxins circulating in the body can saturate receptor sites on cell membranes and can also damage them, thereby making them unavailable for hormones and other essential cellular nutrients. Once receptor sites are damaged or saturated, thyroid hormone circulating in the bloodstream becomes unavailable to the cells in required amounts, producing the symptoms of hypothyroidism. In this case, blood tests may be normal.

One way of testing the effect of the thyroid hormone is the basal temperature test. The temperature is taken using a mercury thermometer, shaken down at bedtime, and placed under the armpit immediately upon awaking in the morning, before getting out of bed and before any movement. The thermometer is kept under the armpit for ten minutes, and the temperature is recorded. Those with temperatures below 97.8 are generally found to have low metabolic function due to an abnormality of thyroid absorption in the cell or inadequate production of T3 from T4.

In all these cases, the use of the natural thyroid hormone (Armour) is most useful since it contains controlled amounts of T3 and T4. Synthetic T4 (Synthroid) will not work if the enzyme required to convert T4 to T3 is not normal. Often patients are placed on Synthroid or a similar drug for low thyroid and feel no different even though the TSH levels become normal. The reason is obvious. Their T4 is not converting adequately to the active T3 hormone, or not enough T3 is getting into cells for whatever reason. The blood test looks great—the patient feels lousy.

Although hypothyroidism can be elusive, some detective work can often clinch the diagnosis so appropriate treatment can be given.

Ralph J. Luciani, DO, M.S, Ph.D., MD (H), practices at the Albuquerque Clinic in New Mexico.

HOW TO DETERMINE IF YOU HAVE A SLOW METABOLISM
by Dr. Joseph Debé

So how can you tell if you have a slow metabolism? We can take advantage of the intimate relationship between metabolic rate and body temperature. A simple, accurate way to gauge your metabolic rate is to measure your body temperature.

To collect meaningful data, follow the protocol below:

1. Before going to bed, shake down an oral thermometer (below 95 degrees) and leave it within arm's reach of your bed.

2. First thing upon awakening in the morning, place the thermometer in your armpit and lie quietly in bed for ten minutes before recording the reading. It is important to take the measurement while at rest, before getting out of bed in the morning.

3. Repeat this procedure for six to ten days.

    Note: Because the menstrual cycle causes fluctuations in the body temperature, women who menstruate should start the measurements on the second or third day of their cycle.

4. After collecting six to ten days' worth of temperatures, determine the average. If it is below 97.8 degrees fahrenheit, you probably have an underactive metabolism. The lower the temperature, the slower the metabolism.

Dr. Joseph Debé practices in Great Neck, New York.

◆ ◆ ◆

Wow! Didn't these doctors go the extra mile with absolutely great information? I am so grateful, as you should be! It is physicians and health care professionals such as these sharing their voices in *Fat and Furious* that should give you hope.

Your part in all of this is to become an information sleuth and gather as much data as possible to present to your health care physician. Remember, the more prepared you are with information and facts, the more likely you will receive support in uncovering your metabolic dysfunction.

This will assist your doctor in uncovering your body's hormonal imbalance. If you're overweight, there is an imbalance somewhere—it's just a matter of locating its origin and how involved it is. Remember, if your doctor seems to be clueless about these hormonal issues or gives you a holier than thou attitude, you already know my philosophy . . . *you are out of there!*

All of these physicians—including their contact information, books, etc.—are listed in the resource guide if you feel that you want to contact any of them.

> *For the resolute and determined there is time and opportunity.*
>
> – Ralph Waldo Emerson

CHAPTER 10

■ ■ ■ ■ ■ ■ ■ ■ ■ ■ ■

Real People, Real Case Studies

Simply listen to the patient. They will eventually tell you what the diagnosis is.

– A wise old professor from medical school

CLINICAL PATIENTS
by Neal Rouzier, MD

Lisa

I can remember a time when I felt absolutely fatigued. I had no energy or drive. I had gained 15 pounds for no apparent reason. I went to several doctors, all of whom prescribed antidepressants for me. I felt even worse on the antidepressants. Even though I felt it was my thyroid, the doctors informed me that my tests were all normal. What I had read still indicated my symptoms were due to a low thyroid condition. I was frustrated with the lack of help or sympathy from my physicians. When I was finally treated with thyroid, it made all the difference in the world. Now I'm better and never look back.

– Lisa, age 39

I have encountered so many people with multiple complaints whose doctors can't pinpoint exactly what ails them. The above scenario is common: the lab tests are always normal, patients are told they are hypochondriacs, and yet they don't improve until they take thyroid hormone. When Lisa was referred to me she viewed me with the skepticism she had developed from her prior health care experiences. Her improvement was not surprising to me, yet it baffled her. How could so many physicians misdiagnose what was wrong and fail to appreciate the correct therapy? I explained that most physicians treat only the lab tests and not the patient. Secondly, most physicians fail to understand that optimal levels of hormones are beneficial and low–normal levels are not. Due to the loss of receptor site sensitivity as we get older, we need higher or more optimal levels of hormones to allow for a beneficial effect. The level of thyroid hormone declines as we get older. Combine that with the fact that the hormone doesn't work as well as it once did leads to ineffective thyroid response. This leads to a whole host of symptoms, low metabolism, and weight gain in spite of "normal" blood tests. As patients realize a dramatic improvement when taking thyroid hormone, it is an easy concept for them to understand. Yet for physicians it is difficult to understand because we focus on lab tests and not symptoms. However, in school we were taught to treat the patient and not the lab test.

Lisa suffered from one of the most misdiagnosed illnesses patients and doctors are faced with daily. I believe that the thyroid may be one of the most misunderstood and most overlooked hormones. More often than not, patients' symptoms are ignored, allowing their low thyroid function to go unaltered. Frequently, symptoms of thyroid insufficiency are misconstrued as normal aging: fatigue, weight gain, low energy levels, and feeling cold, for example. However, thyroid replacement frequently reverses these symptoms. Even more frustrating for women is thinning of skin, nails, and hair. In my experience, thyroid is the only treatment that reverses hair loss in women. Most women over age 45 will suffer hair loss and the only therapy that restores hair growth is thyroid, even though they might not be hypothyroid and have normal levels of hormones. There are over 200 symptoms that may be related to low thyroid function. And since thyroid is the main metabolic hormone, low ineffective levels or poor tissue response increases these symptoms. Increased body fat, elevated cholesterol, cold hands and feet, thinning of nails and hair—all metabolic symptoms—respond to thyroid replacement.

Judy

Judy was a 45-year-old patient who came to me after running out of her thyroid medication. She had changed insurance and hadn't found a physician to prescribe the thyroid for her. After being without her thyroid medication for three months, she noticed a weight gain that would not budge in spite of exercise and diet. Restoring her thyroid levels made it easy for her to lose the weight again. A common complaint that I hear is the inability to lose weight regardless of the amount of diet or exercise. Diet or exercise often actually slow down thyroid production as the body tries to maintain its genetically predetermined weight. The only way to overcome this metabolic shutdown is by metabolic stimulation through thyroid hormone replacement, again in spite of normal thyroid levels.

HORMONE HAVOC
by David Overton, PA-C

In my practice, I strive to treat all conditions with an integrated approach that includes a thorough assessment of symptoms and concerns, diet, and stress handling. Most health problems are caused by a combination of poor diet, stress, unbalanced blood sugar, nutritional deficiencies, poor digestive function, mineral imbalance, essential fatty acid deficiencies, hormonal imbalances (adrenal, pituitary, growth hormone, thyroid, sex hormones, etc.), poor circulation, immune dysfunction due to toxicity or infections, and poor kidney function.

By accurately assessing which combination of problems a patient has, we can develop a personalized treatment plan that treats the patient's specific problems. Most patients and practitioners are not aware that hormones and metabolism are unbalanced by stress, high or low blood sugar, and mineral and fatty acid deficiencies. Many people do not know that toxins unbalance hormones. Most people don't know that hormones are synthesized in the digestive tract and liver. It is simply not sufficient to just prescribe a thyroid or estrogen supplement or drug.

By accurately diagnosing the problem and then treating hormonal imbalances in the proper sequence with an integrated program, we get results by using diet changes, vitamins, minerals, botanicals, homeopathics, natural hormones, and prescription medicines (if needed).

We review blood chemistries to determine how the digestive system is functioning, whether the patient has appropriate mineral and fatty acid balance, and check liver, kidney functions, etc. The single best test to determine carbohydrate tolerance is a glucose tolerance test.

We utilize blood and saliva hormone tests to determine endocrine (hormonal) imbalances. Blood hormone tests are most often imbalanced if a person has a clinical disease. But most people are not diseased. Most people have mild or subclinical hormone imbalances that can be easily diagnosed and treated with *saliva* hormone testing. We utilize hair and other tests to detect and treat toxins. If we suspect parasites or other digestive problems, we utilize a comprehensive stool and digestive analysis to diagnose the problem and then treat appropriately.

I always review a person's diet and perform stress assessments, and develop a personalized diet and stress management plan as necessary.

More important than anything else, we educate our patients.

Every single patient is sent a letter reviewing their lab tests and we schedule time to review tests and decide together on the best treatment options.

The best method I know to demonstrate my approach is to review a thyroid case. Please note how we steadfastly followed an integrated approach, found problems on routine blood chemistries, and confirmed problems with specific saliva hormone tests, glucose tolerance testing, and hair tests. This approach allowed us to determine the proper natural medicines and diet changes needed to restore thyroid hormone balance and *cure* autoimmune hypothyroidism. Most important of all, note how I kept my patient and his parents thoroughly informed at each step about what the lab tests diagnosed so they could understand why Matthew developed hypothyroidism and what he could do to support and treat his thyroid.

Matthew was 16 years old when he came to see me for complaints of fatigue, sluggishness, slow reflexes, and an inability to lose weight. These symptoms were affecting his exercise performance and ability to function. His previous MD had told him his blood tests were all normal. His initial examinations quickly identified multiple endocrine and blood sugar symptoms and a poor diet. The previous blood chemistry tests were decidedly abnormal when I reviewed them. His blood chemistries strongly suggested digestive problems, adrenal dysfunction, fatty acid imbalance, endocrine disorders, toxins, and nutritional deficiencies. Our nutritional assessment questionnaire also strongly suggested digestive problems, mineral and vitamin deficiencies, and blood sugar, adrenal, pituitary, and thyroid symptoms. His glucose tolerance test diagnosed hypoglycemia, and saliva hormone tests diagnosed subclinical adrenal, pituitary, and hypothalamus dysfunction and autoimmune hypothyroidism. Hair testing confirmed mineral deficiencies and imbalances and suggested a toxic burden.

At every step, we sent Matthew and his mother detailed

letters outlining his conditions and how they contributed to his symptoms. We next provided dietary counseling and a treatment program of vitamins, mineral, botanical, and glandular supplements and prescription thyroid medication that completely resolved his symptoms. His tests documented a complete cure and recovery from autoimmune hypothyroidism and he has done very well on a maintenance program combining a true hypoglycemia diet, stress management, supplements, and thyroid medication.

Every week, we repeat this treatment program successfully for a wide variety of metabolic and hormone disorders. It works, because we know the sequence of how the hormones become imbalanced, and we know how to rebalance them. It simply is no longer acceptable to just treat the thyroid or just provide estrogen or testosterone without first testing for hormonal and blood sugar imbalances. All of the hormones interact synergistically.

The standard approaches ignore basic common sense and scientific principles because all of the hormones are affected directly or indirectly by diet, stress, nutritional deficiencies, and blood sugar imbalances. These problems set in place a sequence where the blood sugar becomes too high or low, which stresses the adrenals, which stresses the pituitary and hypothalamus, which causes thyroid or sex hormone imbalances in men and women.

Case Study: Poor Diet Leads to Hypoglycemic with Hormonal and Metabolic Syndrome

Integrated diagnosis combining history, symptoms, physical examinations, standard blood chemistries, diet assessment, and specialty tests (glucose tolerance test, saliva hormone thyroid and adrenal tests, hair test for toxic and essential elements). Integrated and successful treatment utilized diet changes, supplements, botanical medicines, and conventional medicine.

1. Note subtle initial physical findings (integrated conventional, naturopathic, and Eastern examinations).

2. Note poor diet. This diet causes hypoglycemia with endocrine dysfunction.

3. Note initial symptoms suggest blood sugar imbalances and endocrine dysfunction. Note nutritional questions suggest primarily digestive dysfunction, mineral deficiencies, vitamin deficiencies, adrenal, pituitary, and thyroid dysfunction.

4. Note blood chemistries normal, but suggest inability to digest proteins (necessary for stabilizing blood sugar and synthesizing hormones), adrenal dysfunction, risk for developing cardiovascular disease, dysbiosis, endocrine disorder, xenobiotic (toxic) burden, and other issues.

5. Note normal thyroid blood tests. Low–normal TSH suggests subclinical adrenal, pituitary, and/or thyroid disorder.

6. Note saliva short thyroid panel confirms subclinical hypothyroidism and autoimmune thyroiditis (a supposedly irreversible immune disorder).

7. Note fasting blood sugar is normal. Glucose tolerance test diagnoses hypoglycemia. Hypoglycemia causes adrenal, pituitary, thyroid, and metabolic syndromes or dysfunction. Hypoglycemia depletes minerals necessary for metabolism and/or detoxification.

8. Note adrenal dysfunction confirmed with saliva adrenal stress index test. Adrenal saliva hormones diagnose hypothalamus, pituitary, and dysfunction due to hypoglycemia and stress.

9. Note mineral imbalances and probable xenobiotic burden diagnosed with hair test.

10. Note subclinical hypothyroidism and autoimmune thyroiditis corrected (cured) with diet changes, supplements, and low-dose thyroid prescription.

11. All symptoms resolved except obesity, but patient did not commit to stopping diet soda, continuing treatment, and appropriate follow-up testing and examinations.

12. Patient remains at significant risk for cardiovascular disease and metabolic syndrome (Syndrome X), but is satisfied because energy is improved, physical performance is normalized, reflexes returned to normal, and no longer feels sluggish.

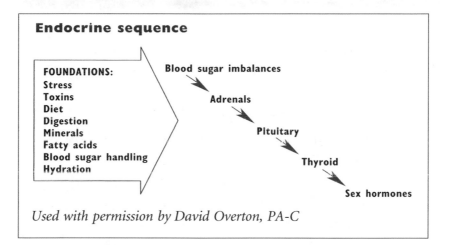

Endocrine sequence

FOUNDATIONS:
Stress
Toxins
Diet
Digestion
Minerals
Fatty acids
Blood sugar handling
Hydration

Blood sugar imbalances

Adrenals

Pituitary

Thyroid

Sex hormones

Used with permission by David Overton, PA-C

Matthew, age 16

Chief complaint: Fatigue. Also complains of sluggish metabolism, coarse hair, slow reflexes, and inability to lose weight. Symptoms are affecting exercise performance.

Past medical history: Elevated cholesterol.

Medications: None.

Initial diet: "Low fat," consumes several diet sodas daily.

Exercise: High school football (symptoms impairing performance).

Family history: Diabetes, coronary artery disease, rheumatoid arthritis, and asthma.

Initial review of symptoms: General—extremely fatigued. Heart—cholesterol controlled by diet changes. Blood sugar handling—excessive thirst, fatigue, and irritability if meals skipped or delayed (strongly suggests hypoglycemia).

Weight and vital signs were refused by the patient.

Nutritional assessment questionnaire reveals (primary concerns):

1. Poor diet.

2. Digestive dysfunction symptoms with probable inability to digest protein and nutrients (see tongue diagnosis below).

3. Mineral deficiencies (contributes to blood sugar imbalances, endocrine dysfunction, heart disease, and immune dysfunction).

4. Vitamin deficiencies (contributes to blood sugar imbalances, endocrine dysfunction, heart disease, and immune dysfunction).

5. Adrenal, pituitary, and thyroid symptoms.

Initial exam: Refused weight. Nail diagnosis—vertical nail ridges (suggests mineral deficiencies and endocrine dysfunction) and white spots (suggests zinc deficiency). Tongue diagnosis—tongue indented (suggests inability to absorb nutrients in digestive tract). Thyroid normal—to palpation. Legs—significant edema (fluid retention) in both legs (suggests endocrine disorder, especially thyroid) and absent ankle reflexes in both legs (strongly indicative of hypothyroidism).

See enclosed reports that follow the Hormone Havoc Endocrine Sequence and how we inform every patient and/or their parents.

10/4/01 Initial Evaluation

Matthew is seen for his initial evaluation. Symptoms, concerns, past medical history, family history, and the initial review of pertinent symptoms and initial physical examination is outlined in the case study.

My initial diagnosis was fatigue due to thyroid disorder and/or adrenal disorder and probable hypoglycemia. In addition, he has a previous history of hyperlipidemia or elevated cholesterols.

He was instructed to complete a three-day food journal for review and his reportedly "normal" previous laboratory tests were reviewed. Those tests showed his cholesterol level and triglyceride level were not normal. In addition, tests suggested digestive dysfunction, adrenal dysfunction, and probable thyroid dysfunction.

He was informed that minimal laboratory testing had been performed. I recommended he repeat his initial thyroid tests, obtain more thorough thyroid hormone testing, and perform adrenal testing and the hair test for toxins and mineral status.

10/31/01 Follow-up Appointment

Matthew was seen with his parents to review his laboratory testing, because they wanted a thorough explanation of all findings before treatment. The high and low values on his previous blood chemistries were reviewed. They were informed that his blood TSH level was low–normal and his saliva thyroid hormones were confirmed subclinical or mild hypothyroidism due to autoimmune dysfunction. In addition, his adrenal saliva tests were reviewed. He was informed that adrenal dysfunction causes thyroid dysfunction and contributes to autoimmune dysfunction. He was asked to schedule an appointment to review his food record and start nutritional supplements.

11/8/01 Follow-up Appointment

After a review of his nutritional assessment questionnaire, Matthew requested integrated natural and prescription medication to treat his subtle digestive dysfunction, vitamin deficiencies, and adrenal, pituitary, and thyroid dysfunction.

Treatments: We used only Biotics Research supplements because they are food based and pharmaceutical grade. Biotics supplements are also certified to be free of toxic metals, chemicals, and hormones.

Digestive support: We started Hydrozyme, one to two tablets with meals, to improve digestion and assimilation of proteins and nutrients.

Multiple vitamin: We started iron and copper-free Bio Multi-Plus, two tablets daily, an excellent multiple vitamin to provide phosphorylated B vitamins and other nutrients critical for thyroid function. Bio Multi-Plus should also support blood sugar stabilization, detoxification, and immune function.

Adrenal support: We started ADHS, two tablets twice daily, a multiple nutrient and botanical formulation to reduce excessive morning cortisol levels and support his adrenal glands.

Pituitary and hypothalamus support: We started Cytozyme PT/HPT, two tablets daily, to support hypothalamus and pituitary function.

Thyroid support: We also started Levoxyl, 0.125 mg every morning, to replenish T4 pro-hormone. He was informed T4 is a pro-hormone with very little biological activity. In addition, we started Meda-Stim, three tablets every morning, a multi-nutrient and botanical formulation which supports the conversion of T4 into T3 (the biologically active thyroid hormone). Matthew was encouraged to improve his diet, schedule a glucose tolerance test to rule out hypoglycemia, and schedule follow-up appointments for monitoring.

He was advised to avoid supplements made from coal tar derivatives as these are poorly absorbed and they often contain xenobiotics. He should not take excessive copper until he performs the hair test to measure copper and other toxic metals.

12/10/01 Follow-up Appointment

Matthew was seen without his parents to review his hair test. He did check his shampoo, hair care products, and supplements, and they did not contain toxins. He was informed his hair test strongly suggested a toxic burden of heavy metals and possibly chemicals. He also had depleted molybdenum and sulfur and imbalanced minerals. I explained to him that toxins deplete molybdenum and unbalance minerals, and that sulfur is necessary for detoxification. This test strongly suggested a xenobiotic burden with mineral deficiencies contributing to his auto-immune dysfunction, metabolic problems, and adrenal and thyroid dysfunction. He opted to perform a DMSA urine flush to confirm the presence of a toxic burden before treatment.

1/7/02 Follow-up Appointment

Matthew reports he is now exercising, following dietary recommendations, and taking his medications regularly. He reports more energy and that sluggishness is improving. He continues to drink diet sodas and is encouraged to stop.

8/13/02 Follow-up Appointment

Matthew finally came in for a personalized diet review. His hypoglycemia was reviewed; again it was pointed out he is consuming junk food, insufficient protein, insufficient healthy dietary fats, hydrogenated and trans-fatty acids, and juice that will cause hypoglycemia.

He was instructed to reduce his refined carbohydrate and starch intake, increase healthy protein intake, decrease his hydrogenated and trans-fatty acid intake, increase his intake of healthy dietary fats, and eliminate his diet sodas. He only agreed to reduce his diet sodas to two per week.

He does not plan to do his urine flush to confirm a toxic burden and wishes just to continue on his treatment program, because all the symptoms are controlled except he has not lost weight.

It was pointed out he will not lose weight unless he exercises and follows a healthy diet. He also needs to recheck his abnormal laboratory tests to confirm his treatment is working. He needs to address stress management because he has neckaches due to stress.

8/15/02 Follow-up Appointment

Matthew now complains of other stress-related neckaches and poor stress handling. We performed Heart Math biofeedback assessment that showed chaotic stress patterns and reproduced neck and shoulder tension and muscle aches and a sensation of butterflies in his stomach. Heart Math treatment resolved all the symptoms and demonstrated coherent stress patterns. He was advised that stress will cause adrenal and immune dysfunction, unbalance blood sugar, and affect metabolism. He was informed Heart Math stress management can be performed at home and is documented to rebalance adrenal hormones and immune function, and prevent heart disease and symptoms.

Our personalized integrated conventional and natural medicine approaches take the best from science and nature and can be learned by patients to restore their health and rejuvenate their endocrine system.

David Overton, PA-C, is the author of FUNCTIONAL & NUTRI-TIONAL BLOOD CHEMISTRY: WHAT THE NUMBERS REALLY MEAN. *He practices at the Natural Medicines & Family Practice in Tumwater, Washington.*

PATIENTS DESERVE TO BE TREATED WITH DIGNITY AND RESPECT, NOT SUBJECTED TO A FIVE-MINUTE DIAGNOSIS
by John G. Hipps, MD

When I first saw JD coming through the door to my private examining room, she came in sideways and just barely made it. Her chin rested on her shoulders just as her abdomen rested on her thighs. She looked the epitome of despair. It was simple enough to see that her sadness was much deeper than what I could see.

She looked at me with tear-filled eyes, saying, "I want, I need your help, doctor." Her face twisted in the pain of mental and physical anguish. "Just look at me. I am so unhappy. Twenty years ago I weighed 185 pounds when I was taking thyroid medication. Now I'm over 400 pounds and my regular doctor tells me my metabolism is normal. He tested my TSH and it was normal."

"Stop taking that thyroid pill," he demanded. "It's not your thyroid and stop eating so much. Get yourself moving more."

"But doctor, aren't you going to talk to me? Don't I need more than a screening test?" she asked. "I am not overeating and I am definitely active. You know I am an all-day child care surrogate mother for up to 15 children of working mothers. Before my last doctor retired, he was treating me for low metabolism and I lost 150 pounds. I know my dose now is not enough. I need testing so I can get back to where I was. I've already gained 50 pounds in the last six months. I feel awful, tired all the time. I can't keep up with the kids. I fall asleep standing on my feet. My skin is rashy just like it was before."

"Look at your TSH number," the doctor interrupted. "It's right in the middle of normal. Your metabolism is all right. Now go see what you can get yourself doing."

By that time, one complaint and five minutes later, JD was even more discouraged than before the visit. She went into deep despair, simply just gave up, and over the following three years her weight continued to go up and her spirit down.

Some months after I arrived in town, she read and heard about my practice and the success many of her acquaintances were having with my approach to helping people with obesity, fatigue, and many other symptoms of many other systems.

JD told me later her doctor saw her for five minutes and was too busy looking at the face of the clock on the wall instead of her own. "I saw him listening to the tick of his wristwatch instead of me."

A glimmer of hope began to glow deep inside her soul after months of wanting and waiting before she made an appointment. It is my custom to allow one hour of appointment time for first-time weight-management visitors to allow for a complete history and physical examination. In doing so, 90% of the time the patient and I can arrive at the probable diagnosis, whether it be for hypothyroidism or not. A physical examination of the remaining 10% usually confirms the diagnosis. Subsequent testing then completes the confirmation.

That testing includes the complete thyroid metabolic panel: T3, T4, TSH, and reverse T3. It also must include thyroglobulin and antithyrophosphatase antibodies, cortisol, DHEA, IGF-1, growth hormone and pregnenolone hormone, a thyroid ultrasound, and an 1123 uptake scan of the thyroid gland. That is, if the doctor practices the art of his or her profession.

For anyone, medical or layperson, who thinks this is over-testing, many years of experience will teach them otherwise. Thyroid metabolism is an extremely complex affair and it is not unusual to find one or more of these tests to be *within the normal range.* It is often the case that just one of all those tests confirms that an individual is, indeed, hypothyroid and agrees with the 99% clinical history of complaints and physical findings. It is not rare that occasionally all tests are within normal limits. It is then when treatment can be successfully accomplished by thyroid medication with regular and careful monitoring of the patient and the symptoms and signs.

I have been told by thousands of patients that the many doctors they have seen over the years had a one-symptom, five-minute visit with them and a physical examination that did not include palpation for the thyroid gland in the lower front of the neck. It is not only fast foods and overeating that are responsible for widespread obesity in the United States; it is the irresponsibility of the health care system as well.

Since my solo practice is unique and unencumbered by third-party payers, I am not the primary care doctor that many people are required to have in order to access medical care through a variety of kinds of managed care. In desperation, nonetheless, these patients are willing to pay at the time of service for the kind of attention they receive from someone like myself. They are also willing to travel great distances to my office in my little community in northwestern Pennsylvania; they come from as far away as Ohio, Buffalo, Boston, New York City, Philadelphia, Washington, Atlanta, and places in between east of the Mississippi River.

One point of significance in this regard is that occasionally an individual is required to see another doctor where they live or who is in their insurance service panel. Occasionally this is a dilemma that the patient and I must deal with. There are times that providers will not or cannot see the sense of my approach to finding out what is going on with an individual patient after an extended two-hour office visit. Therefore, there is unwillingness to cooperate with testing that will confirm what is contributing to the many symptoms these individuals present. The ugly head of managed health care simply taunts them away. Most of the time, with enough effort on the part of the patient and myself, we find a way around such impasses. At the same time, I have had instances where a patient presented with the symptoms and signs of hypothyroidism, was confirmed by testing and treated as indicated to normal thyroid function, then had a necessary occasion to be seen by a managed care physician (and in some instances an endocrinologist) who looked at my previous testing, saw a TSH that was sufficiently within her/his view of "normal," and immediately told the patient to decrease or stop treatment. In such cases, upon return for my follow-up visits, they had not done so.

Forty years ago when I began practice, I remember that the doctor wore a halo of omnipotence over her/his head above an aura of godliness and a pin-striped suit. It is so gratifying in today's information age that people as patients know about their bodies and minds much more than a health provider ever can in a one-symptom five-minute office visit.

JD has been her jolly ol' healthy self, weighing 185 pounds. When she comes to the office now, she literally jumps through the door from the waiting room into the reception room, with an expression of wholesome joy from head to toe.

John G. Hipps, MD, is the author of THE COUNTRY DOCTOR: ALIVE AND WELL *and practices in Emporium, Pennsylvania.*

◆ ◆ ◆

I am grateful that these medical doctors and health care providers have shared with you examples of how thoroughness and some incredible detective work on their part has gotten to the root of their patients' hormonal imbalances. You deserve nothing less than this thorough investigation of your weight issues.

The only gift is a portion of thyself.

– Ralph Waldo Emerson

CHAPTER 11

Replacing Hormones Naturally

The operating statistics that have constituted "normal" have been inaccurate for over 75 years and have not been based on patient evaluations or physical clinical findings. The change in the AACE guidelines will increase the number of people being diagnosed with hypothyroid from 60 million to 100 million.

– Howard Hagglund, MD

Your first and foremost task is to locate a physician or health practitioner who can assist you in getting to the root of your hormonal imbalances. As you can see from the previous chapter, there are medical doctors who are on your side and want you to feel your best. Hormonal imbalances can feel like you are in hell; or as if you are unraveling a ball of yarn to see where the problem begins and where it is going to end.

I have said this before, but it bears repeating: If you are not listened to, or your symptoms are minimized by a physician who gives you a five- to seven-minute "pep talk" on how to eat less and exercise more, or that your fatigue is all in your head, my advice is . . . *Run!* I say get out of that office so fast the doctor will think a hurricane just passed through. Need I say more? You have been abused enough by your own private hell; you don't need shaming ridicule to add insult to injury.

MY TSH LEVELS ARE "NORMAL" BUT I THINK I'M HYPOTHYROID!

by Mary Shoman

The following section is reprinted with permission from Mary Shomon, author of LIVING WELL WITH HYPOTHYROIDISM, *and founder of the website www.thyroid-info.com. For more information, log onto www.thyroid.about.com/library/weekly/aa111097.htm.*

According to the American Association of Clinical Endocrinologists (AACE), doctors have been basing their diagnosis of hypothyroidism on the "normal" range for the TSH test. The typical normal levels at most laboratories fall between the 0.5 to 5.0 range. The new guidelines narrow the range to 0.3 to 3.04. AACE believes that the new range will result in proper diagnosis for millions of people who suffer from a mild thyroid disorder but have gone untreated until now. AACE estimates that the new guidelines may double the number of people who have abnormal thyroid function.

Different laboratories have different ranges for "normal" TSH levels. These ranges are what most conventional doctors use to diagnose this disorder. This is the recurring dilemma that many people have faced in not being correctly diagnosed for hypothyroidism. Though their TSH levels are within a particular doctor or lab's normal range, they are experiencing symptoms of hypothyroidism. Verify what your doctor or lab considers "normal" and double-check this against the new standards AACE has set. You may be one of the millions of people who are considered hypothyroid under AACE's new ranges for identifying this disease.

◆ ◆ ◆

TREATING HYPOTHYROIDISM NATURALLY

If you have been diagnosed with hypothyroid or suspect you are, you will have decisions to make with your doctor.

Those decisions will include what course of treatment you will pursue to regulate your thyroid hormones (and other hormonal imbalances that can be in the mix). Will you take a prescription synthetic drug or try a natural approach? As we've heard, many doctors have spoken out strongly about the ineffectiveness of synthetic hormones. I can't make that decision for you, but I am strongly against synthetic drugs whenever possible. For every drug there is a natural alternative—you just have to investigate thoroughly.

A HYPOALLERGENIC TREATMENT FOR HYPOTHYROIDISM

by Som N. Sok, BS
Western Research Laboratories

Millions of people are unable to lead a fulfilling life because they suffer from a debilitating disease: hypothyroidism. This is a condition resulting from the thyroid's inability to produce enough hormones for it to function properly. These hormones are responsible for helping cells convert oxygen and calories into energy. For this reason, the thyroid is considered the major gland of metabolism. The key hormones produced are triiodothyronine (T3) and thyroxine (T4). Some T3 is produced by the thyroid, but the remainder of the T3 needed by the body is formed from T4 in a process called T4-to-T3 conversion.

When the thyroid is in good condition, it will produce 80% T4 and 20% T3 hormones. The T3 hormone is the more biologically active hormone, because it functions at a cellular level and is several times stronger that T4. There are numerous reasons for the body's failure to produce enough thyroid hormone, including the inability to convert T4 to T3. Western Research Laboratories offers a natural approach to supplementing the body with both of these vital hormones.

Nature-Throid™ and Westhroid™ are natural thyroid hormone products derived from freshly excised and promptly frozen porcine glands. They are hormonally identical. The only difference is the binding ingredients utilized. Westroid is bound with cornstarch, which may cause sensitivities in those with food allergies. Nature-Throid is bound with microcrystalline cellulose, making it hypoallergenic and more suitable for patients who are hypersensitive.

Nature-Throid and Westhroid are prescribed to patients who have been diagnosed with a thyroid disease. These products are measured in grains. Each grain is equal to 64.8 mg containing 9 mcg of T3 and 38 mcg of the T4 hormone. Since it is a prescription hormone medication, patients must follow their doctor's directions to ensure proper treatment.

NATURAL THYROID IN PRACTICE
by Howard Hagglund, M.D

The following article was written by Howard Hagglund, MD, with contributions from Mary Shomon, and originally appeared in THE TOWNSEND LETTER FOR DOCTORS & PATIENTS, *February/ March 2002. It is reprinted with permission. Contact and website information for both authors is in the resource guide.*

Howard Hagglund, MD, is a well-respected authority on thyroid disease with many years of experience treating hypothyroid patients. He is also an author and broadcaster who works to educate physicians and patients about thyroid disease diagnosis and treatment. Dr. Hagglund will now shed some light on the synthetic versus natural thyroid controversy.

I have used natural thyroid because of a very dear mentor and friend, Dr. Eva Wallem. She and most of my colleagues in the alternative medical field insist on natural thyroid. At first it would appear that we are just being a bunch of tree-hugging sentimentalists. But the truth is the natural thyroid contains T1, T2, T3, and T4, and they are not going to be turned away by the immune system of the body. They are ready to be used and adequately survive any barriers of digestion and immune rejection.

The University of North Carolina conducted a large research project comparing natural and synthetic thyroid. They gave concentration and personality tests to those who participated in this study. The patients who were on natural thyroid showed objective improvement in concentration, mood, and well-being. They further reported that they preferred this thyroid to the ones they had taken before. (The article appeared in the *New England Journal of Medicine* in February 1999, for those scholars who need further proof.) I find the natural thyroid gives an even, smooth ride to the equilibration of the thyroid patient. I find that it is very forgiving and will often stand two or three days of forgetting to take the dose.

For those of you who would like my favorite recipe in dosing thyroid patients, I strongly suggest a one-grain tablet in the morning and another again at noon. This is an extremely helpful way to present thyroid to the body for two reasons. One, the T3 will not last longer than four hours, and there is no reason to be taking all of your daily T3 in the morning— spread it around. Take the noon dose for all of the above reasons and it will carry you through the 3 o'clock letdown of the cortisone level in the blood. This cortisone reduction means a reduction in thyroid activity, and you will be well armed to withstand this.

I further want to thank an unknown homeopathic doctor who has given me a good way to monitor this dose of thyroid. Have your patient count his or her pulse every day at rest. If it goes over 90, it's a good idea to remove the morning dose and notify you. Besides this advantage I find my patients will change their dose during the year and according to how their thyroid is performing. I strongly advise that the blood test is frequently in error and of little value when monitoring thyroid dosing.

If you review the standard handbooks of endocrinology, you can find over 46 symptoms of low thyroid. I am frequently surprised at the number of problems that clear up after patients are evaluated and given the proper dose of thyroid and nutrients. Here are some of my major helpers in making the diagnosis of hypothyroidism: thinning hair, cold hands and feet, missing outer third of eyebrow, insomnia, swollen ankles that do not pit, and obesity (but never be misled—thin, beautiful women with great figures are often low thyroid.) I seldom rely on ankle reflexes and depend more on the shape of the torso as another indicator of low thyroid. Most of my low thyroid patients carry their weight in the midsection and their thighs.

If you would like some sneaky little diagnostic tips, check and you'll find the little finger is shorter and does not extend out through the middle of the dip joint. These people also have a history of many maladies and will be in trouble with insomnia, depression, and elevated cholesterol. My most significant helper in diagnosing low thyroid is the physical exam. After that I rely on a saliva test. In fact I recently participated in a large study showing very low concordance between blood tests and hypothyroidism. We have found that there is a very high concordance between the saliva test and the physical findings of hypothyroidism. Be patient, our statistician is still working on that paper, and it is not published. Never be fooled by a normal thyroid blood test—it never was any good and never will be.

On occasion I have used Synthroid but have always been displeased by its ineffectiveness. Check your physiology book and find that T4 must be converted to T3 in order to be effective. This is capricious at best and you will note that the patient's poor nutritional status is the main cause. Synthroid and all other T4s cannot be converted to active useful thyroid if we do not have enough selenium, magnesium, vitamin A, cortisol, vitamin B2, and essential fatty acids. Be further advised that stress produces large amounts of anti-T3. This blocks T4 thyroids from being converted to the useful T3. Do you know anyone who is not under stress seven days a week, 365 days a year?

THE PATIENT EXPERIENCE
by Mary Shomon

Mary Shomon is a highly regarded patient advocate within the hypothyroid patient community. She talked with us about her perspective on natural thyroid medication.

"The best possible thyroid medication is the one on which patients safely feel best," says Mary Shomon, author of *Living Well With Hypothyroidism: What Your Doctor Doesn't Tell You . . . That You Need to Know.* "The problem, however, is that many patients simply do not feel well on levothyroxine—the typical drug prescribed by most conventional practitioners," says Shomon, who receives as many as 2,000 e-mails a week from frustrated thyroid patients. "But the vast majority of doctors don't really understand that hypothyroidism is not always easy to treat with one little pill, as they seem to think."

If Shomon's advocacy and research efforts are any gauge, more than half of all thyroid patients who are taking conventional drugs simply do not feel well, and she believes many could potentially benefit from natural thyroid preparations.

"I receive so many e-mails from people who don't feel well. They've been taking Synthroid for years, and are struggling to even get through the day, much less have any extra energy for exercise," says Shomon. According to Shomon, these thyroid patients get sick with flus, colds, and infections more often. They're depressed, exhausted, and overweight. And the most unfortunate part of the situation, says Shomon, is that "they are told by their doctors that they are receiving adequate thyroid treatment. It's a travesty."

These patients clearly need more than standard therapy—

and that's where natural thyroid can play an important role for many of them. Beyond the need for the T3 found in the natural thyroid, Shomon believes that there are other factors that play a role in making natural thyroid more effective for some patients. Says Shomon, "I've heard from people who tried every possible brand of levthyroxine, even added Cytomel or time-release T3, and still had every hypothyroid symptom in the book. But they switched to natural thyroid, and finally, the symptoms began to clear up — sometimes after years, even decades of chronic illness!"

Some practitioners have suggested to Shomon that there may be nutritional components of natural thyroid that play an as yet unknown role in helping the body absorb or process thyroid hormone more effectively.

"Whatever the mechanism," says Shomon, "the reality is that for some patients, the switch to natural thyroid means they simply feel better, their high cholesterol drops, weight normalizes, depression and brain fog lifts." And, according to Shomon, with those improvements also come reduced risk of future health problems, and a vastly improved quality of life.

Thyroid patients need to be aware of all their options. Despite conventional medicine's bias toward levothyroxine and lack of knowledge of natural thyroid drugs, these natural products deserve greater awareness among both practitioners and patients, as they may offer hope to the millions of thyroid patients who are still suffering with inadequate treatment.

References

1. Food and Drug Administration, "Notice of Requirement for New Drug Application for Manufacturers of Levothyroxine Sodium." http//wwwacess.gpo.gov/sudoca/aces/aacess002.html. Volume 62 (1997).

2. "Effects of Thyroxine as Compared with Thyroxine plus Triidothyronine in Patients with Hypothyroidism." The *New England Journal of Medicine*, February 11, 1999, Volume 340:424–429.

◆ ◆ ◆

Depending on your age, a whole new set of issues (like perimenopause and menopause) comes into play with your hormonal picture. To quote the late Gilda Radner, a hilarious comedian of *Saturday Night Live* fame: *"It's always something!"* If you are struggling with your weight and now entering into the phases of more hormonal changes, your imbalances can really become challenging.

PERIMENOPAUSE AND MENOPAUSE: NATURAL SOLUTIONS

> *Oh honey, I have been in menopause since my divorce ... when I see men ... oh ... do ... I PAUSE!*
>
> – Loree Taylor Jordan

FEMALE HORMONE REPLACEMENT NATURALLY
by Dr. Ralph J. Luciani

Premarin is one of the most popular drugs sold in this country. It contains primarily estradiol derived from the urine of *pregnant mares*, and given to perimenopausal or menopausal women to help alleviate the symptoms of lowered estrogen production by aging female ovaries. Side effects can be numerous, including weight gain, breast tenderness, and even an increased risk of breast and uterine cancer. However, there are options.

The first indication of the need for hormones may not be hot flashes, but may be a change in mood, an increase in sensitivity, crying easily, irritability, and changes in libido and skin tone. In early perimenopause I recommend an initial trial of herbs and plant source phytohormones. Wild yam creams are commonly sold and are good plant sources of progesterone.

Early in perimenopause, use of this type of cream may be adequate to relieve symptoms. In time, however, other supplements—including dong quai, damiana, soy isoflavones, and others—that help stimulate estrogen receptors, may be needed. To help my patients through this life transition in the most natural way, I have developed a supplement pack called Meno-Balance, which contains a combination of herbs and natural substances to enhance libido and alleviate most symptoms of perimenopause. Taking one or two packs daily has proved very successful in achieving this goal. Meno-Balance is available from our clinic.

As perimenopause proceeds to post-menopause, herbs and supplements may not prove to be powerful enough to prevent the symptoms of ever-decreasing estrogen levels. If this occurs I recommend replacement with soy-based natural hormones using estriol as the principal hormone.

There are three major estrogen hormones: estrone, estrodial (Premarin, very potent), and estriol (weaker estrogen). Estriol has been shown to protect against breast cancer, and even in higher doses does not cause weight gain or increase in uterine tissue production. A compounding pharmacist must formulate these soy-based hormones to the physician's specific prescription. We are fortunate to have compounding pharmacies in Albuquerque. I will commonly do blood tests for estrogen, progesterone, and testosterone prior to prescribing a custom formula of these hormones for a menopausal patient. This allows me to know which level we are dealing with prior to the prescription. I will often add natural source testosterone if blood levels are extremely low. Testosterone in females is necessary in small amounts to improve libido and stamina, and along with estrogen can help prevent osteoporosis.

Women therefore have several options as they approach this delicate transition in their lives. Aside from what I've already discussed, a diet high in soy products helps greatly in enhancing any supplementation and can be protective against heart disease and breast cancer. My advice is always try the most natural way to help the body maintain its biological age before resorting to powerful drugs.

Options in Hormone Replacement

■ When is Hormone Replacement Appropriate?

Both the male and female body begin to alter their sex hormone status soon after the age of 40. Yes, men also have a "change of life" — called andropause, similar to the female menopause. This is a natural part of the aging process, but the changes that occur can be devastating both physically and emotionally.

In their early forties, women may notice more emotional irritability with drastic mood swings. Anxiety, depression, sadness, and panic are all symptoms which may occur and may not be obvious to most women as being due to hormone depletion. The usually recognized physical symptoms of hot flashes and menstrual irregularities may not be the first symptoms of a perimenopausal state. It is the emotional component that can be elusive and puzzling. Men, too, can experience mood changes, depression, and decreased libido. All these symptoms can be caused by a decrease in the more youthful levels of sex hormones: testosterone in the male, and estrogen, progesterone, and testosterone in the female.

Anti-aging and rejuvenation therapy have the goal of making us feel like we used to feel when our hormones were more "normal" (i.e., at more youthful levels). The question is, how do we safely replace these hormones that our bodies no longer produce in appropriate amounts? The answer can be complex, since we know that prescription strength estradiol (such as Premarin) is associated with breast cancer in females.

■ Solutions for the Female Hormonal Problem

There are three forms of estrogen produced by the ovaries: estradiol, estrace, and estriol. Estradiol and estrace are potent estrogens that increase the risk of breast cancer. Estriol, on the other hand, is a weaker estrogen that provides anti-aging benefits, but without the apparent risk of breast cancer.

Estradiol is the primary hormone secreted by the ovary, whereas estrone is synthesized from androstenedione and estradiol. A small amount of estriol is secreted by the ovary, but most of the body's estriol is converted from estrone in the liver. Estriol is used extensively in Europe for estrogen replacement therapy, but it is rarely used in the United States. Not only is estriol a safer form of estrogen regarding the risk of breast cancer, but it does not cause endometrial hyperplasia (buildup of tissue in the uterus) as does estrogen.

Estriol is a weaker estrogen, with most women requiring anywhere from 2 to 8 mg daily (compared to 0.625 or 1.25 mg of Premarin). It has been shown to be protective for osteoporosis, as well as giving all the youthful benefits of smooth skin, increased vaginal secretions, and better libido. There is also direct evidence from animal studies, and indirect evidence from human studies, that estriol can actually protect against breast cancer.

If hormone replacement with estrogen is indicated in my patients, I use the formula described by Dr. Jonathan Wright, which is 80% estriol, 10% estradiol, and 10% estrone. This formula can be compounded by a compounding pharmacist into a capsule for oral administration and may also be used as a vaginal or topical skin cream. Only natural plant source estrogens are used in these compounds.

DHEA can also boost estrogen levels, but I prefer not to depend on DHEA in the perimenopausal stage because the production of estrogen or progesterone from DHEA varies from person to person.

If I don't feel that full replacement therapy is warranted, I will initially depend on herbal phytoestrogens or progesterone to help alleviate mild, early symptoms of menopause. These include black cohash, dong quai, wild Mexican yams, and nutrient support with B6 and primrose oil or borage oil. This approach works well early on in perimenopause.

Most importantly in any hormone replacement program is striking a proper balance between estrogens and progesterone. If estrogen is inappropriately unopposed by progesterone, side effects of breast tenderness and mood swings can occur.

■ What About Testosterone?

Believe it or not, women need testosterone, too. It helps prevent osteoporosis but also improves lost libido considerably.

Men's testosterone levels begin to fall slowly during life, and the effects of lower testosterone can be felt more so after age 50. Lower levels can cause decreased energy, depression, dry skin, and decreased libido. Increasing levels of testosterone can improve well-being, libido, strength, and endurance. DHEA again can help produce additional testosterone in males. Testosterone is available by injection, patch, and oral capsules.

One precaution I always take with male hormone replacement is the addition of saw palmetto and pygeum africanum daily to prevent the transformation of testosterone into dehydrotestosterone, which can cause prostate enlargement. All hormones should be replaced judiciously and only after tests have been done to evaluate levels. In summary, hormone replacement can be safely done and can have significant benefits for well-being and health.

Ralph J. Luciani, DO, MS, Ph.D., MD (H), practices at the Albuquerque Clinic in Albuquerque, New Mexico.

❖ ❖ ❖

In addition to working with your physician or health care practitioner, please refer to Chapter 23, Nature's Pharmacy, for recommended supplements and herbs to assist your body in maintaining balance, relieving stress, and giving you optimal nutrition.

Few people can fail to generate a self-healing process when they become genuinely involved in healing others.

– Theodore Isaac Rubin

Can Stress Make You Fat?

The effect of excessive cortical secretion is also present for lean individuals, but overweight and obese people tend to exhibit the phenomenon to a much greater degree—leading several stress researchers to hypothesize that increased cortical production may be one of the primary causative factors in weight gain.

— Shawn Talbott, Ph.D., *The Cortisol Connection*

CORTISOL: THE STRESS HORMONE

We think of the adrenaline hormone (our fight-or-flight hormone) when we think of danger. As a mother of two, I could have turned into The Hulk (minus the green skin of course, and my teeth are much *prettier*) and moved *a house* with my bare hands if my children had been in serious danger. I'm sure you have had an accident or mishap that has just left you physically *shaking in your boots!* Your adrenaline is surging through your body, leaving you with a pumped-up adrenaline rush. Designed to keep us safe from impending danger, our adrenal glands with their biochemical response (adrenaline rush) have become overworked because of overstimulation in our stressful lives.

Along with adrenaline, the adrenals also respond to chronic stress with an excess output of cortisol, known as the "stress hormone." When cortisol levels are chronically elevated like insulin, cortisol increases hunger. High cortisol levels directly stimulate the storage of body fat in your midsection.

I personally don't know anyone who is not under stress—unless they live in a cave with no cell phone or pager. And they definitely are *not* parents. Struggling with life in general can be stressful in itself, but when we add the struggle to lose weight and fighting our own biochemistry, the stakes get higher. All these facts about our hormones are vitally important, because you have a whole biochemical system that is either working for you or against you.

◆ ◆ ◆

The following section is excerpted THE CORTISOL CONNECTION by Shawn Talbott, Ph.D. (and used with permission from Hunter House).

Stress makes a person fat primarily because of an excessive secretion of the key stress hormone, cortisol, along with a reduced secretion of key anabolic hormones, such as DHEA and the growth hormone. This combination of high cortisol and low DHEA causes the body to store fat and lose muscle. Our metabolic rate slows and appetite increases. All of these factors together have the ultimate effect of making a person fatter. Overall, stress makes you burn fewer calories and consume more food (especially carbohydrates)—which increases your stress levels even more! Even the *thought* of food and the *concern* about eating can increase stress—and therefore cortisol levels—in people who have restrained their eating habits and are either dieting or are concerned about their weight. Scientific studies have show that chronic stress clearly leads to overeating—which then leads to fat accumulation, frequently in the abdominal area.

Elevated cortisol levels resulting from chronic stress have been associated with the following conditions:

◆ Increased appetite and food cravings.

- Increased body fat.

- Decreased muscle mass.

- Decreased bone density.

- Increased depression.

- Mood swings (anger and irritability).

- Reduced libido (sex drive).

- Impaired immune response.

- Memory and learning impairment.

- Increased symptoms of PMS (premenstrual syndrome), such as cramps and increased appetite.

- Increased menopausal side effects, such as hot flashes and night sweats.

With increased anxiety during periods of chronic stress, levels of both cortisol and insulin rise and together send a potent signal to fat cells to store as much fat as possible. They also signal fat cells to hold onto their fat stores to use for energy. In terms of weight gain and obesity, the link between cortisol and deranged metabolism is seen in much the same way. These are listed below.

Metabolic Effects of Elevated Cortisol (Related to Weight Gain)

Loss of muscle mass

- Breakdown of muscles, tendons, and ligaments (to provide amino acids for conversion to glucose).

- Decreased synthesis of protein (to conserve amino acids for conversion into glucose).

- Reduced levels of DHEA, growth hormone, IGF-1, and thyroid stimulating hormone (TSH).

◆ Drop in basal metabolic rate (i.e., reduced number of calories is burned throughout the day and night).

Increase in blood sugar levels

◆ Reduced transport of glucose into cells.

◆ Decreased insulin sensitivity.

◆ Increase in appetite and carbohydrate cravings.

Increase in body fat

◆ Increase in the overall amount of body fat (due to increased appetite, overeating, and reduced metabolic rate).

◆ A redistribution and accumulation of body fat to the abdominal region.

◆ ◆ ◆

Remember, the theme of this book is that you have to look at your body as a whole to find the emotional and biochemical imbalances and other factors that may have led to your weight gain. Here are some more issues to consider.

Dr. Joseph Debé, who practices in New York, states:

One of the hormonal imbalances that can persist from in-utero into adulthood is excess cortisol. Cortisol is the body's long-acting stress hormone. It is secreted in higher concentrations in response to pretty much anything that pulls the body out of balance. Mental and emotional stress, and inflammations and swings in blood sugar, are the most common stressors. Cortisol causes biochemical changes that allow the body to adapt to stress, but problems begin if cortisol is chronically elevated. Two of the negative consequences of elevated cortisol are increased appetite and deposition of fat in and around the midsection. A study of women with increased abdominal fat found they reported having more chronic stress. In a laboratory setting, these women were more easily stressed and in response to stress secreted more cortisol. What's the bottom line? Vulnerability to stress can contribute to apple-shaped obesity. Reducing one's reaction to stress is important for weight loss (and health in general).

Another interesting study examined the connection between personality traits and abdominal obesity. Correlations were made between having a fat midsection and cynicism, anxiety, anger, and depression. What's the connection? Possibly, these negative mood states are elevating cortisol levels, which in turn causes fat to be deposited in the middle!

Cortisol is a hormone that is secreted by the adrenal glands. If you are under chronic stress there can be serious negative consequences to your adrenal glands. The street term for this would be "burnout"!

Although the following article is not strictly related to weight issues per sé, we have seen in the previous information that burned-out adrenal glands from excessive cortisol secretion will in fact contribute to hormones being out of balance. Hormones out of balance in turn become weight gain.

ADRENAL FATIGUE IS THE PRICE OF STRESS
by James Wilson, DC, ND, Ph.D.

Dr. Wilson is the author of ADRENAL FATIGUE: THE 21ST CENTURY STRESS SYNDROME. The following article appeared in NEW LIVING magazine, February 2002. www.newliving.com

If you're like most adults, you may have noticed that it's harder to get up and keep going than it used to be. Persistent tiredness is so widespread it almost seems normal but, in fact, it is often the most visible sign that you have a stress disorder call adrenal fatigue. Although it wreaks havoc in the lives of millions of people, conventional medicine does not yet recognize that it is a distinct, diagnosable syndrome. The ability to cope with physical, emotional, or psychological stress depends on the activity of the adrenal glands. They produce and secrete hormones such as cortisol and adrenaline that regulate energy production and storage, heart rate, muscle tone, and other essential processes that enable the body to deal with stress. No matter what the source of stress is, the adrenals have to orchestrate a complex biochemical response.

When you suffer from adrenal fatigue, the output of adrenal hormones has been diminished by overstimulation, usually from the cumulative effect of chronic stress. Resultant biochemical and cellular alterations adversely affect everything in your body from the way it deals with allergies and environmental toxins to fighting infectious agents to dealing with overactive auto-immune conditions like fibromyalgia. These same biochemical changes also lead to other problems such as hypoglycemia and depression. The lower adrenal function drops, the more profound is the effect on every organ and system in the body.

An illness, life crisis, or stressful lifestyle can drain the adrenal resources of even the healthiest person. However, there are certain things that make someone more prone to adrenal fatigue. A diet low in nutrients and high in sugar or refined carbohydrates and hydrogenated oils is probably the single greatest contributing factor. Substance abuse, lack of sleep, and too much pressure exhaust adrenal function over time.

Chronic infections like bronchitis and pneumonia and chronic diseases like arthritis and cancer place demands on the adrenals that can rapidly deplete them. Even a pregnant woman with low adrenal function can predispose her child to adrenal fatigue. Although it's more complex to diagnose adrenal fatigue than something like measles, the best indicators of this condition are the symptoms themselves. Anyone who regularly experiences one or more of the following may be suffering from adrenal fatigue. If you have trouble getting up in the morning even after going to sleep at a reasonable hour, tire for no reason, feel run down or overwhelmed, can't bounce back from stress or illness, crave salty and sweet snacks, experience an "afternoon low" between 2 and 4 P.M. and feel best after 6 P.M., you may have adrenal fatigue.

The most useful lab test for diagnosing adrenal fatigue is the saliva cortisol test. It measures levels of cortisol in saliva at specific times during a 24-hour period. Correspondence between low cortisol levels and symptoms is a good indication of adrenal involvement. Despite the fact that standard blood tests are the first choice of most doctors, they do not easily identify adrenal fatigue.

There are three things you can do about "energy robbers": (1) you can eliminate them, (2) you can change them, and (3) you can change yourself to better adapt to them. Getting rid of some stresses and altering others so they are less draining will lift a tremendous load off your adrenals. However, learning to take the distress out of your remaining sources of stress is the key to staying healthy. Meditation, transforming the way you look at your difficulties (sometimes called "reframing"), laughter, relaxation, exercise, and eating healthful foods are fundamental tools that have profound protective physiological effects on overworked adrenal glands.

Restoring already fatigued adrenals frequently requires certain measures in addition to those mentioned above. Whenever possible, it is best to sleep in until 9:00 A.M. A teaspoon of salt in a glass of water (instead of coffee) can help relieve morning fatigue. Adequate amounts of vitamins C, E, and B complex (especially pantothenic acid, niacin, and B6), magnesium, calcium, and trace minerals are essential for optimum adrenal function. The easiest way to get the necessary nutrients is to take a supplement specifically designed for adrenal support. Adrenal cell extracts and several herbs have also proven helpful in restoring adrenal function. These include licorice, ashwagndha, Korean ginseng, ginger, and ginkgo. The good news is that adrenal fatigue can usually be alleviated through lifestyle and dietary changes you can make yourself.

◆ ◆ ◆

The resource guide to this book contains the resources required to saliva test for all your hormones. Many doctors have suggested to me that they are more accurate than blood tests. Of course, it is a given that you will consult with a physician (maybe even one who has contributed to this book) to assist you with saliva testing.

> *Life was meant to be lived and curiosity must be kept alive. One must never, for whatever reason, turn his back on life.*
>
> — Eleanor Roosevelt

CHAPTER 13

■ ■ ■ ■ ■ ■ ■ ■ ■ ■ ■

But I Can't Live Without My Chocolate!

INSULIN RESISTANCE AND SYNDROME X

A sugar/carbohydrate addict is like a heroin junkie, always on the hunt for their next fix.

— Loree Taylor Jordan

Calling all chocoholics! Come on, you know who you are! Sugar addiction is the world's most socially acceptable addiction, and probably one of the hardest to kick (I speak from experience). Furthermore, you can really overlook your sugar addiction. I am referring to addictions of the refined sugars (such as donuts, cakes, cookies, chocolate bars, etc.) or high-carbohydrate foods (such as bread, pasta, and pizza).

You (like most people) don't want to admit you're addicted (it's called denial), or you might make jokes about handing over the chocolate and no one gets hurt, or you would die if you didn't have your chocolate ... but you are probably unaware of how sugar affects your life negatively. You also might be unaware, as I was, of the long-term effects of sugar addiction. Sometimes the damage may not be apparent until later in life. When I was talking with Jack Challem, co-author of *Syndrome X*, he made the comment to me, "Loree, by the time a person is aware that heavy sugar consumption has affected them negatively (usually in their late thirties or forties) it is already too late—she has created insulin resistance or Syndrome X."

Oftentimes, it is someone close to the sugar addict who recognizes unpredictable mood swings, irritability, hyperactivity in children, or complete personality changes after the ingestion of sugar. Anyone who has witnessed a child who is *bouncing off the walls* after a sugar high knows what I am talking about. I will address the issues of children, sugar addiction, insulin resistance, and the high rate of obesity later on in this chapter.

The symptoms of sugar addiction are real, physical, and often immobilizing. Some people simply seem to feel "knocked out" or fatigued all the time. I call it having a "sugar drunk." You have this knocked-out feeling that leads you to consume more sugar for another high, which then again leads you to an even lower crash. This is a vicious cycle. As a sugar addict you are constantly hungry, or feel shaky, sweaty, and sometimes confused. You complain of low energy, difficulty getting going in the morning, trouble concentrating or accomplishing your normal everyday tasks. You may find yourself subject to angry outbursts for no reason, have trouble getting along with people, or find a great deal to criticize in others. Severe mood swings are common. Many sugar addicts or their family members begin to question their mental stability.

Sugar addiction is a very real, harmful, highly damaging health problem, just as debilitating as an addiction to any other substance. Sugar addicts eat sugar compulsively. It is in control of your life. You go to great lengths to obtain your sugar, and if you don't get it, you experience predictable withdrawal symptoms. If you find yourself wanting to jump the kid walking down the street to get to his candy stash . . . you are a *sugar addict!*

SUGAR OR ALCOHOL . . . CHOOSE YOUR POISON

The only difference between a sugar addict and an alcoholic is that alcoholics drink their sugar and sugar addicts eat theirs. Both change to ethyl alcohol when broken down in the body.

Like alcoholism, sugar addiction is often genetic in origin—it runs in families. People who are overweight and addicted to sugar suffer from a disorder that may not be any more their fault than epilepsy or mental retardation or alcoholism would be. In some ways, treating your sugar addiction is much more difficult than treating a drug or alcohol addiction. With the latter, you can stop the addictive substance completely. With sugar you are constantly at risk of eating the wrong foods—namely sugar-laden foods. There are hidden sugars in *everything!* You may not even be aware of these sugars, making abstinence especially difficult. You have to be a committed label sleuth, reading every ingredient.

I have to be straightforward here on an issue that really bothers me. I absolutely disagree with recovery centers, such as 12-step meetings for alcoholics (I have seen them!), having refreshment tables loaded with donuts, cookies, and sweets. If an alcoholic is truly committed to recovery, then abstinence from consuming sugar is paramount. Many may disagree with me, but consider the facts: eating sugar keeps your body craving sugar. If you balance your body chemistry and your blood sugar levels with proper foods and supplements, your body will no longer be in the craving mode. The addictive craving mode is what makes you walk a mile (in your bare feet . . . *in a hailstorm*) for a mood-altering substance. I don't care if you are reaching for a martini or a donut, your body will still get its mood-altering sugar fix!

You and only you are ultimately responsible for getting to the root of your physical challenges, genetic or not, whether they are physical or physiological or both. I heard one doctor say in a symposium on Syndrome X, and I quote: "The only problem with your genes [jeans] is that they are too tight!" You may be predisposed genetically, but because diet and life-style play a larger part of the picture, this is not an excuse.

CARBOHYDRATE ADDICTION

Carbohydrate addiction: A compelling hunger, craving, or desire for carbohydrate-rich food; an escalating or recurring need or drive for starches, snack foods, or sweets.

Rachel and Richard Heller, in their book *The Carbohydrate Addicts Diet,* conclude the following about carbohydrate addiction:

Carbohydrate addicts recognize that the desire to eat isn't logical, because they know they're not really hungry in the sense of requiring nourishment. But the drive to eat can turn into a compulsion and a cycle of eating, not being satisfied, craving, and eating again. The moral implications of feeling "weak-willed" can really undermine the person's self-esteem when they are not able to control their addictive behavior.

Signs and Symptoms of Sugar/Carbohydrate Addiction

Do you ever experience these symptoms?

◆ A frequent focus on eating.

◆ Do you spend a great deal of time thinking about food, dieting, or your weight?

◆ Lack of satisfaction or the desire to eat again a couple of hours after eating.

◆ Do you get the feeling you aren't really satisfied after eating, no matter what you eat? Are you hungrier two hours after eating than if you hadn't eaten at all?

◆ A sense of fatigue or tiredness.

◆ Do you get a sensation of sluggishness, almost a feeling of being drugged, after eating? Do you feel like lying down, perhaps even drifting off for a nap? Do you put off work or planning activities because you just don't have the energy for them? Do you get hungry or tired in the middle of the afternoon?

◆ An unexplained feeling of anxiety or anger. Do you have a certain unexplained nervousness or irritability? A desire to be alone? Do you find that you are angry with or blaming yourself?

◆ A heightened emotionality.

◆ Do you find yourself feeling sad or weepy without reason? Do you ever experience a feeling of hopelessness, an intense feeling of loneliness, or a generalized feeling of fear? Do you ever go to extremes, with a feeling of euphoria or heightened happiness, only to later feel inexplicably sad or hopeless?

What Causes Carbohydrate Addiction?

Scientists writing in the *New England Journal of Medicine, The Lancet, The Journal of Clinical Investigation,* and many other journals have reported a physiological dysfunction that leads to overweight in many people. This dysfunction results in the wrong amount of insulin in the blood.

In the past, diet experts have failed to treat the problem by reducing the total daily intake of carbohydrates and distributing carbohydrates *equally to all meals.* We know that these strategies *don't work* for the carbo addicts. We have discovered that any weight-loss diet that prescribes three or more small meals each day containing anything more than minor amounts of carbohydrates will ultimately fail with the carbohydrate addict. Such a diet will trigger the insulin response and signal the carbohydrate addict to eat once again.

According to Drs. Rachel and Richard Heller in their book, *The Carbohydrate Addicts Diet:*

A normal person's body releases insulin within a few minutes of eating. *The amount of insulin released is based upon what that person has eaten in previous meals.* When the system is functioning normally, just enough insulin is released to help deliver the carbohydrate energy (in the form of the blood sugar glucose to the liver and to muscle or fat cells throughout the body.)

As the cells take in the glucose, the level of insulin in the blood drops. Upon completing their meal they feel satisfied—their insulin level drops and signals the brain to stop eating.

The carbohydrate addict's body with glucose transport disorder reacts differently to the aforementioned events. A few minutes after eating the body *releases more insulin than is necessary—the body overreacts.* If the carbohydrate addict has recently eaten a meal of carbohydrates, the amount of insulin will be greater still. This is called "hyperinsulinemia." The overabundance of insulin in the bloodstream causes the addict to still experience hunger and not feel satisfied. The failure of the insulin levels to drop in the bloodstream causes the desire and craving for more carbohydrates. This cycle continues into what we call a "carbohydrate addiction."

THE TWO INSULIN PHASES

The body releases insulin in two phases. This applies to normal individuals and carbohydrate addicts alike.

1. The pre-load phase begins within minutes of consuming carbohydrates. The amount of insulin released (regardless of how much carbohydrate is being consumed at the time) is determined by the amount of carbohydrate eaten in the preceding meals.

2. The second phase takes place 75 to 90 minutes after eating and is dependent upon how much carbohydrate was actually consumed at that meal. The body will recognize whether the first phase of insulin was sufficient to handle the carbohydrates consumed. This phase adjusts insulin production and release to the needs of that particular meal. If the amount of carbohydrates consumed requires more than the initial quantity of insulin release, the second measure of insulin will be released.

For the carbohydrate addict:

◆ Too much insulin is produced for the amount of carbohydrate that is consumed.

◆ This excess of insulin results in a decrease in the number of receptor sites (with an accompanying decrease in removal of insulin and glucose from the blood).

◆ Serotonin levels do not rise sufficiently to cause the sensation we identify as satisfaction; the carbohydrate addict does not get the signal to stop eating and continues to eat carbohydrate-rich foods.

◆ Production of insulin rises with each subsequent carbohydrate intake.

◆ Greater and more frequent quantities of carbohydrates may be consumed with no increase in satisfaction.

If you still aren't sure whether you are a carbohydrate addict, there is a test in *The Carbohydrate Addicts Diet.*

For a carbohydrate addict, continuing to eat one high-carb meal after another is like putting gasoline on a fire and expecting it to go out!

INSULIN RESISTANCE—GLUCOSE TRANSPORT DISORDER

High levels of insulin have been observed to coincide with a decrease in the number and sensitivity of insulin receptor sites in muscle and adipose (fat) cells. After many years, cells become so filled with sugar that they cannot admit any more sugar molecules, If your cells are not able to absorb insulin and glucose, you have *insulin resistance.* In short, too much insulin remains in the blood for too long and then less insulin gets into the cells to be burned for energy. This can be likened to a lock and key dynamic. The key has to match the right lock to open the door (see diagram on page 180). Therefore the high glucose turns foods eaten right into fat. *Insulin appears to stimulate fat synthesis and in the simplest of terms . . . you become a fat-producing machine.*

Shawn P. Kellerman, in *The Life Science Resource* (1997, vol. 2 issue 3), explains insulin resistance this way:

> One explanation for insulin resistance is a deficiency of biologically active chromium in a person's system; a result of inadequate dietary supply, excess chromium losses (consumption of sugary foods, age, and stress) or an inability to endogenously convert chromium into the biologically active GTF form. Chromium, acting as a transport mechanism, enables insulin to work more quickly and efficiently to maintain lean muscle mass, help the body burn fat, lower cholesterol, control appetite, and regulate cravings.

Controlling your insulin level is one of the most powerful anti-aging strategies you could possibly implement. The key to this is to follow a low- or no-grain and no-sugar diet, such as the one described in the nutrition plan on Dr. Mercola's website. Following the nutrition plan will automatically limit the foods that will cause your insulin level to rise. Contact information is in the resource guide at the end of this book.

Insulin opens doors

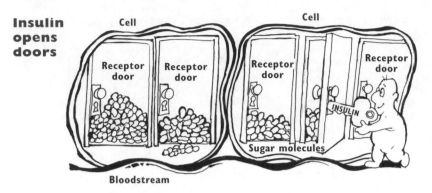

Body cells have numerous receptors for insulin. Think of these receptors as doors through which insulin, the key, enables sugar molecules to enter the cell.

Cell can't store any more sugar

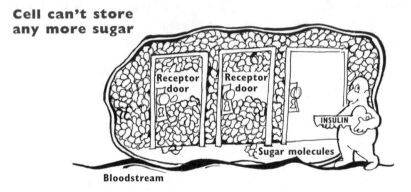

After many years of high carbohydrate consumption, body cells become so filled with energy (sugar) that they can no longer admit additional sugar.

Fewer receptors leads to insulin resistance

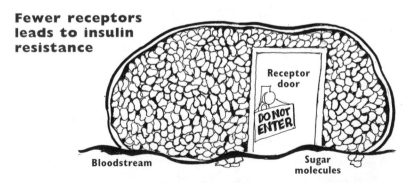

The cells protect against further sugar overload by reducing the number of receptors. The remaining receptors also become more resistant to the actions of insulin.

"Insulin resistance frequently ignored."

According to Dr. Joseph Mercola: *Insulin resistance is probably the single most important dietary factor to consider. It is the one that is most frequently ignored, even in many natural dietary approaches. A simple tool you can use to find out if your insulin level is elevated is to do a fasting serum insulin level. It should be below 10. The lower the number the better you are. I believe an optimum level should actually be 5 or below.*

The many conditions associated with insulin resistance and high insulin levels

Obesity (especially abdominal obesity)

High blood pressure

High blood cholesterol or poor LDL-to-HDL cholesterol ratio

High blood triglycerides

Syndrome X (a combination or all of the above conditions)

Cardiovascular disease

Type 2 diabetes

Polycystic ovary syndrome (PCOS)

Cognitive disorders, dementia, and Alzheimer's disease

Liver, pancreatic, endometrial, breast, prostate, and colon cancer

Nearsightedness

Reduction in the age of female puberty

Source: *Going Against the Grain: How Reducing and Avoiding Grains Can Revitalize Your Health,* by Melissa Diane Smith. Chicago: McGraw-Hill/Contemporary Books, 2002.

SYNDROME X: THE HIDDEN DISEASE YOU MAY ALREADY HAVE

by Jack Challem, The Nutrition Reporter™

The following section was originally published in LET'S LIVE magazine. ©1997 by Jack Challem. All rights reserved.

You may already be suffering from one of the most common—and often overlooked—diseases to strike Americans.

It's not a deadly new virus. Nor cancer.

It's a disease, surprisingly enough, caused by your body's inability to make the most of the food you eat. And one in three people suffer from it.

Doctors call this peculiar condition insulin resistance or, with a bit more mystique, Syndrome X.

If the name doesn't ring a bell, the symptoms might: feeling tired after you eat and at other times when you shouldn't. Gaining a pound here and a pound there—and having diffi-

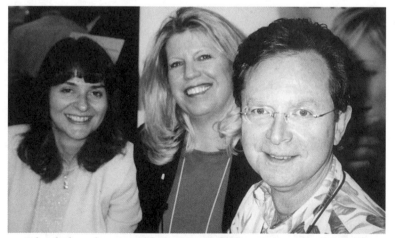

I had the pleasure of meeting Melissa Diane Smith and Jack Challem, co-authors of SYNDROME X, at the Natural Products Expo–West in Los Angeles in March of 2002.

culty losing them. Seeing your blood pressure creep up year after year. And finding that your cholesterol does the same.

Insulin resistance is the chief characteristic of adult-onset diabetes, which affects an estimated 15 million Americans. It sets the stage for obesity and coronary heart disease—even if you're not diabetic.

What can you do about it? The simple prescription is to eat right, take your vitamins and minerals, and exercise—each reduces insulin resistance.

But, as you might imagine, there's more to the story.

Sugar and Insulin: A Double Whammy

Doctors have known about insulin resistance for decades, but only in the past ten years have they gained a clearer idea of exactly how it derails your health.

Insulin resistance is caused in large part by the overconsumption of refined carbohydrates, such as breads, pastas and sugary foods. Eating too much saturated fat (found in beef) and omega-6 fatty acids (found in vegetable oils) and trans-fatty acids (found in margarine and foods with partially hydrogenated oils) also seems to increase the risk of insulin resistance.

Normally, after you eat a meal, your body breaks down carbohydrates into glucose, or blood sugar. The presence of glucose prompts the release of insulin, a hormone produced in your pancreas. Insulin help transport glucose from blood to cells, where it's burned for energy or stored.

When a person eats a lot of refined carbohydrates year after year, a dangerous cascade occurs. Insulin levels remain chronically high, and cells become less responsive—and resistant—to insulin. As a consequence, relatively little glucose gets burned and levels remain high. With chronically elevated glucose levels, insulin resistance evolves into diabetes.

At an American Diabetes Association (ADA) scientific symposium on antioxidants and diabetes, held in November 2002 in Orlando, Florida, numerous researchers implicated elevated glucose as a major source of dangerous free radicals. Glucose, which is a highly energetic compound (and the primary source of energy in the body), spontaneously oxidizes itself and spins off large numbers of free radicals, according to Lester Packer, Ph.D., a cell and molecular biologist at the University of California.

Free radicals, molecules with an unpaired electron, react with normal molecules in the body and oxidize them; this works much the same way heat or oxygen turns butter rancid. When glucose is steadily higher than normal—well above 120 mg/dL—it auto-oxidizes even more readily and spins off still more free radicals. Some of these free radicals, according to Alan Chait, MD, a professor at the University of Washington School of Medicine, Seattle, oxidize cholesterol and set the stage for heart disease.

High levels of glucose cause other problems as well. At the ADA meeting, Richard Ducala, MD, Ph.D., of the Institute for Medical Research, Manhasset, New York, explained that glucose can bind to proteins and "cross-link" them in the process. This is called glycosylation, and is akin to tying your body's proteins, which include your genes, into knots. Like free radicals, protein glycosylation has also been linked to aging and disease.

High levels of insulin create still more free radicals, leading to what researchers describe as "oxidative stress." Ele Ferrannini, MD, of Italy's National Research Council, Pisa, has reported that high insulin levels increase the demand for vitamin E, which quenches free radicals. That's not all. Dean Ornish, MD, of Sausalito, California, recently wrote in the *Journal of the American Medical Association* that insulin helps convert calories into triglycerides and cholesterol, increasing the risk of coronary heart disease.

Insulin Resistance and Heart Disease

Until 1988, researchers studying insulin resistance focused on its role in diabetes. Then, Gerald M. Reaven, MD, of the Stanford University Medical Center, built a strong case for insulin resistance as a cause of obesity, hypertension, and coronary heart disease.

"The fact that an insulin-resistant subject may not become diabetic does not mean that he or she suffers no untoward consequences," Reaven wrote in the journal *Diabetes*. "Indeed, an argument can be made that the more insulin *sensitive* (in contrast to insulin resistant) an individual is, the better off he or she is, and that the attempt to compensate for insulin resistance sets in motion a series of events that plays an important role in the development of both hypertension and coronary heart disease."

Reaven coined the term "Syndrome X" to describe how insulin resistance sets the stage for more serious disease. The syndrome is characterized by six traits: insulin resistance, glucose intolerance, abnormally high insulin levels, high triglycerides, low high-density lipoprotein (the "good" cholesterol), and hypertension. "The common feature of the proposed syndrome is insulin resistance," he explained, "and all other changes are likely to be secondary to basic abnormality."

◆ ◆ ◆

Syndrome X can be diagnosed when two or more of its related disorders occur simultaneously:

- Insulin resistance and glucose intolerance. Elevated or erratic levels of glucose, with insulin resistance. Warning sign: fasting glucose above 115 mg/dl.

- Upper body obesity. Excess body fat around the stomach or chest. Warning sign: a paunch or "pot belly." Lower body, pear-shaped obesity may not be healthy, but it is generally not associated with Syndrome X. Of course the more extra weight a person has, the more serious the problem.

◆ A person does not have to be grossly obese to suffer from Syndrome X. As few as ten pounds of excessive weight can indicate problems, particularly when the extra pounds are also associated with elevated blood fats and high blood pressure.

◆ Abnormal blood fats. Elevated total cholesterol and triglycerides and low high-density lipoprotein cholesterol. Warning sign: total cholesterol above 240 mg/dl and triglycerides above 160 mg/dl.

◆ People with very high triglyceride levels and very low HDL levels—another pattern characteristic of Syndrome X—are 16 times more likely than normal people to have a heart attack.

◆ Hypertension or high blood pressure. Warning sign: consistent blood pressure higher than 140/90.

Insulin resistance and Syndrome X are common forms of prediabetes. If you can catch the problems in time you can correct them before you become diabetic or have a heart attack.

> **It is important to remember that one of insulin's chief functions is to help the body store fat!**

Syndrome X, along with carbohydrate addiction, can be controlled and reversed with diet and nutritional supplements. If weight loss is also the goal, additional nutrition support may be needed for the adrenal glands, the thyroid, and the liver.

Diets for reversing carbohydrate addiction and Syndrome X are provided in *The Carbohydrate Addicts Diet* by Richard and

Rachel Heller; *Syndrome X* by Jack Challem, Burton Berks, MD, and Melissa Diane Smith; and *The Alternative Medicine Definitive Guide to Weight Loss* by Burton Goldberg. See the resource guide for these books.

Much of information in this chapter is from the book *Syndrome X*. The book outlines the following basic diet principles in the Anti-X™ diet. Your diet should be individualized to your present situation.

◆ Avoid refined carbohydrates, including white flour, white rice, white sugar, and other sweeteners.

◆ Eat foods in as natural and fresh a state as possible.

◆ Emphasize non-starchy vegetables as your primary source of carbohydrates.

◆ Keep your intake of nutritious carbohydrate-dense foods moderate or low, depending on your health.

◆ Avoid soft drinks, fruit juices, alcohol, and other highly processed drinks.

◆ Eliminate omega-6-rich vegetable oils from your diet, and use cold-pressed, extra-virgin olive oil instead.

◆ Enrich your diet with omega-3 fats whenever you can.

◆ Steer clear of trans-fatty acids, which are found in deep fried foods, margarine, and foods that contain partially hydrogenated oils.

◆ Eat some protein at every meal and snack.

I don't recommend eating refined sugar at all, especially if you are an addict. It's like telling an alcoholic, "Just have *one* beer." However, I realize that there are going to be times when you are at a special occasion and if the truth were told you are probably going to eat it anyway. Am I right? So if you decide to have some sweetened dessert for a special occasion, then please follow these guidelines according to *The Carbohydrate Addicts Diet:*

- ◆ Eat it with a protein and a low-carbohydrate vegetable.
- ◆ Eat all these foods *within 60 minutes . . . no exceptions!*

If you follow this protocol your body will not overcompensate in the second insulin release (after the 60 minutes). Your body will keep your insulin lower. This is assuming you have been eating a relatively low-carbohydrate diet throughout the day. If you have been carbo loading all day then by all means this technique is not going save your sugar-loving soul!

CHILDREN, SUGAR ADDICTION, AND OBESITY

According to Rob Stein of the *Washington Post* (*San Jose Mercury News,* August 12, 2003):

> Nearly one million U.S. teens suffer from a syndrome associated with being overweight that makes them unusually prone to diabetes and premature heart disease later in life, researchers reported Monday.
>
> In the latest indication of a deepening health crisis because of the nation's obesity epidemic, researchers determined that at least 4% of U.S. adolescents have developed "metabolic syndrome," a constellation of risk factors for subsequent health problems.
>
> "It's frighteningly common," said Michael Weitzman, director of the American Academy of Pediatrics' Center for Child Health Research, who helped conduct the first-of-its-kind research. "It's very, very disturbing. You're talking about people who haven't even become adults yet who are already on the way to cardiovascular disease."
>
> As the nation's obesity epidemic has accelerated, public health authorities have become increasingly focused on metabolic syndrome, which occurs predomi-

nantly among people who are overweight and is perhaps the earliest warning sign of developing health problems.

Teens with the syndrome are believed to be at sharply increased risk for developing diabetes by their twenties and heart disease perhaps as early as their forties.

"Metabolic syndrome is frighteningly common," says Michael Weitzman. "It's very, very disturbing. You're talking about people who haven't even become adults yet who are already on the way to cardiovascular disease."

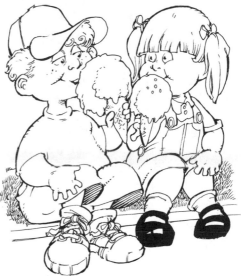

I have personally seen many television and news reports citing national concerns regarding the obesity epidemic in adults and children. The following article expressing this concern comes from the U.S. Surgeon General.

Editorial opinion of the *San Jose Mercury News* (January 13, 2003) states:

> U.S. Surgeon General Dr. Richard Carmona is calling on the public to give [strong] emphasis to obesity. He's calling on Americans to perceive their growing girths and fading fitness levels as a *national emergency*—the fastest growing cause of illness and death, and a tremendous drain on the health care budget.
>
> Carmona spoke out just last week at a conference on childhood obesity in San Diego. He called on parents to

do a better job of ensuring that children eat nutritious meals and get enough exercise. But the research on childhood obesity suggests that it will take more than stiffer resolve by parents. It will take a community effort to turn back the clock—and the scales.

PARENTS AS ROLE MODELS

Parents want to do right by their children, but when it comes to nutrition, "what's right" isn't always apparent. Good nutrition for our children involves more than providing regular meals and keeping the junk food out of the cabinets.

As parents, we have the ultimate responsibility for imparting knowledge about health and modeling healthy behaviors for our children. Our behaviors have an impact on our children, either negative or positive. We know that children practice and imitate our behavior. Whether it is our eating habits or how we communicate, children see and follow the main models they have: their parents' examples.

Probably like you, I did not question or negotiate food choices while growing up in my parents' home. I grew up in my family eating foods that I would not even consider at this point in my life. We had lots of sweets stashed in our house and I was more than willing to eat them. My mother used to store cookies in the freezer. I remember sneaking them, and eating them frozen.

As you read in my introduction, as I was growing up and into adulthood I was a sugar fiend always in search of another fix. It wasn't until my children were already 6 and 8 years old that I started to learn about proper nutrition. By that time they already had many years of bad nutritional habits behind them. Eating too much sugar was one of them. Our dietary makeover to healthier foods was a huge struggle and a major challenge.

My sons would love to tell you (they revel in it actually)

how I tortured them with carrot juice, coconut milk (which I made myself), and healthy snacks. They say they were always embarrassed because their friends would come over and there was "nothing good to eat." Which meant: no chips, ice cream, cookies, etc. I could not expect them to be perfect, so I came up with a plan. We would have "Bojangles Day" in our house. On Bojangles Day my sons would be allowed as much junk food as they wanted within a 24-hour period. What was left over (at the 24-hour mark) was thrown out. What was interesting about this family ritual was that the boys noticed they did not feel well after eating junk foods. They noticed a lack of energy from eating all that sugar. I wasn't thrilled that they wanted to scarf all this junk food, but it was a win-win situation and it kept my sons from feeling completely deprived. The other 90 to 95% of the time their diets were healthy. Becoming a prison warden and expecting absolutely perfect behavior with your children is a set-up for failure and resentment.

This seems to be a blatant contradiction of the *no sugar rule* in this chapter. However, many compulsive sugar eaters (as adults) will tell you that their parents never let them have sugar at all—*ever!* Constant deprivation is a set-up for children to hoard sugar (when they are finally exposed to it) or to completely overdo it by binging on it. I am proposing that we should teach our children balance and moderation. As in the example above, children may surprise you and actually realize the correlation of eating lots of sugar and how lousy they feel. My children did. Your children may learn on their own how to make healthier food choices, such as fruit for a snack.

I agree with Surgeon General Carmona's comments about it taking a community to turn back the scales. Parents have a challenging job fighting the propaganda in the junk food industry. With golden arches and ice cream parlors on every corner, children are bombarded with the excitement of unhealthy choices. We truly are a junk food nation.

Communities and concerned parents need to pull together to institute healthy school lunches and abolish vending machines that offer sodas and junk foods! It is going to take a national approach to this anti–junk food and anti-obesity consciousness.

Feeding our children sugary sweets on a daily basis may seem loving because they want it, but we are setting them up for a lifelong sugar addiction. Teaching children when they are young about the value of healthy food choices will give them a good foundation as adults. Planning family outings that involve healthy exercise sets them up with tools and habits that will stay with them for the rest of their lives.

> *Extreme remedies are very appropriate for extreme diseases.*
>
> – Hippocrates

Detoxify
Your Body!

In DETOX FOR LIFE, *Loree Taylor Jordan's insights into the importance of colon health are presented in a straightforward and entertaining way that will inspire her reader to pursue a more vital and healthy lifestyle.*

– Anthony Robbins, author of *Awaken the Giant Within* and *Unlimited Power*

Information in this section (Chapters 14–18) has been excerpted from *Detox for Life: Your Bottom Line—It's Your Colon or Your Life* by Loree Taylor Jordan, CCH, ID, Madison Publishing, 2003.

Sit down before a fact like a little child. Be prepared to give up every preconceived notion, follow humbly wherever and to whatever abysses nature leads, or you shall learn nothing.

– Thomas Huxley

CHAPTER 14

■ ■ ■ ■ ■ ■ ■ ■ ■ ■ ■

Detoxify Your Colon

Pure, lasting, and abiding health is the result of conscious discipline in cleanliness of body, mind, and spirit. All else is compromise.

— Bernard Jensen, DC, Ph.D., nutritionist

AUTOINTOXICATION

An unhealthy digestive system and impaired intestinal function can have a major impact on your weight. The real importance of removing toxic waste from your bowel, aside from avoiding disease, is to avoid having damaging toxins and byproducts recycling back into other parts of the body. As a certified colon hydrotherapist, I cannot overemphasize to you the importance of detoxifying your body to assist your metabolism in working the way it should. It is one less obstacle in the weight loss puzzle.

Detoxification has been my personal and professional passion for many years. I have studied every book ever published on bowel cleansing. My former husband used to joke at parties that "Most people sit down to read a good novel, but not my wife. She always has her head buried in *The Care of the Colon*." It was true. I couldn't get enough; I read everything in sight on colon cleansing. Who would have known then that I would go on to write my own book, *Detox for Life*, years later!

I am very straightforward about detoxification. I have been

called many things, but *subtle* is not one of them. To serve you, my reader, I have to bring up these uncomfortable bathroom topics, so that you can get a full picture of how your body really works. I am not just talking about weight loss here. I am talking about having a healthy, vibrant body. I have always said that I am *passionate about poop*. Stay tuned to see why!

How much thought do you give to your colon? Probably not very much at all. Most people take the functioning of their digestive system for granted. As long as you feel reasonably healthy, you probably aren't willing to consider the tremendous impact that the functioning of your colon can have on your weight and overall health. You're probably unaware, as I was, that a neglected colon can be responsible for a great many of our diseases. I'm committed to sharing with you the most vital, "kick butt" information about your colon health that you may ever hear. My hope is that the information that follows will be a big, swift, kick-in-the-butt, life-altering event.

WHAT IS AUTOINTOXICATION?

According to the *Colon Health Handbook* (Rockridge Publishing Co.):

> Autointoxication is the process whereby the body literally poisons itself by maintaining a cesspool of decaying matter in its colon. This inner cesspool can contain as high a concentration of harmful bacteria as a cesspool under a house. The toxins released by the decay process get into the bloodstream and travel to all parts of the body. Every cell in the body is affected, and many forms of sickness can result. Because it weakens the entire system, autointoxication can be a causative factor for nearly any disease.

V. Earl Irons, a noted bowel specialist, says: "In my opinion, there is only one real disease, and that disease is autointoxication

—the body poisoning itself. It is the filth in our system that kills us. So I am convinced that unless you clean out your bowel you will never reach vibrant health."

Many of the health problems we live with are problems we can control by getting rid of stagnating and fermenting foods that should have been removed as waste from our body but instead are collecting inside. The possibility of attaining any degree of vibrant health is lost if such fermentation occurs as waste accumulates and is retained by the body. If we are to attain any degree of health, we must not allow our intestines to remain loaded with waste material.

The average person carries around 10 to 15 pounds of fecal matter in his/her intestines. Think about that for a minute: 10 to 15 pounds of disgusting crud rotting in your guts. It has been stated that actor John Wayne's colon weighed an incredible 60 pounds at his death. Can you imagine your colon weighing 60 pounds? It was a known fact that John was a heavy meat eater.

The very best of diets can be no better than the very worst, if the sewage system of the colon is clogged with a collection of waste and corruption.

– Norman Walker, D.Sc., Ph.D.

MEDICAL OPINION

◆ "No harm can result if one to ten days pass without a normal bowel movement."

◆ "The range of normal varies from three movements a day to one every two weeks."

◆ "You may not have a bowel movement for 7 days or 10 days or even 20 days. The material accumulated in your colon is not dangerous to your health. Anticipate and accept twinges and the distended belly that will result. It is worth the wait."

ALTERNATIVE OPINION

Any doctor or health professional who is interested in a natural approach to better health will always place great emphasis on elimination, transit time, autointoxication, and cleansing. Because a difference in opinion exists, I'll let you decide. Even one movement per day means that three meals' worth of waste is still in the colon at all times. How would you feel if two weeks' worth of meals were backed up in your system? That's 42 meals without movement! You decide which is better: eliminating once or twice daily, or once every two weeks.

Autointoxication, or toxemia, is a form of self-poisoning, and one of the most prevalent conditions that acts as a barrier to good health. As such, it becomes the seat of many diseases, according to the clinical studies of many eminent doctors. These physicians include John H. Tilden, MD; Rasmus Alsaker, MD; Frank McCoy, DC; M.O. Gartens, DC; the late Bernard Jensen, Ph.D., DC; the late Norman Walker; and many others whose widely known writings are up-to-date and still available.

In his popular work, *Toxemia Explained*, Dr. Tilden says:

> Without toxemia there can be no disease. All diseases are the same fundamentally. The cause travels back to toxemia, caused by enervation (lack of nerve energy), which checks elimination and induces a toxic state. Every chronic disease starts with toxemia and toxic crisis. When the nervous system is normal, when there is nerve energy, man is normal and immune to disease. Disease begins to manifest only when environments and personal habits use up energy faster than it is renewed.

The late Dr. Bernard Jensen, DC, a natural healer of international renown, summarizes the results of his experience:

> In the 50 years I've spent helping people to overcome disability and disease, it has become crystal clear that

poor bowel management lives at the root of most people's health problems. In treating over 500,000 patients, I learned that it is the bowel that invariably has to be cared for before effective healing can take place. Trying to take care of any symptom in the body without good elimination is futile.

INTERNAL TOXEMIA

The body has a great deal of waste to dispose of through the colon in the form of used-up cells and tissues. These cells and tissues are dead proteins that are highly toxic if allowed to ferment and putrefy in the intestinal system. The body constantly regenerates and grows new tissues and cells, producing toxins through normal, everyday functions that, in turn, continually add waste within our body. Our body has to metabolize this waste. The concern here is with excess intake or production of toxins in the body, or with reduction in the efficiency of the elimination process.

Toxicity occurs when we ingest more than we can utilize and eliminate through the body's designed eliminative channels (bowels, kidneys, lungs, skin, and lymphatic system). The end result can be serious illness and obesity.

DEATH BEGINS IN THE COLON

In 1974, Dr. Bernard Jensen wrote: "The colon is a sewage system, but by neglect and abuse it becomes a cesspool. When it is clean and normal we are well and happy. Let it stagnate and it will distill the poisons of decay, fermentation, and putrefaction into the blood, poisoning the brain and nervous system so that we become mentally depressed and irritable; it will poison the heart so that we are weak and listless; poison the lungs so that the breath is foul; poison the digestive organs so we are distressed and bloated; and poison the blood so the skin is sallow and unhealthy. In short, every organ of the body is poisoned, and we age prematurely; look and feel old; the joints are stiff and painful; neuritis, dull eyes, and a sluggish brain overtake us; and the pleasure of living is gone."

A LESSON FROM LUCY

Our body's digestive and metabolic process reminds me fondly of Lucille Ball. I remember one episode in particular from *I Love Lucy*. The episode shows her at work in a candy factory. Her job is to package candies going by on a conveyer belt, but she cannot keep up with the candies coming down the belt (this was a hilarious skit by a brilliant actress). The candies are piling up and falling off the belt onto the floor. She becomes so overwhelmed that she tries to keep up by shoving them into her mouth. She is trying everything she can, in vain, to keep up with the conveyer belt and manage the backup of candies.

Our bodies are like that factory. The processing mechanism (Lucy and her boxes) becomes overwhelmed by the flow of devitalized foods and metabolic toxins (the candies). Like Lucy, our body can only keep up the race for so long before things start to break down. Our bodies, given their various inherent strengths and weaknesses, can manage quite well with the substances we put into them, and with the activities of work and play that make up our lives if we don't overdo it. But why push it? Give Lucy a break.

NUTRITIONAL ABUSE

Fast food chains predict they'll take in $121 billion selling high-calorie deep-fried lard and salt-based food and sugary soft drinks to Americans this year.

— *Metro*, Silicon Valley's weekly newspaper

Most people will readily admit that they have eaten incorrectly since childhood, and continue their bad habits through adulthood. Usually it is not until a health issue arises—either minor (such as wanting to trim down and lose weight) or life-threatening — that we choose to really examine our eating habits, food addictions, and possible nutritional abuse.

The food that we ingest is basically fuel to operate, maintain, and repair our body. The body was designed to be able to survive and thrive on a long list of what the earth provides for us, but this list does not include everything represented as food these days. Most of us do not live off the land as our ancestors did. Great-great-great-grandpa John did not snack on Twinkies and Doritos while riding in an air-conditioned tractor cab, or come out of the barn with a triple mocha latté made with cream from the farm cow. Our bodies are not designed for the diet we have grown so accustomed to. That is why I believe we are in disease and toxicity crises, and detoxification now is more critical than ever.

Devitalized (processed) food is often "easy" and convenient, but it leads to a devitalized life and a low level of health. The body was not designed to cope with chemical additives, preservatives, artificial colors, flavoring, and so forth, but functions most effectively on fresh fruits, vegetables, grains, nuts, seed, and other foods, prepared in such a manner that their nutrient value is not impaired or destroyed. I say, "Live foods, live body; dead foods, dead body! The whiter the bread the quicker you're dead!"

FIBER FOODS

There are numerous food substances whose ultimate function is to cleanse and remove used-up cells and tissues and take this waste matter to the colon for evacuation from the body. One of these food types is fiber. Fiber is extremely important to the digestive system. Fiber, however, must be composed of roughage, which is found in raw foods. When these fibers pass through the intestines they become, figuratively speaking, highly magnetized, and in this condition they are very helpful in the functions involved in the various parts of the intestines. This fiber acts like an intestinal broom.

In contrast, when "demagnetized" or dead, devitalized foods pass through the body's digestive system, the cumulative effect can be a coating like a sticky, gluey paste on the inner walls of the colon. Over time this coating may gradually increase its thickness until there is only a small hole through the center of the colon. In severe cases this opening can be limited to the diameter of a pencil, through which the feces is supposed to pass. On the other hand, one autopsied colon ballooned out to a measurement of nine inches wide (normal width is 2½ inches), and this woman had professed to be eliminating five times a day!

CONSTIPATION DEFINED

Many of my clients who come in for colonics (you will read about colonics in the next chapter) have expended a lot of energy trying to convince me that they are not constipated, even though they may have only one bowel movement per day. Many years ago I, too, was under that same impression with regard to my, uh, movements. But again, experience has led me to believe otherwise. In my own experience I did not know how a clean bowel should function, and was unaware that according to the definition of constipation, I was actually constipated.

Let's do the math here. If you eat an average of three meals a day and poop only once a day, in the course of a year you are 730 meals behind (no pun intended). Just like Lucy and all the candies backing up on the conveyer belt, you now have 730 meals' worth of foods backing up guess where? You got it: in your intestines. Think of the poor souls who poop only every few days, or go weeks without a bowel movement. Believe me, people like these exist. You may even be one of them!

If you eat three meals a day you should be pooping three times a day. If your digestive system is working properly you should have a bowel movement soon after eating a meal. Anything less than that is considered constipated.

So, really, what is the definition of constipation? The term constipation is derived from the Latin word *constipatus,* which means "to press or crowd together, to pack, to cram." Consequently, to be constipated means that the packed accumulation of feces in the bowel makes evacuation difficult. However, a state of constipation can also exist when movements of the bowel seem normal in spite of an accumulation of feces somewhere in the large intestine. You would not think of diarrhea as being a form of constipation but it is. It is the body's way of trying to get rid of impacted matter further up in the colon.

Proper intestinal management is probably one of the most important things a person can learn in a health-building lifestyle, since some of the most important functions relating to our health take place in the colon.

PRIMARY CAUSES OF CONSTIPATION

Some of the primary causes of constipation are:

Unconscious nutrition. Eating processed, devitalized foods low in natural fiber or bulk does not promote health and well-being.

Ignoring the call to eliminate. Feces or urine contribute greatly to cellular congestion (an accumulation of waste in the cells), autointoxication, and eliminative organ distress. Intestinal constipation causes cellular constipation. It also increases the workload of the excretory organs (the kidney, skin, liver, lungs, and lymph). The functioning of these organs becomes stressed and overworked. The cellular metabolism becomes sluggish, repair and growth are delayed, and the ability to eliminate waste materials is lowered. Instead of being alive and active, the cells become dead and inactive. This process results in a decline of the functional ability of tissues and organs.

Lack of physical exercise/sedentary lifestyle. Lack of exercise results in weak and flaccid muscles incapable of holding up under the demands of poor, inadequate diets and the extra eliminative burden placed on the body. Many people have what is called an "atonic bowel," where the bowel is not performing adequate peristalsis (muscular contractions that move food along the tube of the colon to the rectum). The late Dr. Bernard Jensen referred to this as a "Twinkie bowel." To treat this condition the bowel has to become re-toned and shaped up after years of abuse and inactive lifestyle.

Emotional/mental stress and strain. Stress produces unfavorable conditions in the digestive and eliminative organs, causing them to become tense and underactive. A relaxing environment is essential for adequate digestion.

Consumption of poisons. Poisons (such as tobacco, coffee, alcohol, chocolate, and sugar) have unfavorable effects upon digestion and elimination because they upset gastric secretions and nerve responses.

Some medications also have a very unsettling effect upon these life-giving functions. Medications may cause many afflictions in the bowel or place severe stress on the filtering process of the liver. Laxatives should be considered poisons, because they can be very irritating to the bowel.

Inadequate water consumption. Most people do not drink enough water and are chronically dehydrated. This causes body tissues and fluids to become thicker. The mucus lining in the colon changes in consistency, failing to provide a slick lubrication for the movement of the feces.

Poor living habits. Not following a good dietary health program contributes a great deal to poor bowel function by denying the body regularity and consistency. It never knows what's coming next and can't depend upon a regular routine. It is always on the defensive. The result is a depletion of vital nerve force, and an undermining of the body's ability to set periods of rest and activity.

The late V. Earl Irons, a nationally known colon specialist, defined constipation as the condition in which less than 100% of the food you have eaten in the last 24 to 48 hours comes out when you go to the bathroom. If you are completely healthy and have a completely healthy colon, 100% of the food you eat will come out within 24 to 48 hours of eating. But the big question to ask, he said, is: "Does all the food that is supposed to come out, come out?" In most people, all the food they eat does not come out within 24 to 48 hours after a meal. In many cases, food stays in a person for months and even years. This food will rot and decay and get buried in the crevices and folds of the colon. It can stay in the body for ten years or more.

Healthview Newsletter asked V. Earl Irons if food could actually stay in the body for that length of time. Irons answered: "You are darn right it can. Sometimes even longer. Some people still have a part of the turkey dinner in them that they ate at Grandma's ten years ago. Pieces of the white meat, potatoes, and stuffing are still *stuffed* in them. It might sound funny, but it is not a laughing matter." (Healthview, 1983)

Louise Hay identifies the possible emotional component of constipation as follows (Louise Hay, *Heal Your Body*):

Constipation. Probable cause: Refusing to release old ideas, stuck in the past. Sometimes stinginess. New thought pattern: *As I release the past, the new and fresh and vital enter. I allow life to flow through me.*

Bowel problems. Probable cause: Resent the release of waste. New thought pattern: *I freely and easily release the old and joyously welcome the new.*

DIFFERENCES OF OPINION

I love V. Earl Irons' answer to the question, "Does the medical profession agree with your views that any health problems can be caused by a toxic colon?"

Irons said, "I doubt it. The medical profession knows very little about the colon. Most doctors are ignorant on the subject, totally ignorant. In my opinion, most medical doctors should have their licenses taken away until they start to treat the real cause of most people's problems: a diseased colon."

He went on to say that most of the drugs, medicines, and operations given today have never made any person's colon one bit healthier. If anything, they have only made the situation worse. He stated: "You know, it is interesting that before the turn of the century, most medical doctors did understand something about the importance of a clean colon. Why, today, if you just mention the word colon to your doctor, he will most likely just laugh at you. You can be dead and long buried, and even then your doctor would never admit that your clogged colon had anything at all to do with your ill health." (*Healthview*, 1983)

DENIAL IS NOT A RIVER IN EGYPT
(More About Loree Than You Ever Cared to Know!)

"No way is that toxic stuff inside of me!" you exclaim. If you do not believe this black, thick, rubber-like lining can exist in your body, keep reading. My personal experience will make your jaw drop. If anyone doubted the possibility of such a foul surprise lurking in their system, it was me!

In the summer of 1987, I had the privilege of attending a week-long seminar on iridology given by the late Dr. Bernard Jensen, Ph.D. (world-renowned nutritionist) at his ranch in Escondido, California. All I heard about for a solid week was how Dr. Jensen had helped facilitate healing with 300,000 patients through colon cleansing and detoxification. It really drove home the point that just taking herbs was not enough. Using water through a Colema Board™ (a home colonic unit) or a professional colonic treatment was essential to help strip away the black, gnarly "stuff."

Even though I had completed Dr. Jensen's 7-day cleanse four times previously, I had not yet "dropped my lining" (the black goopy plaque that builds up in the colon) but my assumption at that point was that I was clean inside.

However, after listening to Dr. Jensen's colon detoxification stories I was so hyped and motivated that I went home and decided to keep cleansing until I dropped that lining. I was convinced that it was really there.

I came home and started another cleanse. On the fifth day of my fifth 7-day cleanse, I was shocked out of my mind. I went to the bathroom and this big, long, black, rubbery thing that looked like an alien from another planet slipped out of my body. It was about two feet long! Honestly, if I had seen eyes looking back at me, I would have had a coronary right on the spot! I called my herbalist friend, Marene, and told her my riveting news. She told me if I released any more "stuff" I should take a picture of it like those in Dr. Jensen's tissue cleansing book.

Was that it? Not even close. The next day I put a colander in the toilet to catch any debris so I could actually see how much material was being released. As embarrassing as this is to write about, I will tell you the truth. I dropped buckets full of black, snaky, goopy, ropy material for the next two days. I felt like I was giving birth to an alien child. And yes, I did take pictures of my black lining. The smell was the worst thing I could ever imagine, like a decomposing body. So much for my belief that I had a clean colon! The evidence was more than convincing, believe me.

Talk about a life-changing event. The experience of dropping about ten pounds of the most revolting black material I have ever seen has altered my perspective. There is no substitute for experience. I felt fabulous! But don't just take my word for it. Pick up a copy of *Tissue Cleansing Through Bowel Management* by Dr. Bernard Jensen and study those disgusting pictures of putrid bowel material. It will give you nightmares. Since a picture is worth a thousand words, you will probably be left speechless, your mouth gaping open, but only to gasp or scream. Believe me, there are people just like you who found out (much to their amazed horror) that they were "full of it" and didn't even know it.

MEDICAL OBJECTIONS TO COLON CLEANSING

Medical objection: "The body cleanses itself naturally. There is no need for any special cleansing program. Cleansing the colon is dangerous and completely unnecessary."

My response: Considering the inadequate, devitalized foods most people eat today, there is no way the colon can cleanse itself "naturally." If we ate an adequate diet that consisted of plenty of natural, raw foods, yes, the body would be able to cleanse itself. The real problem here is we can't live a long healthy life with 10 to 15 pounds of fecal matter backed up in the colon.

If the colon cleanses itself naturally, then why do Americans spend more than $400 million a year laxatives? Why do more than 70 million Americans suffer from bowel problems? Why do 100,000 Americans undergo colostomies each year?

If the colon cleanses itself naturally, then why do people rid themselves of pounds of putrid fecal matter and impacted mucus upon completing a bowel cleansing program?

Medical objection: "Wastes accumulating in the colon are not toxic."

Medical objection: The intestinal system (such as the colon) is a porous organ and in fact releases toxins into the entire body via the bloodstream and the lymphatic system.

If you ask the average physician about autointoxication, trust me, he/she will most likely downplay your concerns. The average doctor in general does not have any concept of how to detoxify the body and most certainly does not relate it to disease control. Of course, there are also many doctors who do support detoxification. My intent is not to criticize the medical profession. It provides a great service, but many practitioners are just not trained about new concepts in the field of nutrition and disease prevention through detoxification.

I think V. Earl Irons could not have said it better: "The medical profession labels any form of therapy as quackery if they themselves are not able to administer or control it." I would like to take that comment one step further and say that if there is no financial gain on their part they are really going to shout "quackery."

I believe in detoxifying the body like I believe in breathing air. There is absolutely no doubt in my mind that autointoxication may be a contributing factor to your weight problem and possible ill health. In the next few chapters I will discuss ways to detoxify your body after years of nutritional abuse, and remove accumulated waste material in the colon and other eliminative channels.

A doctor can bury his mistakes, but an architect can only advise his clients to plant vines.

– Frank Lloyd Wright

CHAPTER 15

■ ■ ■ ■ ■ ■ ■ ■ ■ ■

You Want to Cleanse My WHAT? Put Water WHERE?

*Growing up, I wanted to be a beautician. I guess
I got confused and got at the wrong end.*

— Loree Taylor Jordan

I know what you are telling yourself right now: "Stop! Where are you going with this? I didn't sign up for cleansing my colon—I just want to lose weight!" As you have learned in the previous chapter, autointoxication (self-poisoning) can be a contributing factor in metabolic sluggishness and a deterrent to losing weight. Don't shoot the messenger; I'm just presenting the facts. Setting weight issues aside, if you want to live a long and vital healthy life, this is important information.

People always ask me how I got into this line of work: colonics. They ask, "What is a nice girl like you doing in a profession like this?" There I was, practicing colon therapy, when all my life I had dreamed of becoming a beautician! I had promised my mother at a very early age when I loved to style hair that I would become a beautician. I jokingly admit to "being confused and ending up at the wrong end." Perms and hair tints were not to be my destiny. Fate had an entirely different *movement* in store for me!

As I mentioned in the previous chapter, before becoming a colon hydrotherapist I was a voracious reader on the subject of colon detoxification. I was learning so much, I couldn't stop talking about it. Everywhere I went, bowel cleansing was on the top of my list of interesting topics. My friends played along; they listened to my verbal infomercial about the benefits of colonics at every social event. This was such a norm with my friends, they decided they would "give me a taste of my own medicine" by singing a song they had written about me. Four of my friends got up and sang "The Colonic Queen"! The song was very clever, I must say, and absolutely hysterical. We all had tears in our eyes from laughing so hard. That night the Colonic Queen was born, and she is alive and well many years later!

THE REAL SCOOP ON COLON CLEANSING:

THE COLONIC QUEEN TELLS ALL . . .

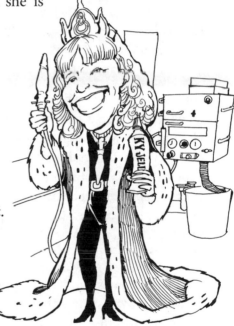

One of the most important and effective ways to cleanse the colon is through colon hydrotherapy, also known as a colonic. Colon hydrotherapy is clean and relaxing. A soothing flow of filtered, temperature-controlled water gently circulates throughout the colon, coaxing your body to release the digested toxins and waste that may have built up inside. Colon hydrotherapy is an ancient, time-honored, gentle water cleansing of the colon, by way of a sterile, disposable rectal tube or speculum. Water and fecal matter are flushed out.

I want to emphasize that the water is inserted into the rectum slowly and gently. Let me repeat that: *slowly and gently.* Honestly, no surprises here. I want to be perfectly clear because imaginations can run wild here. I just imagine my client's sphincter muscle tightening up as they visualize me hooking up the colonic tubing to a fire hydrant outside to flood their colon.

A colonic machine is attached to a wall with piping directly linked to the sewer system (much like a toilet would be.) A clear, contained tube (no smell or odor) allows viewing of the waste material before it goes into the sewer system. A colonic is facilitated by a trained colon hydrotherapist who administers and regulates the flow of water into the bowel. Most clients say that a colonic is more comfortable than they had first imagined. Other adjunct therapies you could receive during a colonic are foot reflexology, massage of lymphatic areas, heat lamp treatment, and aromatherapy oils to aid the body in releasing toxins. The entire treatment lasts about 45 to 60 minutes.

Unfortunately, with misunderstandings and preconceived ideas, controversy continues to surround colon hydrotherapy. Historically, we recognize two unequivocal conclusions. First, many health professionals and patients strongly believe in the benefits of this treatment. Second, because of lack of professional control (such as licensing by the state as opposed to certification by accredited colon hydrotherapy schools) and lack of study by most physicians, colon hydrotherapy has never received the attention and recognition it justly deserves.

With today's modern technological advancements in colon hydrotherapy instrumentation, particularly with regard to safety, along with better educated and skilled hydrotherapists, colon hydrotherapy has become a valuable tool to physicians in treating disease. Yet colon hydrotherapy is still misunderstood in this enlightened era. Some articles in popular magazines continue to tout the dangers of colon hydrotherapy.

> **Q: What if I am too embarrassed to go in for a professional colonic?**
>
> **A: Get over yourself.**

REAL MEN GET COLONICS

I'm not trying to give men a bad rap here. They are great clients and, I must say, usually the most entertaining. It is just getting those macho guys into the office and then into those backless, bun-exposing gowns that seems to be the problem. If I told you all the funny jokes and comments men come up with regarding the insertion of the speculum and this whole colon cleansing process, this book would be X-rated. It's a good thing I have a sense of humor, or I never would have survived all these years in this profession.

I once had a new male client in my office who was just hysterically funny with all his barbs and jokes about his vulnerability on my colonic table. He was so funny I couldn't resist playing along with him. His main concern seemed to be how he would know when he was full of water, and how I would know when to shut the water off. I looked at him calmly and said, "Well, usually you can tell your intestines are full when water shoots out your ears."

"Oh my God!" he said.

I just smiled at him. When he realized I was kidding and giving him a dose of his own medicine, he relaxed. He had a great colonic session and felt wonderful when he left. In all seriousness, male clients make up about 30 to 40% of my practice and they are a joy. Keep up the good work, guys!

Colonics are becoming fashionable in Hollywood. Many actors and actresses have made references to using colonics in their weight loss and health-building regimens. I've seen a number of movies and TV sitcoms referring humorously to colonics, and of course I get a grin on my face like the Cheshire cat.

FOR BULIMICS

It's very important at this juncture to point out that many people who have eating disorders such as bulimia have repeatedly abused laxatives and enemas as a way to purge their bodies after eating binges. As a responsible health educator, I am in no way suggesting it is acceptable to use colonics or enemas to eliminate large amounts of food you have eaten in a binge.

If you are currently, or have in the past, abused your body this way, my suggestion is that you talk with a colon therapist and have him or her assist you in cleansing your body in a healthy, nonaddictive way. Please don't set yourself up for a self-abusive cycle.

POWERPOOPIN'

In my many years as a colon hydrotherapist I have developed several colon cleansing programs to assist the body in removing unwanted debris. Taking herbal supplements will help to pull that debris off your colon wall. Remember my own colon cleansing story? Those incredible results were possible with the assistance of herbs, supplements, and the Colema Board (home colonic unit). I'm going to suggest a two-week gentle cleansing to start you off.

What Should I Eat When on a Cleansing Program?

Foods to eliminate while cleansing:

- Coffee. (Forget it! It kills all the *good* bacteria in your intestines.)

- Dairy products that are mucous-forming (for example, milk, cheese, and butter).

- Sugar in all forms (including alcohol).

- All junk and fast foods.

- Sodas and caffeined drinks.

- Red meats, pork, fatty meats such as bacon.

- Fried foods.

Foods to increase while cleansing:

◆ Lots of pure water and herbal teas (at least a gallon a day).

◆ Fresh fruit and vegetable juice (invest in a good juicer and make your own).

Other suggestions for your cleanse:

◆ Eat lightly, such as salads (hold the goopy dressings) and soups.

◆ Keep starchy pastas and breads to a minimum or, better yet, eliminate them altogether.

◆ Don't overload your digestive system.

◆ Eat five to six small meals per day instead of three large meals.

◆ Stick with light meats, such as chicken and fish.

◆ Increase your raw foods (fruits and vegetables).

During this two-week period you will be removing all the acid addictions mentioned above. This is the time when you might get what is called a cleansing headache, and withdrawal symptoms. You may have been indulging in some powerful addictive substances—such as chocolate, sugar, caffeine, and alcohol—and your body may struggle giving them up, but try to persevere. In only three to seven days you'll be feeling on top of the world.

Here is another component of the two-week cleanse. This prepackaged program, along with the healthy diet you will be following, will assist in removing toxins.

Two-Week CleanStart® Cleanse

CleanStart® comes in 28 prepackaged packets to be taken twice daily. Please refer to Chapter 23, Nature's Pharmacy, for the herbal ingredients in this program. It is recommended:

◆ Drink the contents of one cleansing packet 15 to 30 minutes before breakfast and 15 to 30 minutes before dinner.

◆ Mix cleansing packet in eight ounces of juice or water. Shake, blend, or stir vigorously and drink immediately. Drink an additional glass of water immediately after cleansing drink.

◆ Take the contents of one capsule packet (three capsules) with breakfast and dinner (twice daily).

This cleanse is so simple. The prepackaged packets make it easy to take with you even if you are traveling. I love this program!

Should I get colonics with the CleanStart program?
I generally suggest a series of three to six colonics during the CleanStart program to really get things moving. The colonics will help remove the fecal material that is being loosened up by the cleansing packet and supplements. Then I suggest a colonic at least once or twice a month thereafter for maintenance and to monitor your progress, which could take up to a year. Please note, this is just a suggestion. Follow the advice of your colon therapist who knows your health history.

Can I work during this cleanse? Won't I have to stay near the bathroom all day?
Absolutely! (You can work!) I never take time off work when I cleanse. In the beginning of the CleanStart you can have more copious bowel movements during the first few days or so, and then it will taper off. Your body will be playing catch-up with the backup of fecal matter but you will not have explosive, urgent diarrhea. This program is balanced with herbs that cleanse but also re-tonify and build your intestinal system. You will *not* have to camp out in the bathroom.

Do I have to use your cleansing products, or can I use my own?

These programs have been designed to work synergistically. I do not recommend picking and choosing different supplements or herbs in the program. I will be pretty blunt here — are you surprised? — either do the programs as designed or don't do them at all. Let me tell you why. If I gave you the recipe for a casserole and you left out some of the ingredients, it would not taste as good as if you had made it correctly. The cleansing program is designed the same way. If you take out the capsule packet, for example, and just do the cleansing drink, you run the risk of having your intestines bloat up because the powdered psyllium (in the cleansing drink) does not have laxative herbs to move the bulking agent through the intestinal system. This is just one scenario. Everything in the program is there for a purpose — do not pick and choose.

Another success tip is to partner with a knowledgeable colon therapist. They can work with you over a period of time and learn your medical history and concerns. Many colon therapists have also designed their own programs with products they are familiar with. There are many cleansing products available either through health practitioners (such as colon therapists) or in health food stores. I recommend that if you use products suggested by your colon therapist, then follow their instructions carefully, stick with their program in its entirety, be committed, and be persistent.

When I did an herbal cleanse (with my former husband) in the early years of my marriage, I just about blew up my former husband's intestines! I don't intend to scare you, but I assure you, *I did not follow instructions.* I am the kind of person that if one pill is good, two is better, and when you are dealing with such a delicate area the instructions are law. Can you see it? We interrupt this programming to bring you a special news bulletin .... *Wife blows up husband's intestines with an herbal bowel cleansing program ... film at 11 ... Oops!*

Will the CleanStart make me sick?

The herbs won't make you sick, but the toxins being circulated in your bloodstream and lymphatics may make you sick. If you get sick, it is because you brought it on yourself with incorrect eating habits, use of drugs, etc. That is why colonics are recommended during this process to minimize the toxins being circulated.

Is it really necessary to cleanse my colon?

Go back and re-read the previous chapter!

After your two-week cleanse you will feel so good you will probably want to continue. You'll feel great, but this is only the beginning stage of detoxifying. If you want to get a little more aggressive, in *Detox for Life* read about *Loree's Kick-Butt Bowel Blaster Clean-Out-the-Crud Cleansing Drink* and the *7-Day Boot Camp Cleanse*. These programs really detoxify the waste material in your colon. I have successfully used these cleanses with my clients for over 15 years. The results have been astonishing.

All the cleansing products in this chapter are listed in the resource guide for you to order.

> *You cannot create experience . . .*
> *you must undergo it.*
>
> – Albert Camus

CHAPTER 16

■ ■ ■ ■ ■ ■ ■ ■ ■ ■ ■

Removing Parasites Can Reverse Weight Gain

Make no mistake about it, worms are the most toxic agents in the human body. They are one of the primary underlying causes of disease and the most basic cause of a compromised immune system.

– Hazel Parcell, DC, ND, Ph.D.

In her books, *Cure for All Diseases* and *Cure for All Cancers*, Hilda Clark maintains that all diseases have their start with parasitic infestation and environmental toxins.

DID YOU SAY PARASITES?

This chapter will be a bitter pill to swallow and by far the most shocking. Just the idea of parasites and worms crawling around in your body is enough to send you into denial. All I can say is, take a deep breath, keep an open mind, and review the facts. I know that I am pushing the envelope with this chapter but I have got to go there. Trust me! I have shown you the significant importance of detoxification to assist your body in weight loss, but there is another critical component. I am going to open Pandora's box right here and now. Hold tight because this information is not for the weak-kneed.

To add insult to injury, as your body is working overtime to handle, digest, and clean up your own wastes, worms and parasites find a perfect breeding ground between the thick mucus coating and your colon wall. And as they eat your food, their excrement becomes a source of toxic poisoning that goes right into the bloodstream and overloads the liver. Yes, you heard me right. As if black, goopy snakes coming out of the colon are not grotesque enough, now you can add worms and parasites to the list.

With the filth and toxins you have created in your body from years of nutritional abuse and poor living habits, you may have provided a perfect environment for the invasion of parasitic scavengers. I always say that maggots cannot live in a clean garbage can. Parasites cannot live in a clean, healthy body.

Parasite infections are often thought to cause weight loss but the truth is that they can also lead to chronic obesity. Parasites can cause weight gain by damaging the body's detoxification system, particularly the liver and lymphatic system (more on how to cleanse these areas in another chapter.) Parasites can also lead to hormonal imbalances, which in turn lead to weight gain.

WHAT YOU ABSOLUTELY HAVE TO KNOW ABOUT PARASITES

You must educate yourself. Ignorance is not bliss with this epidemic. I have had people squirm in their chair or make awful faces when I even suggest how parasites may relate to their health challenges. The typical comment is something like, "I don't want hear about it." One man said, "What would it hurt if I don't know? What harm can parasites possibly do? We all have them, don't we?" I calmly replied, "They can kill you." I may sound overboard on this, but all passions are strong. I must emphatically state to you that parasites can and will cause diseases that can lead to your death or the death of someone in your family. Saying anything less than that would be professionally irresponsible on my part.

I learned a lot about parasites from Ann Louise Gittleman's classic, *Guess What Came to Dinner*. In this book (which was first published in 1993 and updated in 2001) I discovered that the word "parasite" is from the Greek word *para* (meaning "beside") and *sitos* (meaning "food"). A parasite is described as an organism that derives its food, nutrition, and shelter by living in or on another organism. A parasite lives off the host—that is, off you or me. Americans today are host to more than 130 different kinds of parasites, ranging from microscopic organisms to foot-long tapeworms. Parasites show no socioeconomic boundaries, and may be found in all climates. Practically every imaginable kind of exotic parasitic disease has been identified in our country. Parasites are an insidious public health threat in the U.S. today. They are insidious because so very few people are talking about parasites, and even fewer people are listening. They are insidious because many physicians don't recognize classic symptoms of parasitic infection.

I was totally amazed to learn from *Guess What Came to Dinner* how parasites are the great masqueraders. Some of the symptoms of parasitic involvement are constipation, diarrhea, gas, bloating, irritable bowel syndrome, joint and muscle aches and pains, anemia, allergy, skin conditions, granulomas, nervousness, sleep disturbances, teeth grinding, chronic fatigue, and immune dysfunction. The most common symptom is no symptom at all. Of course, the first place your mind wants to go with this information (after the shock wears off) is: "How can a parasite or worm live in my body without my knowing it's there?" *Trust me, it can!* Ross Anderson, MD, says, "It never ceases to amaze me, when I hear of an adult passing a worm in total surprise, that they could have had such a creature living inside of their body for possibly years."

In *Alternative Guide to Weight Loss*, Burton Goldberg describes a man who was in his late seventies with a fluctuating weight problem in his gut. His distended abdomen was very firm to the touch. His nutritionist was Ann Louise Gittleman, and she immediately suspected parasites. After being on an herbal antiparasite program for four weeks, his bloated abdomen started to soften, and the distention eventually disappeared completely. This patient's weight stabilized again at his normal weight after weighing as much as 200 pounds.

About six months ago I was watching one of the late night talk shows and one of my favorite actresses and singers of all time, "The Divine Ms. M," Bette Midler, was talking about all the weight she had recently lost. She said she had been sick for about four months and it was finally discovered that she had a parasite in her intestinal system. She didn't go into all the details of symptoms, just that she couldn't eat. She joked about how all her friends wanted to know where they could get one! All kidding aside, we don't want to get a parasite for weight loss or for any other reason!

SHOULD I GET TESTED FOR PARASITES?

In my opinion, you should save your money. If you are tested by a doctor for parasites (though chances are your physician won't suspect parasites in the first place), the results are most likely to come back negative. Does this mean that you are free from parasites? Unfortunately, medical testing procedures—besides being expensive—detect only about 20% of the actual cases of parasites. According to Dr. Ross Anderson, "Although more than 1,000 species of parasites can live in your body, tests are available for only approximately 40 to 50 types. This means that doctors are testing for only about 5% of the parasites and missing 80% of those. This brings the ability to clinically find parasites down to 1%. Now, if I had a 1% chance of winning in the stock market I don't think I would invest." Another point to consider is that only 30% of parasites are living in the lower intestinal tract. The other 70% are living in tissues, organs, and muscles, and are undetectable by a stool sample.

With the statistics being what they are, save your money on all the fancy-schmancy testing, and just assume that you do have parasites. Get out of denial, realize that you are probably

Parasites outrank cancer as man's deadliest enemy on a worldwide basis.

It is believed that 90% of the population is infested with worms.

Over 100,000 Americans die annually due to parasitic diseases.

not one of the 5% of the population that is not infected with parasites (unless you've been living in a protective bubble all your life), and follow a simple herb program. End of story. Let's not make this any more difficult than it needs to be.

Parasites are the most unsuspected source of ill health and suffering on the planet today. Make no mistake about it: nearly eight out of ten Americans are carrying one or more "uninvited guests" somewhere in their body.

According to nutrition expert Ann Louise Gittleman, ND, MS, CNS:

> Unfortunately, many of us suffer or know others who suffer from mysterious maladies that affect our feeling of well-being and for which neither our doctors nor we can find a curable cause. Parasite infections can cause fatigue, hypoglycemia, skin problems, depression, upper respiratory tract infections, environmental illness, PMS, and gastrointestinal problems. Parasites can also be the cause behind chronic weight problems.
>
> Some treatments or medications help for a while, but the condition never entirely goes away. We frequently continue to have sensitivities, intolerances, or allergies to various foods, often accompanied by depression. Our body is telling us that something is physically wrong, but we are not listening!

Ann Louise Gittleman gives us the following symptoms to look for:

- Obesity or trouble losing weight.
- A craving for sugar.
- Gas, bloating, or burning sensation in the stomach.
- Unclear thinking and forgetfulness.
- Itchy ears, nose, or anus.
- Female problems with PMS and menstrual cycle.
- Male sexual dysfunction.
- Lethargy.
- Loss of appetite.
- More appetite than normal but still feel hungry.
- Grinding teeth while asleep.
- Bed-wetting.
- Drooling while sleeping.
- Blurry or unclear vision.
- Chronic fatigue syndrome.
- Cancer.

Ms. Gittleman sums it up well: "If you have been suffering from symptoms you simply cannot get rid of with even the best diet, exercise, or stress relief program, chances are parasites are the underlying cause."

SOURCES OF PARASITIC INFESTATION

How has this parasitic epidemic taken place? A quick look at the means of transmission of parasites will give us some answers.

- Airborne. Some parasites are airborne and you can breathe them into your body. Remember, we all have to breathe. (Don't deny it: I've seen you.)

- Food/restaurants. Have you ever eaten in a restaurant? You could be exposed to parasites. Improper washing of foods or the food handler's hands can cause parasite infection. When I read Ann Louise Gittleman's *Guess What Came to Dinner*, I was so paranoid I wouldn't eat in restaurants for *months!*

- Raw fish, sushi, or sashimi, and undercooked fish carry fish tapeworms.

- Raw beef and rare steaks or hamburgers carry beef tapeworms, toxoplasmosis, and possible trichinosis.

- Raw lamb can carry sheep tapeworms and toxoplasmosis.

- Raw pork carries pork tapeworm, toxoplasmosis, and trichinosis.

According to Gittleman (*Guess What Came to Dinner*, 1993): "In the *New England Journal of Medicine*, researchers have reported finding a new parasite that is transmitted to humans from fish. The eustrongylides worm had been thought to be found primarily in fish-eating birds. In the case reported in the journal, the 24-year-old student complaining of severe pain in his abdomen underwent surgery for appendicitis. The surgeons found a normal appendix. They also found a ten-inch pinkish-red worm, which crawled out onto the surgical sheets. The student was a once-a-month sushi and sashimi eater and most recently had eaten sushi at a friend's home."

(After reading this, becoming a vegetarian was sounding better all the time.)

Gittleman identifies these factors that have contributed to the parasite epidemic:

Water. In California, for example, the Sierra Nevada waters are contaminated with guardia lamblia, an amoeba. This water

> *We have a tremendous parasite problem right here in the United States—it's just not being identified.*
>
> – Peter Weina, Ph.D., Chief of Pathobiology,
> Walter Reed Army Institute of Research

travels down to the Bay Area and often contaminates the local drinking water, especially with cysts (parasites lumped together into balls) which may not be filtered out at the water plant. Home water filtration units should specify that they filter out cysts. Rivers and lakes may be contaminated with amoebas and protozoa. Swallowing water when swimming, skiing, kayaking, etc., can be another source of parasitic infection.

Day care centers/institutional care. Imagine that a day-care employee unknowingly gets fecal matter under her fingernails while changing a baby's diaper. She washes her hands very well (though she may not have used antibacterial soap), but residue remains. She then changes another diaper or two, or ten. She can very easily infect herself and other children by passing parasites from one child to another.

Other people. Parasite cleansing programs should be done by the whole family, not just one member. Sexual contact and certain sexual practices (better deworm your spouse or significant other) may also spread parasites. We are not just talking condoms here. You can contract parasites just from kissing your partner.

Traveling abroad. We used to think that parasites were a third-world country problem, but in a "global village" formed in part by widespread international travel, parasites are a fact of life everywhere, even in your hometown.

Animals/pets. Owning and living with pets involves many opportunities for parasitic infections. You must become very conscious of poop-scooping in your yard, using antibacterial soaps after cleaning up or touching your pets, scrubbing under your fingernails, etc. Washing hands after handling pets is a very important habit to instill in children. Ninety percent of cats have toxoplasmosis. Cuddling up to your cat places you at great risk, as does emptying its litter box. Wearing a mask when cleaning out litter boxes will prevent breathing in the litter dust and ova (eggs), but you'll have to use your own discretion when it comes to cuddling.

I know you love your dogs, but let's avoid swapping doggie saliva. Dogs can carry tapeworms in their mouths. When I see a child—or even worse, an adult—allowing a pet to lick their face and mouth while kissing them in return (even in dog food commercials), it makes me crazy. I absolutely want to scream. I am serious. It is not cute; it's insanity. I mean, *puh-leeze!* Do not, under any circumstances, allow or encourage your children to let pets lick their face—or share their food. You know the old "let the dog and child share the ice cream cone" scenario. Also, please emphasize the importance of proper cleansing of hands and face after handling pets.

Let's really be blunt here—you should be used to that by now—should you allow any creature that has just licked its anus to lick a bit of food off your plate? I mean, come on. Unless you use special sterilization techniques, simply washing the dishes (even in a dishwasher) isn't going to cut it. The average dishwashing liquids do not kill parasite eggs. You might as well drink out of a toilet. Of course, the obvious prevention is to deworm your pets on a regular basis with parasitic herbs, but also to have the utmost cleanliness with them. And if you develop a little paranoia over parasites, all the better—your pets will feel better, too.

When I first read Gittleman's *Guess What Came to Dinner* I just about flipped. I had known about parasites for years, but knowing and *KNOWING* are entirely different things. I went on a week-long cleaning frenzy that included every square inch of my house and pet quarters. I was an advocate for rescuing abandoned pets from animal shelters, cleaning them up, and finding them homes. So I was especially paranoid about what parasites these animals (bless their little homeless hearts) were bringing into my family's living environment. I was bleaching dog runs and pet dishes and blankets like you would not believe. (Bleach kills parasites and eggs.) My husband's chin hit the floor when he saw me flying through the house like the proverbial white tornado, disinfecting everything (and I mean everything). I would have thrown our bed mattress and box spring in the washing machine if I could have made them fit! I bleached every nook and cranny imaginable. I consider myself a very fastidious housekeeper but the thought of parasite dust floating around my house just made my skin crawl.

I did that for a while, then I took a deep breath and calmed down. You can't live in a plastic bubble or disinfect everything you or your family touches. I can only speak for myself here, but God forbid that I would not keep pets (they are a true joy in my life) for fear of parasites.

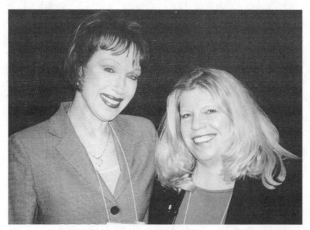

Ann Louise Gittleman and I during the Natural Products Expo–West in Los Angeles in March of 2002. She has been very supportive of my work and I truly admire her dedication to the field of alternative health.

PARASITES CAN EAT HUMAN BODIES

There are two major categories of parasites:

Large parasites are primarily worms large enough to be seen by the naked eye. Some worms can be 10, 12, or even 15 inches long and in most cases cannot travel to other parts of the body except the digestive tract. In *The Essentials of Medical Parasitology,* Thomas J. Brooks says, "Tapeworms are among the oldest parasites of the human race. Indeed, some species have become so well adapted to live in the human intestine that the host [man] may be entirely asymptomatic."

The fish tapeworm is the largest of the human tapeworms, reaching a length of 33 feet or more. There can be 3,000 to 4,000 segments in a single worm. One worm can produce more than a million eggs a day. Dr. Bernard Jensen's book, *The Science and Practice of Iridology,* contains a picture of a 20-foot-long tapeworm passed by a patient who had absolutely no idea she was infested.

Smaller parasites, mostly microscopic in size, include protozoa and amoebae. Despite their near invisibility, they can be very dangerous. Don't take their small size lightly. One type of tiny parasite that infects the colon is called entamoeba histolytica. This type of infection can also be found in the liver, the lungs, and the brain. The disease form is called amoebiasis, and is often transmitted via contaminated food or water.

MORE ABOUT PARASITES

Once worms or parasites are established in the body, these invaders do the following, according to Ann Louise Gittleman:

1. Worms can cause physical trauma to the body by perforating the intestines, the circulatory system, the lungs, liver, and so on. Put quite bluntly, parasites can turn your organs into Swiss cheese. When chyme is released into the perforated

intestines, it then oozes into the lymph system. Some parasites invade the body by penetrating the skin, producing dermatitis.

2. Worms can also erode, damage, or block certain organs. They can lump together and make a ball, or cyst. The size and weight of the parasitic cysts— particularly if they are located in the brain, spinal cord, eye, heart, or bones—produces pressure effects on these organs. Obstruction, particularly of the intestine and pancreatic and bile ducts, can also occur.

3. Parasites have to eat, so they rob us of our nutrients. They like to take the best of our vitamins and amino acids and leave the rest to us. They grow healthy and fat while our organs and skin starve for nutrition. Many people become anemic. Drowsiness after meals is another sign that worms are present in the body.

4. The presence of parasites in the body irritates the tissues of the body, inducing an inflammatory reaction on the part of the host. They destroy cells in the body faster than cells can be regenerated, creating an imbalance that results in ulceration, perforation, or anemia.

5. The presence of parasites depresses immune system functioning while activating the immune response. This can eventually lead to immune exhaustion. Certain parasites have the ability to fool the body of the host into thinking that the worm is a normal part of the body tissue. Therefore, the body will not fight the intruder.

6. The most important way these scavengers damage us is by poisoning us with their toxic waste. In other words, they poop in our bodies. Not only do we have

to worry about our own poop, we have to worry about parasite poop, too. Each worm gives off a certain metabolic waste product, which our already weakened body has trouble disposing of. The poisoning of the host with the parasite's waste is a condition called "verminous intoxication." It can be very serious for the sufferer, and it is difficult to diagnose. The host (that's you and me) now has to work twice as hard to remove both its own waste and that of the parasite.

Gittleman goes on to say: "Parasites depress immune system functioning by decreasing the secretion of immunoglobulin A (IgA). Their presence continuously stimulates the immune system, leaving the body open to bacterial and viral infections."

BEEN THERE, DONE THAT

Let me tell you my own worm story. Of course I do have a worm story. This is another more-about-Loree-than-you-ever-cared-to-know story! I wouldn't challenge you with your own health issues if I didn't have my own. Embarrassing as it is, here goes.

A few years after my bowel cleansing events, I had been taking a lot of garlic and black walnut herbs for an antifungal condition (these herbs are also historically known for their antiparasitic properties). Well, out of the blue, when I turned around to flush the toilet I saw this six-inch-long white "thing" floating in the toilet. Again, I almost went into cardiac arrest in my bathroom. Was this what I thought it was? A worm? *Oh my God,* I'm thinking. I fished it out of the toilet and took it in a jar to my herbalist friend Marene, praying that I was just overreacting or imagining things. We compared it to the ascarsis parasite picture in her book and confirmed that indeed I had passed an ascarsis worm. Marene asked me if this was my specimen, but my face had already given it away. I was as white as a sheet. I was in shock. I just passed a worm, and the proof (whether I liked it or not) had been floating in my toilet and visible to my very own eyes.

My kids got a kick out of showing their dad when he got home. "Look at mom's worm in a jar!" Thank God they didn't want to take it to school for show-and-tell.

A WORD ABOUT TAPEWORMS

The book, *Medical Parasitology*, by Markell and Voge, points out that therapy to remove tapeworms from the small intestine is successful only if the whole worm is expelled. If the head remains, the worm will grow back.

My friend Marene and I heard, direct from the Dr. Bernard Jensen, about a way to remove tapeworms. This surefire method involves using warm milk and honey. You better sit down for this one. He said that with other methods the tapeworms will come out of the body, feel the cold air, and break off—leaving the tapeworm head still inside. Since your goal is to get all of the tapeworm (including the head), you need to sit with your butt in a pan of warm milk with honey in it so the tapeworm will be drawn out of the anus. The whole tapeworm will come out of the anus because the warmth (of the milk) and the sweetness (from the honey) draw it out.

I assure you I am not making this up! I looked at Marene in total disbelief. I remember making some comment to her like, "Our clients already think we're a few clowns short of a circus. This suggestion will definitely cinch it."

REMOVING PARASITES FROM OUR BODIES

A parasite's only goal in life is to live and reproduce at our expense. So how do we get these creepy-crawly parasitic creatures out of our bodies? Treatment of parasitic infection must be geared to eradicating the parasites rather than relieving the symptoms of infection. If the parasites are not eradicated, the infection will continue to cause untold damage to the system. Given a proper environment, a parasite colony can flourish to sometimes fatal proportions. Our goal here is to remove the parasites from the system in conjunction with a bowel and gastrointestinal cleansing program. Many parasites become embedded in the intestinal wall, and no herb treatments can effectively reach them until the mucous and encrusted waste matter overlying the worms are softened.

Talking to other practitioners (and my clients) over the years, I have heard many testimonials from people who have had worms crawl out of their eyes (tear ducts) and nose when starting a parasite cleansing program. Dr. Ross Anderson shares the experience of a woman who, after only two days on an herbal cleansing product, felt a poking sensation in her lower abdomen and a wiggling sensation in one of her legs. The next day she passed an eight-inch worm, and since then has passed many different sizes and types of parasites. Are you still with me here? Hopefully you haven't thrown down this book and gone running for God knows where. This is important information you must hear.

Let's talk about some of the herbs that are historically used for parasitic infestation. Remember when I told you I was using garlic and black walnut and subsequently passed a six-inch ascarsis parasite? Well, garlic has been used for centuries to treat parasites.

Garlic is one of the most effective herbs for killing and expelling parasites. It is effective against toxic bacteria, viruses, and fungi, and is known as the "poor man's penicillin." Garlic contains more germanium, an anticancer agent, than any other herb. It has a detoxifying effect on all the body systems and many other valuable properties for the body, but for the moment we will limit our discussion to its antiparasitic properties.

Black walnut is most commonly associated with killing and

expelling parasites, internal and external. It is effective on the malaria parasite and on tapeworm. Black walnut also helps to burn up toxins, which can then be carried out of the body by laxative herbs.

Nutritionist Ann Louise Gittleman has tried every parasite cleansing program, herb, and homeopathic on the market to get rid of these critters. Consistently, her clients report the most lasting results with the Verma and Para Systems from Uni Key for general parasite removal. The Verma System (Verma Plus and Verma Key) is an all-natural cleansing system designed to help eliminate intestinal worms. The Para system (Para Plus and Para Key) is a broad-spectrum natural cleanser used to help eliminate invasive microscopic parasites. When you don't know exactly what you may be carrying, she recommends the Verma program first, followed by the Para program.

Verma Key is for worms and flukes. The capsules contain black walnut, wormwood, balmony, wormseed, cascara sagrada, slippery elm, garlic, and cloves. Verma Plus, a liquid tincture, is also for worms and flukes. It contains black walnut, worm-wood, centaury, male fern, orange peel, cloves, and butternut. Use the Verma products simultaneously for about two months and then for about a week each month thereafter.

The two Para products are for the one-celled critters like amoeba, giardia, blastocystits, and cyrptosporidium. Para Key capsules contain cranberry concentrate. Use the Para products simultaneously for two months and then for about a week each month thereafter.

After the parasites are removed from the system, Gittleman suggests a state-of-the-art general detox product called the Super GI Cleanse. This product is the best antiparasite mainte-nance because it contains mild antiparasitic herbs for daily use and targets the liver, kidneys, and lungs, as well as the intestines. Just remember to keep a plunger close to the toilet.

You will be removing so much fecal matter after taking the Super GI that it is best to be prepared. Gittleman told me she is thinking of having Uni Key provide a plunger with each Super GI order!

Another herbal product that I have been using for myself and my clients for years is Clear™. It is a Mediterranean recipe that has been on the market for seven years now, producing incredible results. Clear contains green and black walnut, black seed, cloves, cramp bark, fennel seed, hyssop, pumpkin seed, peppermint leaves, gentian root, thyme, and grapefruit seed.

Clear is typically used in a 90-day treatment program as part of a digestive and colonic aid. It is taken early in the morning with no food for one to two hours. Parasites are very resilient and have been known to survive under many conditions. To eradicate them completely, you must be consistent with your herbal program.

Many people, including myself, choose to stay on a maintenance dose of two Clear capsules per day indefinitely for more vibrant health. We can be exposed to many things that affect our immune system on a daily basis. If you have a lifestyle of high exposure you might want to stay on a maintenance dose of Clear, black walnut, or garlic herbs.

So the protocol you want to follow is to:

- ◆ Build the immune system with herbs, vitamins, and mineral supplementation.

- ◆ Heal and cleanse the intestinal tract and bowel. This can be accomplished with herbal remedies. Sometimes the intestinal tract can be completely ripped up by parasites gripping into the intestinal tissue with their sharp teeth. Hookworms especially bite and suck on the intestinal wall, which can cause bleeding and necrosis (death of the tissue).

◆ Administer effective substances such as herbs, garlic, homeopathy, etc., to eliminate the parasites.

◆ Re-colonize the gastrointestinal tract with friendly bacteria such as acidophilus, bifidophilus, etc.

◆ Follow a preventive program to prevent reinfection.

A word about parasite drugs or medications versus herbal programs. If you were given a prescription drug for a certain type of parasite, the drug would be parasite-specific. This means that it would kill only the parasite it was designed for. You have read the statistics. Finding the type of parasite you are dealing with is like finding a needle in a haystack. Herbs, on the other hand, kill all types of parasites in the body. So wouldn't it make sense to just use a nontoxic herbal program and keep this whole matter as simple as possible?

Ordering information for the herbal products is given in the resource guide at the end of this book.

Remember, it is vitally important to treat the whole family for an infection or for prevention. People who live together can infect one another when making food for each other, sharing bathroom facilities, kissing, being sexual, etc.

CHAPTER 17

■■■■■■■■■■

Staying in the Cleansing Flow: Water, Kidneys, Lymph

The success of any fat/weight loss regimen is only as successful as your commitment to take in adequate amounts of water.

Loree Taylor Jordan

Toxins in your body can be making you fat. One of the most simple and often overlooked ways to continually flush the body's cells as it is metabolizing wastes and body fat is with water. Water is one of the most significant components of any successful weight loss regimen.

Water:

♦ Helps control appetite.

♦ Participates in the biochemical process that metabolizes fat.

♦ Alleviates fluid retention and edema by alleviating the body's desperate need to hold onto water.

♦ Flushes out toxins that reside in fat tissue and are released into the bloodstream when fat is metabolized.

♦ Improves the metabolic activity of cells, as a co-factor in the energy metabolism processes.

Excerpted from *Water: The Foundation of Youth, Health, and Beauty* by William D. Holloway, Jr. and Herb Joiner-Bey, ND.

THE CLEANSING POWER OF WATER

*In health and in sickness, pure water is one of
the choicest blessings. It is the beverage given by
God to quench the thirst of man and animal,
and to cleanse the poisons from our system.*

— Byrne

I cannot overemphasize the importance of super-hydrating your body with liberal amounts of water on a daily basis. Water is the largest single component of the human body. Our brain is 85% water. Water is the essence of life. Blood, digestive juices, perspiration, tears—the list of water-based solutions that make our bodies function goes on and on. Every bodily function is designed and monitored around the efficient intake and flow of water. This water distribution is the only way of making sure transported elements such as hormones, oxygen, and nutrients reach our vital organs. We depend on water to hydrate our cells. We absolutely cannot survive without water.

F. Batmanghelidi, MD, states in *Your Body's Many Cries for Water:* "One of the unavoidable processes in the body's water rationing phase is the complete cruelty with which some functions are monitored so that one structure does not receive more than its predetermined share of water. This is true for all organs of the body. Within these systems of water rationing, the brain function takes absolute priority over all the other systems. The brain is 1/50th of the total body weight, but it receives 18 to 20% of blood circulation. When the ration masters in charge of body water reserve, regulation, and distribution become more and more active, they also give their own alarm signals to show that the area in question is short of water, very much like the radiator of a car giving out steam when the cooling system is not adequate for the uphill drive of the car."

It is suggested to take in your body weight in ounces of water every day (for example, if you weigh 150 pounds, drink

150 ounces daily). During any weight loss program I suggest about a gallon of water every day. Water is the cornerstone for detoxifying all the organs and cells of the body and assisting in weight loss. By drinking liberal amounts of water we reduce the acid buildup that has been stored in various organs such as the heart, liver, and colon, as well as connective tissue and joints. Let us take this one step further and say that this overacid condition accelerates degenerative disease and the aging process.

WATER, NOT SODAS

When I consult with my clients I cannot believe how many people think that fluid and water are synonymous. Water is water, anything else is not. I am talking about pure water— not coffee, tea, sodas, and all the sugar-laden manufactured beverages that unfortunately serve as substitutes for water for many people. It is true that these beverages contain water, but they also contain dehydrating agents. Dehydrating agents, like those in coffee and sodas, *deplete the body of its water reserves.*

Now, to add insult to injury, one of the main components of most sodas is caffeine, an addictive drug. If you don't think so, just go cold turkey from coffee or caffeine sodas and you will get a migraine headache you will never forget. I used to be a Diet Pepsi addict. When I did my first colon cleanse cleansing for three long days, I thought the top of my head would explode! There are soda pop junkies who are addicts just like alcoholics, drug addicts, and cigarette smokers. Drinking soda is more socially acceptable but can also be deadly.

Children are the worst victims of nutritionally uneducated parents. They are brought up at a young age on manufactured juices and soda drinks, and they become addicted. I have actually seen, more than once—I am telling you the absolute truth here—young toddlers with soda pop in their baby bottles. I had not completely embarked on my nutritional path at that point in my life or God knows what I would have said to those parents. *Soda* in a baby bottle???? *Don't get me started!*

In *Your Body's Many Cries for Water,* Dr. Batmanghelidj says, "Caffeine's addictive properties are because of its direct action in the brain. It also acts on the kidneys and causes increased urine production. Caffeine has diuretic properties. It is physiologically a dehydrating agent. This prime characteristic is the main reason a person can drink so many sodas every day and never be satisfied. The water does not stay in the body long enough. At the same time, many persons confuse their feeling of thirst for water; thinking they have consumed enough water that is in the soda, they assume they are hungry and begin to eat more than their body's need for food."

Along with caffeine, sugar, and aspartame (sweetener in diet sodas) we must also consider the effects of phosphoric acid. According to John Thomas, author of *Young Again,* "The side effects of soft drinks loaded with phosphoric acid are incomprehensible and go beyond just our pH level. When we ingest phosphoric acid, our body is forced to draw on bone calcium to buffer the acid introduced into the bloodstream, which skews the calcium phosphorous ratio and grossly alters body physiology. When the side effects of aspartame sweetener are added, it's a wonder we don't just die!"

Okay, you say you are convinced now that chronic cellular dehydration is detrimental to your overall health and is necessary for weight loss. You agree that drinking adequate water is not a should but a *must* for optimal health! So, is all water equal in its benefits to the body? Just as with food sources, you could choose a greasy hamburger or a fresh salad. Both are considered food, but do they have the same benefit to the body? A hamburger is a dead, devitalized food devoid of enzymes. A salad is fresh food with enzymes intact. The body will utilize and break down these two foods differently. So it is with water. Water can come in two forms: live water or dead water.

LIVE WATER VS. DEAD WATER

I could recite a lot of scientific mumbo jumbo, but let's just keep this simple and to the point. The goal in drinking water is to get that water to the cellular level for energy and to hydrate the cells rapidly. If the water is not able to get deep down into the cells themselves, then the body will not completely benefit from receiving it. Let's consider how water that is molecularly restructured can handle this issue. We will see that all water is not created equal.

In choosing a water source, we should look for a water that is molecularly superior for our optimal health. One water that I use and can recommend is Penta-Hydrate,™ produced by Bio-Hydration Research Lab in San Diego, California. It is the third generation of "3G" performance-enhancing water after bottled water and "oxygenated water." Penta Hydrate energizes the body faster by hydrating cells rapidly. The following is taken from their product report which the company agreed to allow me to pass on to you, my readers.

Bio-Hydration Laboratory, in an experiment to remove dissolved solids from water, discovered that their test water maintained its clustered molecular state, which, under normal circumstances only happens for a short, unsustainable period of time. In the human body, water resides in one of two molecular states: bound and clustered. Bound water is attached to other molecules, ions, and free radicals, making it thicker and prohibiting it from moving through cell walls via osmosis. In other words, bound water simply cannot hydrate cells. Unfortunately for the water drinker, water exists in this bound state 85% of the time.

The importance of this discovery is paramount because water in its clustered state is another story. Clustered water passes through cell walls effortlessly because it's smaller and unbound from the molecules

that weigh down bound water. But due to water's com-
plexities and instability, clustered water only exists for
short periods of time and in very small amounts. At
any given moment, only 15% of the water we drink is in
this clustered state.

So, simply put (I like to keep things simple . . . chemistry is
not my forte), water can penetrate the cells only in a clustered
state. So a live water such as Penta-Hydrate that is molecularly
restructured to stay in this clustered state solves this problem. I
was introduced to Penta-Hydrate water at Life Mastery with
Tony Robbins and noticed a very different taste immediately—
it is very smooth. I personally drink it, and I love it.

THE KIDNEYS

According to Dr. Bernard Jensen, the kidney is one of the
most abused organs in the eliminative chain, largely because
most people do not drink enough water throughout the day.
The kidneys must also accept toxic material from the liver, the
bowel, and any other eliminative organs. During a fast or an
extreme elimination diet, the kidneys are placed under additional strain from the intensified elimination of toxic material.

I use the team player analogy to explain organ and body
systems. If someone on the team (an organ or system) is lagging
(as my sons would say), then another team member (organ or
system) has to pick up the slack to eliminate toxins. This can
cause a domino effect on all the eliminative channels in the
detoxification process.

Many people think that if they drink lots of water they will
get edema or retain water. Actually the opposite is true: if you
fail to drink adequate amounts of water (at least a gallon a day)
your kidneys will actually hold onto and try to store the water
that they have. For your kidneys to process wastes and stay in
what I call "the flow," water should be a top priority for you.

Drink the juice of ½ lemon in a glass of warm water first thing each morning to gently cleanse your system. Also, drinking cranberry juice and apple juice is beneficial to the urinary system. In Chapter 23, Nature's Pharmacy, there are many herbs listed that will assist your kidneys in strengthening and repairing your urinary system.

Again, we need to look at toxic emotions to assist the body in its healing work (Louise Hay, *Heal Your Body*):

Kidney problems. Probable cause: Criticism, disappointment, failure, shame, reacting like a little kid. New thought pattern: *Divine right action is always taking place in my life. Only good comes from each experience. It is safe to grow up*

Kidney stones. Probable cause: Lumps of undissolved anger. New thought pattern: *I dissolve all past problems with ease.*

THE LYMPHATIC SYSTEM

The lymph system is part of the body's internal plumbing, helping it dispose of wastes and debris generated by muscles and other body tissues. A variety of factors can cause lymph fluid to become heavy and thick, which restricts its flow and causes it to back up in the body. Such blockages not only cause excess body weight but a number of other serious diseases.

— Burton Goldberg, *Alternative Medicine Definitive Guide to Weight Loss*

Aside from eliminating excess weight, it is vitally important to assist our immune system and eliminative channels by keeping the lymphatic system healthy. The lymphatic system removes wastes and toxins via a clear liquid that runs through lymph nodes and keeps our immune system healthy. You must have an adequate water intake to maintain a healthy lymphatic system.

The lymphatic system can be thought of as being responsible for waste disposal—it's a "metabolic garbage can of the body." It moves cellular waste from the cells to be eliminated from the body. As with all of the eliminative channels of the body (colon, kidneys, lymph, liver), you can get into trouble when your toxin levels are more than the organs can handle. A domino effect causes toxins to spill over into other areas of the body. Overloaded lymph nodes can result in many health problems, including excess weight gain.

CELLULITE

Lymphatic congestion and slow drainage result from excess wastes being generated by an inefficient metabolism. The lymph system can become stagnant and lead to excess weight. When you are overweight and your lymphatic system is also sluggish, wastes can accumulate beneath your skin, causing that dimpled "cottage cheese look" of cellulite. In her book, *The Fat Flush Plan* (McGraw Hill, 2002), Ann Louise Gittleman quotes a study conducted at Brussels University in Belgium and cited by Elizabeth Dancey, MD, in *The Cellulite Solution*, which found that women with cellulite showed lymphatic system deficiencies.

The most common place that fat accumulates in our bodies is directly beneath the skin, in fatty areas of the body (ladies, you know where I am talking about)—for example, buttocks, thighs (saddlebags), and upper arms. I am sure you know the feeling of that three-way tell-all mirror in the Macy's dressing room that shows every disgusting dimple detail. You hear a loud horrified scream as you are getting undressed and then realize it came from your own lips! If you want dimples, I'm sure you want them on your facial cheeks, not your butt cheeks!

My sister and I, in one of our funnier moments, talked about getting her husband's belt sander from the garage and doing a little cellulite planing on our butts and upper thighs to smooth out those dimples! Of course we were hysterical with laughter, but there for a minute it did not sound like a bad idea.

Seriously, increasing lymphatic flow, removing internal trapped toxins, and flushing your body with adequate amounts of water all assist the body in reducing cellulite.

The lymph system does not have a pump like the heart. Therefore, the fluid is moved through muscular contractions to "pump" the lymph. Only by movement (yes, that means exercise) can the lymph detoxify itself. The best overall aid to a congested lymph system is exercise. I know you want me to say that you can get these health benefits, lose weight, and reduce cellulite by sitting on the couch like a couch potato or something ridiculous like that, but no can do. Circulating the lymphatic system takes movement, exercise, and effort. Get up and start moving. Find an exercise you like so you will stick with it, and get going!

Please refer Chapter 23, Nature's Pharmacy, for some herbal strategies for cleansing lymphatic congestion.

> Lymph congestion. Probable cause: A warning that the mind needs to be re-centered on the essentials of life: love and joy. New thought pattern: *I am now totally centered in love and the joy of being alive. I flow with life. Peace of mind is mine.*
>
> – Louise Hay, *Heal Your Body*

CHAPTER 18

■ ■ ■ ■ ■ ■ ■ ■ ■ ■ ■

Love Your Liver:
Flushing Away the Pounds

More than ever before in the history of mankind, human beings need to have healthy livers to break down the thousands of toxic chemicals that have insidiously crept into our environment and food chain. The liver is the gateway to the body and in this chemical age its detoxification systems are easily overloaded. Plants are sprayed with toxic chemicals, animals are given potent hormones and antibiotics, and food is processed, refined, frozen, and overcooked. All this can lead to destruction of delicate vitamins and minerals, which are required for the detoxification pathways in the liver.

– Sandra Cabot, MD, *The Liver Cleansing Diet*, 1996

A tired, toxic liver can be a hidden saboteur in your body's attempt to lose unwanted pounds and inhibit your metabolism from burning fat. In this chapter, I want to show you how to cleanse your liver for weight loss and for optimal health.

Your liver is your body's most important organ, functioning as a filter for your own metabolism and the detoxification of foreign chemicals and drugs. The liver also metabolizes proteins and regulates hormonal balance, so proper functioning is essential to your overall health.

Ann Louise Gittleman explains the role that the liver has in metabolism as follows (*The Fat Flush Plan,* McGraw Hill, 2002):

A fat-burning machine

Each day your liver produces about a quart of a yellowish green liquid called bile that emulsifies and absorbs fats in the small intestine. Bile contains water, bile acids and pigments, cholesterol, bilirubin, lipids, lecithin, potassium, sodium, and chloride. The liquid is stored near the liver in the gallbladder, from where it is transported to the intestine as needed during digestion.

Bile is the real key to the liver's ability to digest and assimilate fats. It can be hampered from doing its job because of a lack of bile nutrients, congestion, or even clogged bile ducts, which hamper bile flow and result in less bile production. If there is not enough bile produced, fat cannot be emulsified.

If you have a roll of fat at your waistline, you may have what is commonly called a "fatty liver." Your liver has stopped processing fat and begun storing it, for reasons I'll explain in a moment. Only when you bring your liver back to full function will you lose this fat.

An efficient metabolizer

The liver metabolizes not only fats but also carbohydrates and proteins for use in your body. The organ has a triple role in carbohydrate metabolism. First, it converts glucose, fructose, and galatose into glycogen, which it stores. Second, when your blood sugar level drops and new carbohydrates are available, the liver converts stored glycogen into glucose and releases it into your bloodstream. Third, if your diet is regularly low in carbohydrates, the liver will convert fat or protein into glucose to maintain your blood sugar levels.

The liver converts amino acids from food into various proteins that may have a direct or indirect impact on your weight. Many proteins, for example, transport hormones through the bloodstream; hormone balances are crucial to avoid water retention, bloating, and cravings, as well as other health problems. Proteins also help transport wastes—such as damaged cholesterol and used estrogen and insulin, to the liver for detoxification and elimination through the kidneys.

◆ ◆ ◆

Typically, when I mention liver cleansing to my clients, they are surprised and, quite frankly, have never thought of it before. Let's think about how your car would function if you never had an oil change. Your liver filters toxins from the body like the oil filter keeps impurities from your car engine. If my clients treated their cars the way they have treated their bodies (and never provided any maintenance) they would all be walking for transportation. Just think of detoxification as preventive maintenance. Research suggests that by the of age 40 the average person's liver is only operating at only 30% capacity because 70% of the liver is toxic.

A healthy liver can deal with a wide range of toxic chemicals, drugs, solvents, pesticides, and food additives. Your liver also has amazing powers of rejuvenation, continuing to function when as many as 80% of its cells are damaged. Even more remarkable, the liver can regenerate its own damaged tissue. You owe it to yourself and your liver to detoxify and help your liver take a "deep breath" from years of toxic abuse.

Here is another opportunity to get real honest with yourself about past eating behaviors. Overeating and binging is a form of toxic abuse. If, for example, you are or have been a *sugaraholic,* you have loaded your body with *toxins from sweets!* If your diet has not been healthful, you may high toxicity in your liver—

you just don't know it yet. Your stubborn weight problem may be another one of your clues.

THE ROLE OF THE GALLBLADDER

As the liver processes toxic byproducts, either metabolic or foreign, it also helps in the process of digestion by producing bile salts, which are stored in the gallbladder. When hormonal signals come from the stomach, the gallbladder constricts to squirt bile into the duodenum in order to digest food, mostly fats. The bile may thicken, eventually turning into stones, which can leave the gallbladder painfully inflamed, particularly after a fatty meal. Most people suffering from this condition are obese. The thickening of the bile is a warning signal of a hyperinsulemia or pre-diabetes condition.

YOU NEED TO DETOXIFY YOUR LIVER AND GALLBLADDER

I want to be perfectly clear here that even though you do not have a perceived problem with your liver or gallbladder it is still necessary to initiate cleansing and detoxification. If you are walking around the planet, breathing, eating, using chemical cleansing agents, soaps, and drugs, you need to cleanse your body's filtering system (the liver). Even with the liver's incredible regenerative abilities you don't want it to become so exhausted that it loses its ability to detoxify itself.

In my opinion, cleansing and detoxifying the liver and gallbladder is one of the most powerful procedures you can do to improve your body's health and become successful in weight loss. Since these organs work in tandem I am going to discuss them together.

A WORD ABOUT GALLSTONES

For many people, including children, a critical issue of the liver and gallbladder is that the biliary tubing can be choked with gallstones. That is why natural health practitioners (including myself) advise a targeted cleansing of the liver and gallbladder twice a year for gallstones. I firmly believe that if people would cleanse these organs, emergency surgeries would be greatly reduced or avoided altogether. In *Cure for All Cancers,* Hilda Clark states that you should cleanse until you remove 2,000 stones from the gallbladder. Just a note here: If you have had your gallbladder removed you still need to cleanse because the liver will make gallstones.

Many people will be shocked at what comes out of their liver and gallbladder even when they don't have any diagnosed problems. I *especially* encourage you to consider the liver and gallbladder flush outlined in my book, *Detox for Life,* if you have had problems with your gallbladder or if you are (or have been) extremely overweight.

In the book, I share my personal story of my liver and gallbladder flush. This gallbladder flush rendered lots of stones out of my gallbladder. So imagine my surprise when a recent ultrasound in a hospital emergency room revealed gallstones in my gallbladder. Guess who had a gallbladder issue? You guessed it: *me* . . . and right at this book deadline too.

I am telling you, I don't *do* emergency rooms! But I was having pain in my ribs on the upper right side of my back so severe that every time I moved, it felt like someone was knifing me in the back. I was in severe pain so I had to check this out. I had gone to my massage therapist and he could not relieve it, so I ruled out any muscular involvement.

Of course, the emergency room doctor recommended I see a surgeon in two days to schedule gallbladder surgery . . . oh, I don't think so! I will handle this naturally, and surgery for me is not an option.

I was very perplexed that this could happen when I had been so diligent about cleansing my liver and gallbladder.

When I spoke with a fellow health practitioner, nutri-path Stephen Heuer, to obtain some supplements to start a gallbladder flush, the first thing he asked me was if I had been on a low-fat diet recently. I told him I was on a low-fat program from my trainer, until I rebelled and started adding more fats and oils back into my diet. Stephen was convinced my training diet is what prompted this gallbladder hoarding of cholesterol and subsequent gallstones. Who really knows what tipped the apple cart and created stones in my gallbladder?

I will just deal with it and move forward, but I honestly believe that if I had not done *any* previous cleansing I would have been signing surgery approval forms for gallbladder surgery. I would have been whisked off to the operating room so fast it would have made my head swim.

I am currently being treated with herbs and acupuncture to heal my gallbladder, and there is not a surgeon in sight! I am out of pain and doing well. But it's not over yet—it will take some time to completely heal. Look for my upcoming book, *The Saga of Loree's Gallbladder!* I am just playing with you, but it would not be a bad idea. Maybe an upcoming episode for *ER*?

I figure that everything happens for a reason. The reason this came up for me now was so I could write about it and share this vital information with you. Stephen passed the following article on to me from Dr. Cowan.

CHOLESTEROL DEPRIVATION CAN CAUSE GALLSTONES

The following is excerpted from the newsletter WISE TRADITIONS: DOCTOR'S CORNER *written by Tom Cowan, MD.*

The gallbladder is a reservoir or holding tank for bile salts, which the body uses to digest fats. When we eat fat, the body releases bile into the digestive tract to break down into absorbable fatty acids.

Bile salts are made of cholesterol. Gallstones are a sign that your body had "decided" to increase its reservoir of cholesterol. Why would it do this? The obvious answer is that it has become "afraid" that the supply of cholesterol is low, therefore it uses the strategy of storing extra for a rainy day.

Give your body what it needs, in this case more cholesterol. Once your body is convinced that you are serious and will provide it with a steady stream of cholesterol, which it desperately needs to stay alive, it will give up the flawed strategy of storing extra. The stones will dissolve, and you will be well again. I know of two people who adopted this strategy, and within a year their stones completely dissolved. Actually, you might want to thank your gallbladder for devising such an innovative strategy for keeping you alive until you learned how to eat in a way that provides your body with the materials it needs to be healthy.

The best way to provide your gallbladder with cholesterol is to eat plenty of animal fats. If you eat a lot of vegetable oils and trans-fats, the gallbladder is likely to become inflamed. If you are on a low-fat diet, the gallbladder atrophies because it does not have enough work to do.

◆ ◆ ◆

Dr. Cowan brings up a very important point about low-fat diets. Many personal trainers subscribe to the theory that fat makes you fat, so their diets restrict the intake on fats. I had even been told to use only egg whites because eliminating the egg yolk cuts down on fat grams. I don't agree.

I have been working with a personal trainer and in the beginning I followed his food plan for months, thinking his formula would do the trick for fat loss. It just felt too restrictive on this dietary fat issue. I began to debate this with him and said that *our bodies need fat!* I don't mean trans-fat like French fries, but essential fats.

I believe that we should have olive oil, flax seed oil, essential fatty acids, omega fish oils, and even pure raw butter. We kept going round and round about why I was not losing weight (even though I was building strength). His theory was I was *cheating too much!* His idea was that eating an egg yolk or having olive oil on my salad was "cheating."

My theory was that I was not "cheating" by having an egg yolk or olive oil, but was giving my body essential nutrients. I also feel that since my metabolism was still in the repairing mode and hormones were still balancing themselves out, losing weight was not in the cards at that moment in time.

TOXIC EMOTIONS

It is important to mention that organs in the body are associated with certain emotions. The liver is associated with anger and rage. I once had a consultation with a male client and his wife regarding some health issues. My analysis and muscle testing led me to ask this man, "What are you so angry about?" He was flabbergasted that I directly asked him that question with firm eye contact, but his liver (and some intuition on my part) led me down a different path than my original nutritional concerns. Our bodies speak volumes—we just need to know how to listen.

In Chapter 3, Feelings Buried Alive Never Die, I shared with you core, primitive pain that the body can expel in healing itself. The rage and anger come from a cellular level, from not being able to protect oneself from violence or abuse. I believe the cellular vibration of that abuse can sit embedded in the liver as toxic residue (like ashes after a fire) until released.

Here are some thoughts from Louise Hay (*Heal Your Body*):

Gallstones. Probable cause: Bitterness, hard thoughts, condemning, pride. New thought pattern: *There is joyous release of the past. Life is sweet, and so am I.*

Liver problems. Probable cause: Resistance to change, fear, anger, and hatred. The liver is the seat of anger, rage, primitive emotions, and chronic complaining. New thought pattern: *My mind is cleansed and free. I leave the past and move into the new. All is well. Love and peace and joy are what I know. I choose to live through the open space in my heart. I look for love and find it everywhere.*

If I were reading this book, the first question I would ask is, "If this author is knowledgeable about detoxification, how could *she* have a weight problem?" My response would be: "Great question!"

First, I want to say, if I had not participated in colonics, colon cleansing, and liver and gallbladder flushes as I have, my weight issues might have been more chronic than they are. When I started cleansing at the age of 29, I was not overweight. Second, my weight issues later in my life, as you will see, were more hormonal imbalance as a latent result of a long-standing sugar addiction (insulin, thyroid, and perimenopause) than toxic overload.

In the last few chapters, I have shared with you vital information about cleansing and detoxifying your body for optimal health and weight loss. Your body has many pieces of a weight loss puzzle that ultimately must fit together just right. Detoxification is another critical piece of that puzzle on your way to a lean and fit body.

Information in this *Detoxify Your Body* section (Chapters 14–18) is excerpted from *Detox for Life: Your Bottom Line—It's Your Colon or Your Life* by Loree Taylor Jordan, Madison Publishing, 2003. Please see the resource guide to order, or visit www.DetoxforLife.net.

Physical Mastery: Exercise, Diet, and Nutrition

As a nation we are dedicated to keeping physically fit—and parking as close to the stadium as possible.

— Bill Vaughn

You gain strength, courage, and confidence from every experience in which you really stop to look fear in the face. You are able to say to yourself, "I lived through this horror. I can take the next thing that comes along."... You must do the thing you think you cannot do.

– Eleanor Roosevelt

CHAPTER 19

■ ■ ■ ■ ■ ■ ■ ■ ■ ■

Training Day with Mr. Universe

Whenever I feel the need for exercise, I go and lie down for half an hour until the feeling passes.

— Will Rogers

Ed Corney was a featured guest on my San Francisco radio show. Aside from a great interview, we had instant chemistry and rapport as friends. I was completely impressed with his accomplishments in the world of bodybuilding.

At the pre-interview I learned that not only was he considered a primary player in the field of bodybuilding and fitness, he was also a highly recognized celebrity in the sport. Ed had performed in various films featuring bodybuilders; he could even be seen in the bodybuilding classic *Pumping Iron* with Arnold Schwarzenegger. He had received prestigious awards such as Mr. America, Mr. Universe, and Mr. Olympia Over 60.

I knew all this, but when he walked into the radio studio the visual of him—*wow!* Was it hot in there or was it just me? I was looking—okay I was staring, I admit it—at this gorgeous hunk during our interview wondering if he might be the one to help me train and get back into great shape. I proposed the question to him after our interview and we set up a meeting to discuss the possibility of training together. He had trained with the celebrities. Why would he want to train with me, a bodybuilding nobody? The only competition I was interested in winning was the one with the zipper of my jeans!

At our lunch meeting, we discussed a training schedule, diet, and my expected outcome of success. Ed asked me to commit to three months of training with him as a condition of working with me. I committed to the process. I explained to Ed my frustrations with my yo-yo weight, and my ongoing struggle with sugar addiction. I wanted to be strong in my body but I also wanted to be strong in my spirit. Ed said to me, "Loree, when I get done with you, men will be falling all over themselves, lined up to take you out. You will look so good your ex-husband will want to kill himself!" That worked for me so I told him, "Let's get started!"

WEEK I
Saturday, Oct. 31, 1998

I am very excited but nervous about starting my personal training with Ed Corney. I have wanted to do this for such a long time, I know in my heart that I will have to be fully committed. I went to a party tonight . . . Oh my God . . . the food. A huge long table of food. It was hard to resist since I knew that many of these foods would not pass my lips again for a long time—probably for the rest of my life. So I gave myself permission to eat whatever I wanted, knowing full well that I would have to confess my sins to Ed the next day. I savored each bite knowing it would have to last a lifetime. God it was good! That chocolate mousse was out of this world.

Sunday, Nov. 1, 1998

Up at 8:00 A.M. to get ready for my first day of training. I feel like a kindergartner at the first day of school. I am excited but also scared to death. Ed and I meet at the gym. We are both in good spirits. However I must admit I don't feel on top of the world because I have a carbo/sugar hangover from partying the night before. We start with cardio on the treadmill, followed by chest and abs. I joke with Ed and tell him I am out in the dating world competing with the young perky breasts crowd. So let's get my breasts up at least above my kneecaps. He laughs.

I follow Ed around the gym at his direction like a little lost puppy, listening to all his instructions. I have to say Ed really earns my respect that first day watching him train. I have already made a promise to myself that I will not whine even though I may truly feel like it. Ed says that he is just getting me in pre-condition. Little do I know that in a few weeks the party will be over and we will be down to real hard work. It feels good to be back at the gym.

During our workout session I look at Ed and confess my dietary sins of the night before. As I am detailing my long list of dietary indiscretions he is lifting his eyebrows with amusement and disapproval. When I finally tell him about the chocolate

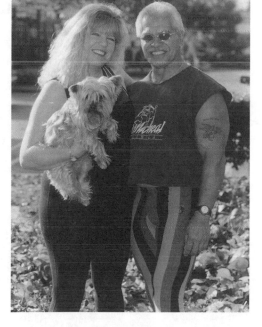

mousse he rolls his eyes. "Ed, I feel like crap today for eating all that garbage and junk food." His response: "Well, it sounds like you have learned a valuable lesson and I hope that you record how you feel in your journal." Oh yes, here it is . . .

"Mr. Universe" Ed Corney with me and the late Ms. Wookie

Friday, Nov. 5, 1998

I rush home from San Francisco after taping my radio show, change my clothes, and rush to the gym to meet Ed. This is my last training day of the week. I am so tired I just want to take a nap . . . I am pooped. I made a commitment so I must follow through. I can feel a little soreness but I am not incapacitated, just fresh enthusiasm in my muscles. I tell Ed that I know myself very well. If I was not committed to meeting him, I would have totally blown off working out because I am so overcommitted with running my business and my radio show. This is why I need a committed training partner: so I will follow through until I am strong enough to be committed on my own.

Some of my observations this first week of training were the camaraderie, friendship, and support from everyone at the gym. Ed introduced me to everyone as we were setting up for our workouts. If you want to go to the gym and blend into the scenery and not be noticed, don't take Mr. Universe with you.

I also noticed that all the women wore workout clothes that accentuated and showed off their physiques. I, unlike them, showed up in baggy T-shirts with my arms and body covered up. So what does that tell you? I was not exactly proud of how my body looked. It was bad enough that I had to look at my own body. I didn't want to impose that on anyone else. I remember what Ed had said to me in our first meeting. He told me, "Stand in front of a mirror [ouch, do I have to?]. If you like what you see, great . . . If you don't, do something about it . . . change it . . . get angry . . . get into action." I was a far cry from being fit and sexy. I can just hear Anthony Robbins' voice now in my head as he would say, "When the pain of where you are [in my case overweight] is more than the pleasure [of eating] you will have to move into massive action to change it." Well . . . hiring a trainer for me was massive action. It was a total commitment both in time and money.

As I looked at lists of errands, endless phone calls to return, and work piling up, I was feeling as if my life was controlling me instead of me controlling it. After I went to the gym I felt much better—more mentally prepared to return phone calls, run errands, and just participate in my life. All that "stuff" was still there waiting for me when I got home from the gym but I saw it with a much more positive attitude. I am grateful, and I am also proud of myself for taking action.

Saturday, Nov. 6, 1998

God, all I want to do all day is *eat*—even the wallpaper is looking good. What is wrong with me? All I can think about is food today. *Help! I have munchies like you can't believe!* I stay home all day because if I leave the house I know I will eat something undesirable. I will blow it, I can just feel it. I go to bed early. I just want this day to be over and get to the next day.

WEEK 2
Sunday, Nov. 8, 1998

This is my first photo shoot to take my pre-training photos. I know that I will look at these pictures and freak out because I will see that I look *too fat!* Ed, Juan (the photographer), and I get to the gym for the photo shoot and also for a real-life workout. We have a great workout; I just try to pretend that Juan is not even there taking pictures. I have to say that Ed is a great sport about all this and a support to me during this whole process.

Monday, Nov. 9, 1998

Got a late start at the gym but had a great workout with legs. Ed says, "Loree, now the party is over and we are really going to work." The leg squats are difficult—excruciating actually (God, I hate squats)—but I know I have to work hard to get the results I want. Ed also increases all my reps from 12 to 15. He asks me during the workout if I noticed he has increased the reps. I tell him that I might be blonde but I can definitely count. Later on I insist that we have done three sets already when he assures me we have only done two. I stand corrected, I tell him—maybe I can't count after all. We also increase the abdominals which feels good . . . after we are done of course. I ask Ed what if I am doing an exercise and I really feel that I cannot complete what he asks me to do? He tells me that he has selective hearing (personally I think that is a man issue, really). He says that he will listen and tell me to do it anyway. Boy, I can tell I am going to feel those leg muscles tomorrow. Yikes!

Thursday, Nov. 12, 1998

After my workout I attend a business meeting with my ex-husband. Since I am at the meeting a little early I go clothes shopping at a nearby shopping mall. My natural tendency is to eat something but instead I reward myself with a few new lingerie items instead of food.

Friday, Nov. 13, 1998

Woke up this morning with the headache from hell. My neck is so out of adjustment I can barely move. I am stressing about doing my radio show this morning with this headache. But the show must go on so I get out of bed and start moving.

In the afternoon I meet Ed at the gym at our appointed time. My head is throbbing. Let me tell you, if I were not committed to a trainer I would be home lying on the couch telling myself all the reasons I couldn't work out. Ed is pretty pleased that I am able to get my abdominal exercises up to 60 reps in a set when only a week ago I was at 12. This is progress. I feel good about myself—that I am able to follow through, increase my reps, keep my commitment to myself, and reach my goals even when it isn't easy. Right after my workout I go to my chiropractor and get my neck adjusted. He says my cervical spine (neck) is out of alignment by a mile.

Monday, Nov. 14, 1998

I still have a headache because I am fighting off an illness. I go to the gym not really feeling very well, a little queasy in the stomach. I tell Ed that I am not feeling very well but I want to complete my workout. We are doing legs; I feel that I can handle it. It is a little tough . . . I can't feel very energetic but I am committed to being there. At one point I feel nauseous during the set. Ed tells me that it is perfectly okay to vomit *after* the set, just not during (don't you just love him?). Of course, he just loves to tease me. I respond with one of my looks . . . the "look that can kill" stare. He always laughs at me when I give him *the look!* But that is why he is there: to push me farther than I think I can go. Now, to tell you the truth, if I were deathly ill I would have not been at the gym. I have common sense and Ed would have told me to stay home if I was vomiting. I don't want you to think I have the trainer from *hell.* He actually did cut me some slack on the abs that day so I know he has a heart under all that muscle.

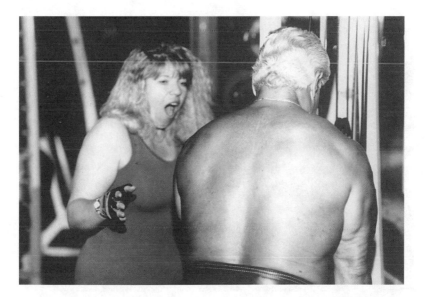

"Oh my God, Ed, how do I get muscles like that?"

Thursday, Nov. 17, 1998

I find myself becoming increasingly frustrated and upset as the day progresses. By noon I am in tears with frustration. I need to have a real good cry. I am watching my reaction which is to use food instead of process my feelings. I actually go to my bedroom, throw myself on the bed (real dramatically . . . you have got to be dramatic, it feels better) and begin to sob. I just feel so overwhelmed by life at this moment. Even though I am thrilled with my new radio show (my show has changed to a new time and is going from a one-hour program to a two-hour program), I am feeling the intense stress of it. I just lie there . . . think and cry . . . cry and think . . .

I have got to get up and met Ed at the gym . . . Damn it! *I don't want to go!* I just want to cry and lie on my bed like a blob. Well, Loree, that may have been your pattern before, but not now. We are doing things differently and making better choices. Besides, I know that exercise will change my mental state and make me feel better. So I get up, get dressed, and meet

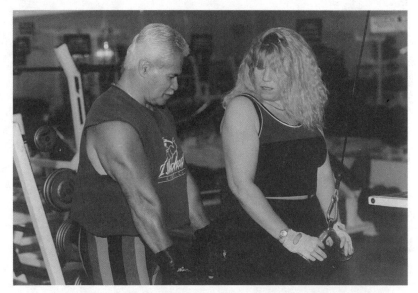

"Say what? How do I do that tricep pull again?"

Ed at the gym with tear-stained cheeks. He can tell that I am upset. I tell him that I just don't want to be there. His reaction: "Okay, great! Well, let's go slam some weights to get all that anger and frustration out!" (If he wasn't so cute I would choke him.) I am thinking to myself, I hope he doesn't think he has some drama queen as a client. Well, we slam weights and I leave feeling like a new woman. I improved my mental state and there was no chocolate involved . . . Oh what a feeling!

Friday, Nov. 18, 1998

I find myself in better spirits today. This is the last Friday of my one-hour radio show. My new radio show starts next Wednesday. I decide to spend some time talking on my show today about the emotional aspect of weight and eating. It feels good to be that vulnerable with my audience about using food for love, sex — everything imaginable except just for nourishment of our bodies. Several listeners call to share their insight when I mentioned that we are all teachers here to teach each other. If we open our hearts and share our experience, our lessons, and our pain — much like I am doing in this book — we become each other's teachers and students. One woman calls me after the radio show to say that she never listens to my radio station but heard me talking about the pain I was going through in my marriage before it broke up and felt like she was hearing her own story. I say there are no accidents. If my voice and story spoke to her on the air, maybe this book will speak to you in your heart and in your soul.

On the lighter side I also stated that I had Mr. Universe on my team as a great supporter of my efforts and if I didn't succeed Ed would *kick my butt!*

Met Ed for training in better spirits. I felt light in my heart after sharing on the show this morning. Had a great workout. This is the end of my second week.

Saturday, Nov. 19, 1998

A rest day from training. *Thank God!* At the video store I pick up a few movies to watch while I fold laundry. I decide to rent Oprah's video, *Making the Connection.* I was extremely moved by the openness and the vulnerability of Oprah and the women contributing: they were sharing their pain for the whole world to see. I mean, think about this for a moment. Think of the pain and shame we have all felt in struggling with our weight issues. We feel that our family and the whole world is watching us fail, again and again. But what if the whole world was watching us, literally? I think of Oprah and Delta Burke, who have carried the burden of their weight issue in front in the public eye. Can you imagine how painful it would be to see the tabloids having a field day with every pound you have gained, to have the public scrutinize you mercilessly about every bite going into in your mouth? I guess not being famous can have its good points.

WEEK 3
Sunday, Nov. 20, 1998

Had another photo shoot. We just wanted to get some alternative shots. And yes . . . my reaction when I see the previous photos is, "Oh my God! How did I get this fat?" Really, do I know myself or do I know myself? But there it is recorded, for the world to see, my rolls and bulge—the true story. I look at my butt and think Juan has made a mistake, used his wide-angle lens and taken a picture as wide as the state of Texas! Or is that *Tex-ASS?* All you can do is get a reality check and say, "God I hate this." Just own it and say that is my butt! Let's face it. How many times do we see ourselves from behind? We should do it more often, we would probably think twice before shoving something in our mouth. When you do see your butt in the dressing room mirror, you can excuse it as the bad lighting, or the mirror, or the planets not being aligned in your horoscope that morning. If you think hard enough you can come up with an excuse, anything other than owning that this is *your own butt!*

This is the first time that I am doing squat lunges. Oh Lord have mercy—have you noticed how religious I have become during this training process?—I hate these. My quadriceps are absolutely shaking and quivering, feeling like they are barely able to support my weight. Little do I know that for the rest of the next week I am going to need a wheelchair because I can't walk . . . I am so dramatic, am I not? I don't really get a wheelchair, I just *feel* like I could use one. I moan and groan every time I have to walk. Not that I will get any sympathy from Ed pray tell. When he gives instructions to me and I question him on the weight he is asking me to get or the reps he is asking me to perform, he just laughs and says, "Hey, did I stutter?" Which in training language from Mr. Universe, trainer to trainee, means "Get a move on missy. Let's get to it!"

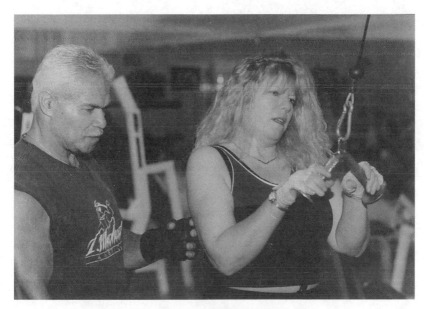

"Yeah, yeah this is fun."

Thursday Nov. 26, 1998

Whew, what a week! I meet Ed at the gym at 9:00 A.M. to get our workout in before the holiday fanfare. I am impressed that the gym is bustling with members training on the Thanksgiving holiday. I am now starting to feel that I am a part of the gym family: I'm starting to get to know everyone at the gym, the regulars. Did I mention the handsome hunks? I mean, who cares if I get in shape or not, the stud muffins in the gym are worth the membership fee alone. I have been known to have my attention wander between sets because the male scenery is just a little too delicious. You guys have got to know that muscles are very sexy.

Ed starts the day by telling me that we are going to do five sets of all the exercises. I just stare at him. All I can do is groan. Oh God! "Really?" I ask him, "Five sets instead of three?" Here I am, thinking that we will coast a little on the holiday. What

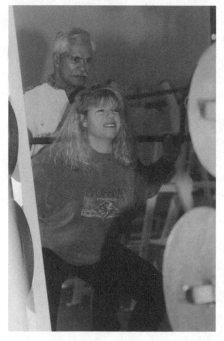

was I thinking? His reply to me is, "Loree, did I stutter?" and we all know what that means. I just roll my eyes and say *"Yes, Master"* in a southern drawl. Other gym members laugh at us.

I may joke about our conversations but there is a very valuable lesson here. Weight training is challenging. If you stop every time it gets hard or uncomfortable, guess what? You'll never progress. Believe me, Ed has had me doing weights and reps that I would have said, "No

**Our quadriceps workout.
"Ed, are we done yet?"**

way will I be able to do it."

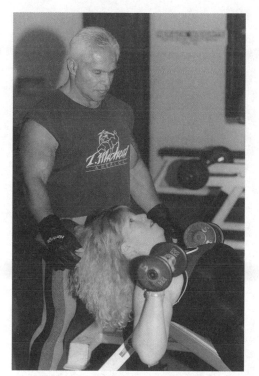

Body form is absolutely essential for each repetition. Ed doesn't miss a beat!

Well, guess what? I am doing much more than I ever thought possible.

I jokingly tell Ed that I think he is trying to make my biceps so sore that I won't be able to pick up my fork and lift it to my mouth. At my turkey dinner I have little bits of everything, trying to fill up on green salad and protein, so Ed won't shoot me tomorrow. I do have a small (I can hardly taste it) piece of pumpkin pie. I would say I was on the right track, but I wasn't perfect.

Friday, Nov. 27, 1998

Ed tells me at our workout how much I have progressed in my strength and my reps. I ask him if he is just saying that to make me feel good. His reply: "No, Loree. I really mean it. Your strength has greatly improved and this is just in a few weeks." Also I had measured and I have lost a few inches. I can't wait to see what happens in a few months. I am tempted to staple my bikini up on the gym wall for incentive, but I think management would have a problem with that.

I am excited to go car shopping after my workout today. I tell Ed that I think I need a new black Mercedes to go with my new body. It's funny how our self-esteem gets caught up in what we feel we deserve or don't deserve. I have wanted a black on black Mercedes for years. But for some reason I am still struggling with my worthiness to actually go buy it for myself. What will people think? They will think I have great taste, that is what they will think. I look at a certain sport utility as well; it is just hard for me to say to myself that it is okay to have what I want. Even my son says to me, "Mom, get yourself a nice Mercedes. You deserve it." Well, gotta go. I have to go car shopping.

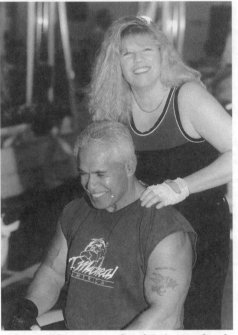

I am the one who just worked out and the trainer gets a neck massage? What is wrong with this picture?

WEEK 4
Sunday, Nov. 29, 1998

Can you believe it? Week four. I have made it a whole month. *Yahoo!* I am telling you, I love it. I am up at 6:45 A.M. to get ready for training at 9:00 A.M. Something valuable I learned on Friday morning. I ate too close to my workout (less than two hours) and promptly got nauseous. So that's why I am up at 6:45 A.M.—to have my breakfast in plenty of time to digest before my workout.

Today is our leg day, so no cardio. I am hoping Ed will forget about lunges today (fat chance.) *I hate lunges with a passion!* No such luck. I think about throwing myself on the gym floor in a screaming tantrum, like a two-year-old, but think better of it. We do lunges, braced on a bar lunging forward to get a maximum stretch. I am really having a hard time getting my balance; every time I lunge forward I feel off balance and feel like tipping over. It reminds me of learning how to ride a bike when even the smallest of movement feels like you're going to tip over. "It is a good thing that I never had aspirations to become a ballerina" I tell Ed, as I am going through killer lunges looking like a drunk trying to stay straight on the line.

Ed just keeps giving me instructions . . . bend deep, lift your back foot, etc. I am not liking this man today . . . grumble . . . grumble. We then go to the leg press, where he puts me through five grueling sets. Three of the sets are done in succession, with very little rest in between, and higher weights. I can really feel my quadriceps quivering and shaking when I get off that leg press.

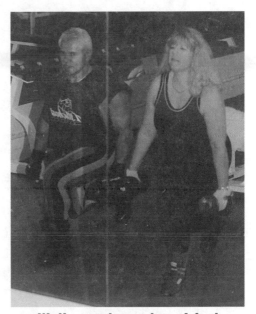

Well, you know how I feel about lunges!

A personal success tip from me to you: Never, I repeat, *never* wear thong underwear to the gym, especially for a leg training workout. Guess what is stretched and pulled when you are training your legs? You guessed it: your buns! You will feel as if you could floss your teeth with your thong, it will be pulled up so high! You will find yourself begging for a paramedic with the *jaws of life* to remove that thong wedged in between your butt cheeks. Or you may even require thong extraction surgery . . . *ouch!*

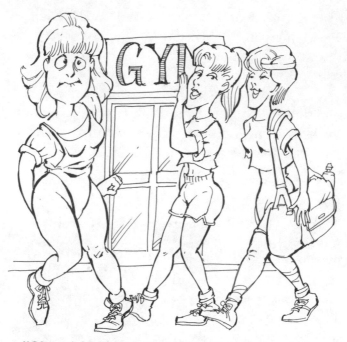

**"Oh no! I think Loree forgot to leave her
thong underwear at home again."**

I have never been so grateful to hear those beautiful few
words: *Keep going. This is your LAST ONE.* I tell a couple working
out next to us (who know Ed) that I have been kidnapped at
gunpoint and brought to Gold's Gym against my will, and that
they should call the police. "Please help me," I plead with them.
"Help me!" We all laugh. Ed is a good sport and he teases me
just as much, believe me.

The next challenge of the day is the donkey press to work
the calves. When I see Ed put the weight at 120 pounds, I immediately protest. "Ed, last week I only did 60 pounds. How can
you raise me up to 120 already?"

"I was hoping that you wouldn't remember," he quips. We
agree that I will start at 80 pounds. I set the weight myself;
in my haste I set it at 100 pounds. (He is never going to let me

live this one down.) Of course I do not realize this until after my set. When I go to remove the pin I realize that I have just done 100 pounds and am now required to go to 120 pounds for my next set. Just a few minutes ago I vehemently protested that I could not do it. Of course Ed is grinning from ear to ear, with that I-told-you-so smirk of his (I want to slap him) because, as usual, I did more weight than I thought possible. By the end of the third set I pumped 15 reps of 140 pounds, but ask me and I would have insisted that I could not do that. All that whining and at the end of our third month of training I am pumping 400 pounds on the donkey press!

Once again I hear Anthony Robbins' voice in my head saying, "If you can't . . . you must." Well, I thought I couldn't and guess what: I did! Here again I was getting a lesson about underestimating myself with my limiting beliefs. We had a great workout today. I feel proud of myself, proud of my progress, and grateful for all the support I am receiving.

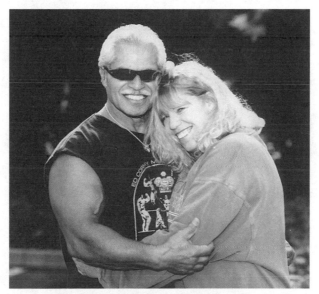

Okay, I admit it, Ed kills me at the gym but I still love him.

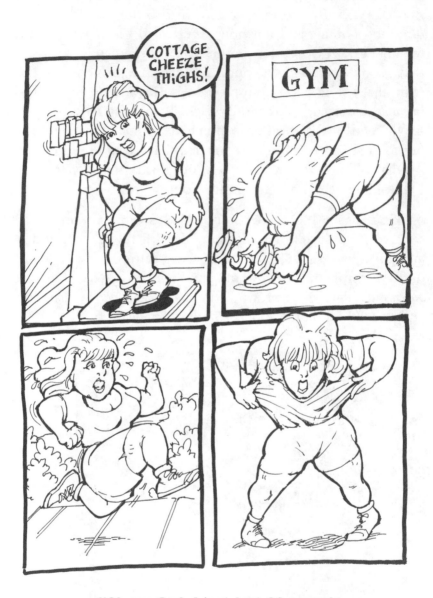

"Oh my God, I just lost 20 pounds.
Where are my boobs?"

Loree's Progress Report from Ed

We are beginning our second month of training together. Loree has shown a profound commitment and determination to get in shape. The primary objective, of course, is to tone, firm, and lose weight. In so doing, the improvement reached within four weeks has been absolutely incredible. Keeping within her repetitions — of no less than 12 and no more than 15 — her strength, endurance, and recovery time between sets have improved tremendously.

I must add that I certainly bring out the hidden side of her determination, which was nonexistent prior to our teaming up. Although the entire body is worked over four days weekly, our flexible schedule allows her to also balance her work and training schedule quite nicely.

I have concentrated more effort on cardio, abdominal, hips, and thighs. Loree will sign up for either kickboxing or spinning classes, which will further enhance her cardio program and burn more body fat.

I must add that it's a pleasure to have a client with a very determined and positive attitude to improve.

– Ed Corney

❖ ❖ ❖

I trained with Ed Corney for three months, as agreed. I followed his diet plan. I have to say in those three months I was getting toned and very strong (I probably could have lifted a car). I did lose a few inches here and there. However, I still did not lose very much body fat, especially around my waist. My fat was hanging on for dear life.

I was still fat, furious, and very frustrated. I had been working very hard, training and dieting, but my metabolism was fighting me at every turn. If Mr. Universe could not turn this around I was at a loss for an explanation. I considered training with him longer, but he was scheduled for a minor shoulder surgery and would not be able to train for several months. Unfortunately, Ed had a major stroke during surgery and almost lost his life. I remember sharing Ed's condition with my morning radio show listeners, breaking down in tears on the air. I became very fond of Ed during our training together. I visited him often while he was recovering. He is doing well now, progressing and back at the gym working out. I believe that his tremendous physical condition is what pulled him through this ordeal.

In retrospect I did not know that my insulin was most likely still high, and my thyroid underactive at that point. I was following Ed's diet but it allowed enough carbohydrates to keep me in a non–fat-reducing mode. Ed added more cardio training but that still wasn't reducing my body fat. Hidden metabolic issues that I was unaware of were underlying my failure to succeed at fat reduction and clouding my outcome. It would take five more years before I would get to the real root of this ongoing challenge.

*Never underestimate your power to change yourself;
never overestimate your power to change others.*

– H. Jackson Brown, Jr.

CHAPTER 20

■ ■ ■ ■ ■ ■ ■ ■ ■ ■ ■

Exercise, Training, and Metabolism

If you want to achieve true fitness and vitality, you have to stop beating your head against the wall. You have to understand the rules of nature's game and learn how to bend them in your favor. It's not willpower; it's METABOLISM. It's not motivations; it's BIOCHEMISTRY. It's not your attitude; it's your HORMONES.

– Stephen Cherniske, MS, *The Metabolic Plan*

Many of you will turn to personal and fitness trainers in an attempt to reach your weight loss and physical goals. Just as with any health or medical professional, you need to find a compatible match, someone who can assist you in achieving your goals and understand your physical challenges and limitations.

In the preface, I shared meeting Dr. Pataki in 1997, and developing a professional friendship with him. Over the years, I have been grateful to Dr. Pataki for the wealth of knowledge he has imparted to me. At first I was intimidated by his powerful accented voice, his athletic persona (just imagine Arnold Schwarzenegger—minus the shades and black leather jacket), and his scientific dialogue. I have since come to realize that the sports scientist behind the powerful voice is a very patient and gentle soul who thrives on teaching others.

I interviewed Dr. Pataki for *Fat and Furious*, not because any of you are training for the Olympics but because his philosophy of physiology meshes very well with the advice given in this book. He is very centered in his philosophy of training and does not approach working out with the extreme and compulsive behavior that has gotten many of us into trouble.

AN INTERVIEW WITH LADISLAV PATAKI, Ph.D.

Dr. Ladislav Pataki has a background of scientific work that includes not only two Ph.D. degrees, but the high rank of Independent Scientist of the Academy of Sciences of the SSR. A trainer of numerous Olympic and elite athletes, both in the Soviet Bloc and in the USA, he is recognized as an expert on the theory and practice of athletic achievement.

In his fifties, Dr. Pataki has had years of commitment to sports performance and physical mastery. He is also living proof that as one becomes older, one doesn't have to decline physically. Dr. Pataki currently holds several world records in master's track and field, and through proper nutrition and training has improved his body's condition and his athletic performance every year between the ages of 50 and 55. He is the author of *Winning Secrets: Confessions of a Soviet Bloc Sports Scientist.*

Many of you have sought or will seek the advice of a personal trainer to help you reshape your body. I asked Dr. Pataki some of the deciding factors for choosing a personal trainer or athletic coach for assistance in physical performance. We also covered some of his philosophies on training in general.

Why would someone want to hire a personal trainer rather than working out on their own?

DR. PATAKI: Loree, many people have a hard time staying motivated in their training schedules. Having to commit to a workout training schedule with a trainer is a great benefit to those inclined to miss workouts. Conversely, a trained professional will give advice to assist you in avoiding the pitfalls of overtraining. Many people overtrain and therefore do not get the results that they are after. On their own they may become depressed from what they perceive as lack of progress. A trainer will give them realistic expectations and avoid injuries. A trainer will also monitor their diet for optimal energy, progress, and fat loss.

What qualities should a person look for in a training professional?

DR. PATAKI: My suggestion would be to really check into a potential trainers education and experience. What are their work ethics? Can you talk to their other clients for references? How long have their clients been with them? Are they sensitive to the client's goals and physical limitations, and not just their own agenda? Has the trainer ruled out any existing health conditions that would inhibit training?

What would be the average time one could expect to see results from strength training?

DR. PATAKI: I would give a strength training routine at least six months to see really good results. Without a trainer some people would give up if they don't get instant results.

◆ ◆ ◆

I asked Dr. Pataki to address my concerns regarding exercise and training, and the concept of overtraining and its effects on what I call the "metabolically challenged." Dr. Pataki explains:

> Let me first explain the theory of anabolic and catabolic metabolism as it relates to exercise and training. Anabolic metabolism is the rebuild, repair, and restore activity of your body. Catabolic activity refers to breakdown and degeneration. Anabolic and catabolic are both essential processes of life.
>
> At every stage of your life, your health is determined

by the ratio of damage to repair. Degeneration associated with aging and loss of physical energy is caused by decline in anabolic repair, and the accumulation of catabolic damage.

You want to exercise regularly, which takes discipline and dedication. Whether you are motivated to lose body fat, tone your muscles, improve your heath, or become a competitive athlete, one of the main determining factors in your success is the hormonal balance in your body.

We know from research and experience that "hypertrophy," or muscle growth, is induced by the release of growth hormone DHEA. After the first 15 minutes of exercise and lasting for approximately an hour, the body releases a maximum amount of this substance. If an athlete exercises for a much longer time, however—such as three to five hours—something quite different occurs. The organism begins to protect itself through the production and release of cortisol into the system. Cortisol is a catabolic hormone. It tears muscles down rather than building them up. This phenomenon places a limit on the appropriate length of effective training sessions. Training in short sessions as often as five times a day is preferable to training in one extended session five times as long.

Now, of course I am referring to athletes training for competition events. You are not going to work out five times a day. But the theory is the same. By decreasing workout lengths we increase our anabolic metabolism for tissue repair and reduce catabolic metabolism.

The two main hormones I am referring to, which are secreted by the adrenal glands, are DHEA and cortisol. One of these hormones, DHEA, has an anabolic effect on the body, whereas cortisol has a catabolic breakdown effect on the body. The key here when exercising and training is to achieve the proper balance between the production of these two hormones. Chronic stress can raise the body's cortisol level and conversely decrease DHEA production.

It is important to understand that overenthusiasm and overtraining when the body is in a catabolic state with high cortisol levels can be perceived by the body as *stress*. Overexercise can easily produce a cortisol/DHEA imbalance.

Amino acids are the building blocks of proteins, which are the foundation of the cellular structure. If the body has a high cortisol level in relation to DHEA level, protein synthesis slows, with the result being reduced muscle mass.

As with athletes, many people are so wrapped up in their training or fat loss goals, they miss that they are overtraining. In my years of coaching Olympic athletes some have realized that they have wasted time and effort—sometimes months—before realizing they were overtraining. During overtraining, not only did they fail to advance towards their goals, they also regressed in their physical conditioning.

My recommendation in this instance is not to cease training altogether. The central nervous system of any-one accustomed to a regular training schedule becomes tuned to that schedule, both biologically and neuro-psychologically. If workouts stop for long, the inactivity creates stress and depression. This in turn will cause your body to secrete cortisol, which as I have discussed earlier results in catabolism, the breakdown of muscle tissue. Your best remedy is to keep training, but decrease your training intensity to around 65%.

However, on the other hand, perhaps you've been careful not to overtrain. You have varied the intensity of your workouts, allowing sufficient time for recovery. Yet you feel fatigued, and may experience chronic insomnia as well as repeated injuries. These symptoms suggest that you should take a deeper look into your general health and metabolic profile. You could have a serious illness or you could well be experiencing a nutritional imbalance, perhaps a mineral deficiency or hormonal imbalance.

A CELEBRITY LEGEND

A perfect example of a celebrity who has mastered anabolic metabolism is an incredible exercise legend, Jack LaLanne. I grew up with Jack LaLanne and I loved watching him on television. Jack has been known to do 900 pushups *in a day!* He was born in 1914 but you'd never know it by looking at him.

I had the tremendous privilege of meeting Jack in Los Angeles where we were both speakers at the Natural Products Expo–West in the spring of 2002. *Dateline* was filming a documentary on Jack and everywhere he went in the Expo (cameras and all) he was such an admired celebrity. This man looks like he is in his fifties and has the attitude and spirit of a thirty-year-old. I can say from personal experience, *whew, is he feisty!*

Stephen Cherniske, MS, explains in detail in his book, *The Metabolic Plan:*

> Jack has discovered the secret of anabolic metabolism, which is that the brain—which controls every cell in your body—doesn't know how old you are. It doesn't really care, because chronological age is not nearly as important to survival as biological age.
>
> When Jack LaLanne's brain checks in for updated information (so it can operate his body in the most efficient way possible), his muscles report that they just performed 900 push-ups. The brain concludes that the body is superbly fit and quite capable of surviving. It then sends anabolic instructions to every tissue in the

body to maintain peak immunity, vitality, bone mass, high metabolic efficiency, mental acuity, and a positive attitude. Included are instructions to convert every morsel of food he eats to energy, so that Jack LaLanne will never—even if he lives to 120—have to count calories.

MONITORING YOUR METABOLISM

Your metabolism is the body's process of converting food and stored fat into energy. This energy is used to stay warm, move around, and keep vital organs functioning. Metabolism is typically measured in calories. Total metabolic rate represents the calories needed to maintain body functions, daily activity (work and lifestyle), and exercise.

Your resting metabolic rate (RMR) represents the number of calories required by the body in 24 hours to maintain vital body functions (such as heart rate, brain functions, and breathing). In simple terms, it is the number of calories a person would burn if he or she were awake but at rest all day. RMR can account for up to 75% of a person's total energy expenditure.

Metabolism is impacted by unique characteristics such as gender, age, weight, body composition (amount of muscle versus fat), level of fitness, physical activity, eating, stimulants, emotional excitement, stress, and gaining and losing weight. A knowledge of RMR is important in managing caloric needs. Traditionally, it has been difficult and expensive to accurately measure RMR, so people have used estimates, which are inaccurate on many people.

Because metabolism is different among individuals and influenced by many factors, it should be measured regularly during a weight management program. Your metabolism can vary from day to day and within the same day. That is why it is important to measure your metabolism under similar conditions to get the most accurate reading of your resting metabolism.

Your resting metabolic rate can be influenced by:

- ◆ Body weight
- ◆ Body composition (amount of fat to muscle)
- ◆ Age
- ◆ Gender
- ◆ Hormones
- ◆ Stress
- ◆ Use of stimulants such as caffeine

For information on how to get your metabolic rate tested please consult the resource guide.

OVEREXERCISING TO LOSE BODY FAT QUICKLY IS NOT AN OPTION

Jogging is for people who aren't intelligent enough to watch television.

– Victoria Wood

I can honestly say with confidence and some certainty that if you have been on the road to weight loss, exercise and extreme dieting have been part of that equation. If you are anxious to lose weight, you have been told that to rev up your metabolism you need to get to the gym, hire a trainer, or sign up for a marathon. That is all commendable, but first things first.

I am addressing this book to those I call "metabolically challenged," not your average run-of-the-mill person who cuts out ice cream for a few weeks and loses five pounds. If you can gain five pounds in a day just by reading this book and breathing air, or by driving by a donut shop, then you are the one I am speaking to. Your metabolism and hormones are out of balance. That is why you are overweight in the first place, end of story.

It is physiologically impossible to burn off more than one to two pounds in a week without doing extreme damage to your metabolism. With all these possible hormonal challenges you are facing you should get on your knees and thank the heavens above if you can even lose that much in a week. There were weeks where the only weight loss that would show up on my scale was if I shaved my legs and plucked my eyebrows that morning!

If your metabolism is in need of rebalancing and repair, hoping, praying, starving, and running a marathon are only going to cause your metabolism more damage. It is very tempting to get into extreme exercise to burn up more calories, build muscle mass, and try to get your metabolism moving faster. I have three words for you . . . *Get over it!* I know it is what you have been taught, it's what your doctor or your trainer told you: exercise more, increase your metabolism, you'll burn more fat. Wait! Stop! Hear me out!

It is true that exercise builds muscle mass and is your backbone to your metabolic rate. Muscle mass uses more energy than the rest of the tissues. The more muscle mass you have, the higher your metabolism, and the less muscle mass, the lower your metabolism. But to the person (that's you and me) who is struggling in hormonal hell, the body perceives all this exercise as stress and overexercising.

Overexercising damages your metabolism. Overexercising as a way to pump up your metabolism and burn more fat actually leads to more hormonal imbalance that directs your body to use up its functional and structural biochemicals more than rebuild them. Think of what we learned earlier: if the body perceives exercise as stress it can release the hormone cortisol, and too much cortisol can lead to fat storage—the opposite effect of what you are trying to achieve.

If your body and hormones are in a state of imbalance, exercise activity that is perceived as normal for someone else may be overexercising for *your* metabolism. I am not giving anyone (myself included) the excuse to become a couch potato and not exercise! On the contrary, what I am saying is work with your health care provider and trainer and follow the recommendations that will benefit your body's metabolic condition. You have to follow your gut. You'll know what is overexercising for your current health condition.

Let me give you one example (there are numerous that could be applicable) just for argument's sake. Let's look at a recovering sugar addict with a high-stress lifestyle. Let's call this person Mary. Mary thinks she is making a positive lifestyle change and is all hyped up to exercise. She hits the cardio machines at the gym every morning without fail before her high-stress job. Mary may very well have burned-out adrenal glands from excessive sugar consumption and her stressful executive job. So guess what? Cardio/stimulating exercises leave Mary feeling drained and exhausted after her exercise instead of invigorated.

Should Mary stop exercising? Absolutely not! But she may need balancing, rebuilding, and repair of her metabolism before this type of exercise is appropriate for her. She might find under the guidance of her health care provider that nutritional supplements, hormonal support, and a program of walking are more suitable for her metabolism at this time.

Exercise is important. It is healthy. We should all do it daily (unless otherwise advised by your physician). If you are not up for weight training or aerobics, taking a walk every day is soothing to your soul. My dogs, Briggs and First Officer Riley, and I enjoy our time together walking, breathing the fresh air (of course sniffing and peeing on every tree on the planet), and observing what nature has to offer. If you don't know what to do at least you can walk every day.

Your metabolism can be likened to your car. If your car runs out of gas and stalls in the middle of the street, your yelling, screaming, kicking the tires, and throwing a hissy fit are not going to get the car moving again. The car needs *gas!* Not *attitude!* The only way the car will get moving is if you give it gas. Your car has a gas gauge, you were *warned* before it sputtered to a stop, but you chose not to pay attention.

Getting yourself to the gym and pumping out more cardio when *your ass is dragging* on the ground is about as effective as yelling at the car stalled in the street. If you have a trainer who is pushing you beyond your physical limitations (there is pushing for effective training and there is *pushing)* and he or she is not willing to understand your limitations, you have my permission to kick him or her to *the curb!* You can only fight your biochemistry for so long. If your metabolism is dragging and your gas gauge (low energy and hormones) is blinking, do something about it before you have to be *towed* to the physician's office.

If you have some respect for people as they are,
you can be more effective in helping them to
become better than they are.

           – John W. Gardner

CHAPTER 21

■ ■ ■ ■ ■ ■ ■ ■ ■ ■

A Word About Diet

No matter what kind of diet you are on,
you can usually eat as much as you want
of anything you don't like.

– Walter Slezak

Here is the real challenge for you. *What in the heck do you eat to lose this weight?* I am going to answer you honestly . . . I don't know! I don't know, because I am not your metabolic physician with your chart in front of me, looking at your hormonal profile. It would be very arrogant of me to suggest a detailed diet plan for you without knowing all these variable circumstances. I have given you general guidelines to use at your own discretion with the help of your health professionals.

The physicians in this book have discussed many hormonal imbalances that may have contributed to your weight gain. They have stated over and over that everyone is biochemically unique and *one size* or *one diet does not fit all.* Chapter 8 by Dr. Robban Sica, If Your Diet Doesn't Fit You, How Can Your Clothes? can serve as a reminder to you of all the factors that go into an individualized diet plan. Just a few of these factors are carbohydrate sensitivity, insulin resistance, thyroid function, hormone balance, food allergies, metabolic type, blood type, and age. There are many more!

At the heart of the whole weight issue is balancing your foods in proper combinations of fats, proteins, and carbohydrates for *your* metabolic profile. I will say that again for emphasis: *your* metabolic profile, *not* someone else's. Dr. Sica also addressed the importance of the right kinds of fats. Many of you have become fat phobic! The right kind of essential fats will *not* make you fat. You need fat to produce and balance your hormones. Fat is not the enemy!

Later in another chapter I will address what to do to find Dr. Right to assist you in a weight loss diet specifically for you. What you can do in the meantime, while you are searching for Dr. Right and getting your strategy in place, is get started on *The Fat Flush Plan* by Ann Louise Gittleman (McGraw-Hill, 2002) to start detoxifying your body. You can think of this as a positive action plan to move your body in the right healthy cleansing direction as you begin your weight loss journey. Whatever diet strategy you ultimately end up with (from Dr. Right, of course!) you will be that much further ahead by detoxifying your body.

Several years ago Susan Powter, a blonde woman with a shaved head, bounced around the infomercial stage (like she was high on cocaine) screaming, "Stop the insanity" and promoting her book by the same name. This woman was pushing the "no fat" theory and promoting eating lots of bagels, rice, and high-carbohydrate—but in her words, "no fat"—foods. She did lose weight (I am happy for her), but someone who is carbohydrate intolerant would not lose but *gain weight* on this regimen.

My suggestion is that you enroll a physician who specializes in metabolic medicine and follow his/her diet recommendations for you. I suggest that you keep a lifestyle diary of your daily habits, including everything you eat (yes, every morsel), your exercise schedule, energy, and sleeping habits. Take this to your physician to assist them in determining your metabolic profile.

Please promise me you will not get sucked into the latest diet scheme. The diet industry is a multi-billion dollar industry. Desperation can really push you to grab that credit card and purchase your next "diet program" of hope. True, there are nutritional supplements to balance and support your hormonal system and help your body lose weight (many are in this book) but they are not a quick diet fix. Think of the popular weight loss shake that is *blank*-fast (I don't want to get sued). You can lose up to two pounds of body fat per week *only. There is no fast.* That is it! End of story. Patience and persistence wins the weight loss race.

This is a *take it one day at a time* plan. It is a *take responsibility for what goes into your mouth*, and *eat to heal your body and your metabolism* plan.

One doesn't discover new lands without consenting to lose sight of the shore for a very long time.

– André Gide

CHAPTER 22

■ ■ ■ ■ ■ ■ ■ ■ ■ ■

Balancing Body Chemistry for Weight Loss

ACID/ALKALINE BALANCE IN WEIGHT LOSS

Balancing your pH will save your life, though I would be absolutely shocked if you told me that a physician, when addressing your weight concerns, asked you for your pH values. This information is going to take you right back to science class, but the bottom line is, if your body is too acid it prevents you metabolically from losing weight. I am going to show you how to monitor your body's chemistry by taking a simple pH test with your saliva and urine. This is so simple a child could do it.

> *The term pH, which means potential hydrogen, represents a scale for the relative acidity or alkalinity of a solution. Acidity refers to a pH of 0.1 to 6.9, alkalinity to a pH of 7.1 to 14, and neutral pH is 7.0. The numbers refer to how many hydrogen atoms are present compared to an ideal or standard solution. Normally, blood is slightly alkaline, at 7.35 to 7.45. Urine pH can range from 4.8 to 7.5, although normal is closer to 7.0.*
>
> *– Alternative Medicine Definitive Guide to Cancer,*
> Future Medicine Publishing, 1997

Balanced body chemistry exhibits what is called proper alkaline-acid ratio. We are going to talk about your body's pH balance and the effect it has on gaining and losing weight. A healthy body usually keeps large alkaline reserves to meet the demands of too many acid-producing foods. When these are depleted beyond a 4:1 ratio, health can be seriously threatened. If we eat too many acid-producing foods we become over-acid, our immunity to disease is weakened, and our weight loss potential can be compromised or cease altogether. High acidity can affect all major body systems, especially the digestive, intestinal, circulatory, respiratory, and immune systems. It is now believed that one of the basic causes of disease is acidosis, or over-acidity.

Those who have unbalanced pH and are considered "acidic" may have many health conditions. Acidosis forces the body to borrow minerals—including calcium, sodium, potassium, and magnesium—from vital organs and bones to buffer the acid and safely remove it from the body. This process can weaken these organs and bones over time. It is also vitally important to understand how your emotions can affect your body's chemistry. Anger and emotional upset will cause your tissues and cells to become instantly acidic. Acidosis may affect body systems and lead to serious health concerns such as:

◆ Weight gain.

◆ Cardiovascular weakness.

◆ Bladder and kidney concerns.

◆ Acceleration of free radical damage.

◆ Structural system weakness, including brittle bones and hip fractures.

◆ Joint discomfort and other discomfort associated with lactic acid buildup.

◆ Low energy.

A recent study conducted at the University of California, San Francisco, on 9,704 post-menopausal women showed that those who have higher acidity levels (also called chronic acidosis) from a diet rich in animal foods are a greater risk for lower bone density levels than those who have "normal" pH levels. The researchers who carried out this study hypothesized that many of the hip fractures prevalent among older women correlated to higher acidity from a diet rich in animal foods and low in vegetables. The body apparently borrows calcium from the bones in order to balance pH, and this calcium borrowing may result in a decrease in bone density

– American Journal of Clinical Nutrition,
Jan. 2001, Vol. 73, No. 1

HIGH ALKALINITY IN THE BODY

Though relatively uncommon, high alkalinity in the body causes many of the same kinds of mineral problems as acidity. It often takes longer for a person who is "alkaline" to achieve balance than one who is acidic. Alkalinity may lead to:

◆ Digestive system sluggishness.

◆ Intestinal system concerns, including poor elimination.

◆ Respiratory system compromise.

◆ Immune system weakness.

◆ Nervous system exhaustion.

A pH-balanced environment maintains proper metabolic function and allows the body to function optimally. In order to keep the acid-alkaline ratio in balance, Dr. Ragner Berg, the world's foremost authority on the subject, says we should eat about 80% alkaline-producing foods and 20% acid-producing foods. Alkalis help to neutralize the acids when one does become over-acid or ill. Eating more alkaline-ash foods helps the body regain its balanced chemistry.

ACID/ALKALINE SELF-TEST: HAVE YOU CHECKED YOUR pH TODAY?

Water is neutral with pH of 7.0. Any reading with pH below 7.0 is acid, while any reading with pH above 7.0 is alkaline. The ideal range for saliva and urine is 6.0 to 6.8. Our body is naturally mildly acidic. Some people will have acidic pH readings from both urine and saliva; this is referred to as "double acid."

Urine pH

Urine testing indicates how well your body is assimilating minerals, especially calcium, magnesium, sodium, and potassium. These are called "acid buffers" because they are used by the body to control acid levels. When acid levels begin to increase, the body becomes less capable of excreting acid. It must either store the acid in body tissues, or buffer it—that is, borrow minerals from organs, bones etc., in order to neutralize the extra acid.

If your urinary pH fluctuates between 6.0 and 6.4 in the morning and 6.4 to 7.0 in the evening, your body is functioning within a normal range.

Saliva pH

The results of saliva testing indicate the activity of digestive enzymes in your body, especially the activity of the liver and the stomach. They reveal the flow of enzymes running through your body and show their effect on all the body systems. If your saliva stays between 6.4 and 6.8 all day, your body is functioning within a normal range.

The Body's Acid Management System

Acids do not stay in the blood. The body manages acids as follows:

♦ Excretion of acids—colon, kidneys, lungs, skin.

♦ Buffering of acids—calcium, magnesium, sodium, potassium.

♦ Storage of acids—tissue, joints, muscles, arteries.

♦ Minerals are used to buffer acids.

The reference section of this book includes books on acid/alkaline balance. They can assist you in adjusting your diet to bring your pH balance back to normal. Alkaline-forming foods should be consumed when the body is too acidic (pH under 7.0). Acid-forming foods should be eaten when the body is too alkaline. Low-level acid and low-level alkaline foods are almost neutral.

Although it might seem that citrus fruits would have an acid effect on the body, the citric acid they contain actually has an alkaline effect on the system, converting to carbon dioxide and water. To treat acidosis, start with small amounts of citrus fruits and gradually add larger amounts.

It is vitally important to self-test your pH levels for optimal health. Weight loss pH balancing is at the foundation of your weight loss and health-building program. In the privacy of your own home, you can determine your pH factor quickly and easily. The resource guide in this book tells you where you can order a pH testing kit.

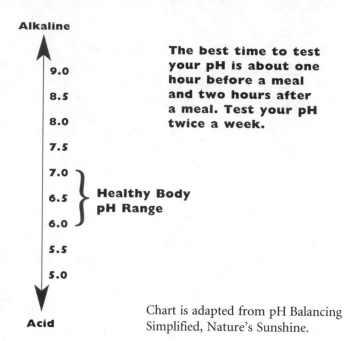

Alkaline

9.0

8.5

8.0

7.5

7.0
6.5 } **Healthy Body pH Range**
6.0

5.5

5.0

Acid

The best time to test your pH is about one hour before a meal and two hours after a meal. Test your pH twice a week.

Chart is adapted from pH Balancing Simplified, Nature's Sunshine.

Some Common Acid Addictions

- Coffee
- Soda
- Sugar
- Alcohol
- Cooked meat
- Refined carbohydrates
- Synthetic medicines
- Chemical drugs
- Anger and stress

ENZYMES ASSIST THE METABOLIC PROCESS

Another important factor in balancing the body's chemistry for optimal weight loss is to consider how the body's enzyme pool is kept replenished. Life could not exist without enzymes. Enzymes are essential, but each person is born with a limited enzyme potential. Therefore, maintaining an adequate supply of enzymes is vital to support your body's health. Enzymes are a part of every metabolic process in the body, from the working of our glands to the proper functioning of our immune system. Enzymes not only play a role in digestion, but are also active to fight diseases and assist with other metabolic processes.

WHAT ARE ENZYMES?

Enzymes are complex organic substances produced in plants and animals that catalyze (speed up) chemical reactions in cells and organs. There are many digestive enzymes in the body. Working with body fluids, they help to break down large chemical chains into smaller particles. The body is able to absorb these smaller particles and utilize them. Without enzymes, the body functions would be too slow to sustain life.

Your body gets enzymes from two main sources: it produces some and it gets some from outside the body. Every cell in

Life's demands drain your enzyme supply.

Day-to-day living puts a tremendous demand on your body's supply of enzymes. Emotional or mental strain can also adversely influence enzymatic action. Try thinking of your enzyme supply as a bank account. Skimpy deposits of enzymes (processed, dead, devitalized foods) and heavy withdrawals (chronic stress, strenuous exercise, illness) are just some of the things that can put you into eventual bankruptcy of your enzyme bank account. If you spend your enzymes rapidly, your life does not last as long as it would if you use your enzymes more frugally. The body is under a great daily burden to produce the volume of enzymes necessary to run efficiently. Unfortunately, we are not conscious of this or we would be extremely concerned about how enzymes are dispensed, and less likely to waste them.

your body is an enzyme factory. Unfortunately, the number of enzymes each cell can produce is limited. In addition, it is possible that some of us are either not born with, or lose the ability to make, certain enzymes. If we have abused our bodies with unhealthy lifestyles it is likely that deficiencies in enzymes will occur.

To prevent a premature shortage of enzymes, include rich sources of enzymes in your diet whenever possible. Every bite of raw food provides your body with enzymes. Enzyme supplements taken with every meal will also add to your enzyme supply. Get in the habit of carrying supplemental enzymes with you for meals eaten outside the home. A good digestive enzyme supplement will also attempt to re-stimulate natural production of HCL (hydrochloric acid) in addition to supplementing it.

Common Digestive Supplements

papain	bromelain
lipase	bile
pepsin	pancreatin
protease	glutamic HCL
amylase	betaine HCL
lactase	

Over-the-counter digestive supplements contain other enzymes, which serve various aspects of the digestive process. The papaya fruit has long had a reputation for its protein-digesting enzyme papain. Papain is found in the unripe papaya fruit and leaves. Bromelain, derived from pineapples, is another tropical fruit enzyme that helps break proteins apart into amino acids.

Dr. Howell's research suggests that the rate of enzyme depletion in the body is a determining factor in longevity.

Enzyme-depleted food robs your body of its enzyme potential and may reduce your lifespan. When you add enzymes beyond what your body can produce, you can begin to rebuild your enzyme pool. Remember to keep adding generous deposits to your enzyme bank account, thus staying young and enzyme-rich for life.

Food enzyme deficiency and its aftermath must be recognized as the most serious and profound oversight and omission in nutrition.

– Dr. Edward Howell

Much of this chapter is excerpted from *Detox for Life* by Loree Taylor Jordan, CCH, ID, Madison Publishing, 2003.

CHAPTER 23

■ ■ ■ ■ ■ ■ ■ ■ ■ ■

Nature's Pharmacy

There are no known side effects from herbs used knowledgeably and wisely. Knowledge and wisdom are the key words. Herbs should not be used indiscriminately, without knowledge, any more than food should. We must use common sense, fortified with a basic knowledge of the properties of herbs, in order to use them effectively.

— Stan Malstrom, *Own Your Own Body*

Herbs and supplements from nature's pharmacy will assist your body in losing weight, supporting your glandular system, and giving you vital nutrition. Poor dietary habits, consuming lots of sugar (be honest here . . . Oreos is not a food group!), smoking, and other unhealthy indulgences have depleted your body of vital nutrition.

Well, that was then and this is now! The past does not equal the future. You couldn't change what you didn't know. You are now ready to embark on a different path of knowledge and empowerment. For this purpose I will describe some of the commonly used herbs, supplements, and herbal combinations for losing fat, restoring glandular health, detoxifying your body, removing parasites, and regenerating your nervous system.

BOWEL DETOXIFICATION

Bowel Detox. A key product containing nutrients that support proper digestive and intestinal function. It promotes healthy, regular elimination of waste from the colon. This formula provides betaine HCI, pepsin, pancreatin, and bile salts to aid digestion in the upper gastrointestinal tract. Each capsule also contains 200 mg of psyllium hulls, plus kelp plant and chlorophyll to provide needed bulk, encourage proper flow of waste, and detoxify the colon. This combination comes in a base of phylum hulls, algin, cascara sagrada bark, bentonite, apple pectin, marshmallow root, parthenium root, charcoal, ginger root, sodium, copper, chlorophyllin, vitamins A, C and E (d-alpha tocopherol), beta-carotene, betaine HCL, bile salts, pancreatin, pepsin, selenium (amino acid chelate), and zinc (glaciate). (Nature's Sunshine Products)

CleanStart.® Helps protect your body from common colon toxins that deplete and degrade your health. This two-week program strengthens the waste-filtering process, supports natural toxin elimination, and subsequently improves energy and promotes a feeling of well-being. CleanStart is easy to take and is balanced for more compete results. It also tastes good. Each program contains 28 daily drink packets and 28 capsule packets. Each drink packet contains psyllium hulls, bentonite clay, aloe vera juice, chlorophyll, potassium, stevia, and natural cinnamon or citrus flavoring. The fiber in citrus CleanStart is half psyllium hulls and half modified maltodextrin for a smoother taste. Each capsule packet contains Enviro-Detox and LBSII. The program delivers ten grams of fiber per day, plus the additional cleansing benefits of bentonite, aloe vera, and chlorophyll.

Ingredients in CleanStart and their benefits:

Bentonite. A natural clay that comes from volcanic ash. Taken internally, it supports the intestinal system in the elimination of toxins.

Cascara sagrada. Known as "sacred bark," this is one of Nature's Sunshine's most popular herbal products. As a nutritional support for proper waste elimination, the bark has been used by cultures around the world.

Cascara sagrada acts as an herbal laxative, influences intestinal contraction, and supports a clean, healthy colon. Nature's Sunshine offers the herb individually or in many combinations.

Chlorophyll. The green pigment in plants that harnesses the sun's energy in photosynthesis. Chlorophyll performs metabolic functions in plants such as respiration and growth. Interestingly, the chlorophyll molecule is chemically similar to human blood, except that its central atom is magnesium, whereas that of human blood is iron. Liquid chlorophyll may help deodorize the body and help cleanse the blood of impurities.

LBSII® Lower Bowel Combination. This herbal laxative supports proper waste elimination and encourages a clean colon. The herbs in this popular combination are a source of calcium, crude fiber, magnesium, phosphorus, and sodium. It contains cascara sagrada, buckthorn, licorice root, capsicum fruit, ginger root, Oregon grape, turkey rhubarb root, couch grass herb, and red clover tops.

Psyllium hulls. Provides bulk to the diet. The hulls absorb several times their weight in liquid. Psyllium has high amounts of indigestible fiber that have a mucilaginous quality.

Enviro-Detox. Environmental pollutants and toxins can build up in the body, slowing the body's natural cleansing processes. Enviro-Detox is a combination of 13 nutrients selected for their ability to provide ongoing support to the body's five main detoxifying organs: liver, kidneys, lungs, bowels, and skin. It contains burdock root, dandelion root, fenugreek, ginger, marshmallow root, pepsin, red clover flowers, sarsaparilla root, yellow dock root, echinacea purpurea root, lactobacillus sporogenes, cascara sagrada, and milk thistle concentrate. All have a long history of folk use. Each nutrient in this exclusive formula has been carefully selected to provide maximum nutrition for individual body systems and the body as a whole. The beneficial bacterial lactobacillus sporogenes helps populate the intestinal tract, as cleansing may cause a flushing of friendly flora. Unlike other strains of the organism it does not need to be refrigerated to maintain viability. (Nature's Sunshine Products)

BLOOD SUGAR AND GLANDULAR BALANCE

In the beginning it may seem impossible to balance your glands and balance your blood sugar levels, but it does get easier. Eating frequent meals to keep blood sugar stabilized is one of the keys to success. Eating complex carbohydrates, overall good nutrition, and regular exercise will help you to reach a healthier goal. Remember, it is healthier to get your "high" on feeling good rather than a false rush from sugar.

Complex carbohydrates such as fruits, vegetables, whole grains, nuts, seeds, beans, and legumes enter the bloodstream slowly and do not trigger extreme fluctuations in the blood sugar level like refined sugars do. Even though fruits are complex carbohydrates, sometimes it is necessary to eliminate them completely for a short time while trying to bring the blood sugar and hormonal balance back after a history of sugar addiction.

Adrenal, Desiccated. Provides bovine adrenal gland and carrot root to promote endocrine health and normal cellular function. The use of glandular therapy, in which specific animal organ and gland tissues are ingested for the concentrated nutrients present in them, has a long history of use across a variety of cultures. Bovine tissues like the adrenal are combined with carrot powder in Adrenal Desiccated to provide concentrated nutrients that are especially supportive to their parallel tissues in the human body. Carrot powder provides concentrated antioxidants and vitamins, including vitamins A and C. The vitamins and minerals contained in Adrenal Desiccated enable enzymes and hormones to function properly, contributing to the healthy maintenance of the adrenal, nervous, endocrine, and immune functions, as well as other control functions for the body. (Standard Process, Inc.)

Adrenal Support. A synergistic blend of vitamins, minerals, enzymes, and adaptogenic herbs designed to support and strengthen the adrenal glands. Adrenal Support is also formulated with an adrenal glandular substance from New Zealand. Scientific evidence suggests that the ingredients in Adrenal Support may offer help in supporting adrenal functions and maintaining health. The B vitamins, for example, support bioavailability and biological-terrain-friendly forms of these vital nutrients. Each capsule contains bovine adrenal glandular substance, vitamins B1, B2, B6, pantothenic acid, and vitamin C, plus zinc, potassium, magnesium, protease, borage (borago officinalis) oil powder, licorice root (glycyrrhiza glabra), and schizandra (schisandra chinesis) fruit. (Nature's Sunshine Products)

Adreset.™ Features extracts of Asian ginseng, rhodiola, and cordyceps-adaptogens that support an appropriate and healthy response to stress by promoting balanced hypothalamic-pituitary-adrenal axis function. Adreset is designed to enhance stamina and energy, providing exceptional support for those who are stressed and tired. (Metagenics)

Alpha Lipoic Acid. Often called the universal antioxidant. It is both fat- and water-soluble and can cross any membrane in the body. Consequently, alpha lipoic acid can protect the integrity of the cell membrane as well as offset cell stress. It also promotes mitochondrial activity to help keep your body and its tissues young, enhances the efforts of other antioxidants, helps support the body's natural removal of toxins, and offsets oxidative stress. In addition to its antioxidant properties, alpha lipoid acid directs calories away from fat production and toward energy production, supports blood sugar levels already within the normal range, and enhances the nervous and cardiovascular systems. Nature's Sunshine's alpha lipoic acid is formulated with turmeric, a liver-protecting antioxidant. (Nature's Sunshine Products)

Ayurvedic Blood Sugar Formula. This formula, developed by Indian Ayurvedic masters, provides nutrients necessary for optimal glandular and digestive system function. It supports the liver and pancreas and blood sugar levels already within the normal range. Each capsule contains a blend of gymnema sylvestre leaf and concentrated extracts of the following herbs: momordica charantia fruit bark, pterocarpus marsupium gum, aegle armelos leaf, enicostemma littorale herb, andrographis paniculata herb, curcuma longa rhizome, syzygium cumini seed, azadirachta indica leaf, picrorhiza kurroa root, trigonella foenum-graecum seed, and cyperus rotundus tuber. (Nature's Sunshine Products)

AS with Gymnema. Formulated to support the body's efforts to lose weight and decrease consumption of sugary foods. It contains gymnema leaves, marshmallow root, and psyllium hulls. Gymnema is said to slow the absorption of sugar in the intestines. Psyllium hulls provide essential dietary fiber to increase feelings of fullness and help move dietary fat out of the body before it is absorbed. (Nature's Sunshine Products)

Cataplex® F. It is often necessary to supply a source of iodine when increasing essential fatty acid (EFA) intake, since additional EFAs increase the body's need for iodine proportionately. A strong functional and interdependent relationship exists between this vitamin and the thyroid gland. As fats are metabolized, the thyroid gland works to meet the demands, and iodine is essential for thyroid function. Cataplex F helps the thyroid meet this demand with the addition of iodine.

This is a proprietary blend of carrot (root), bovine adrenal, bovine liver, magnesium citrate, dried alfalfa juice, mushroom, dried buckwheat (leaf) juice, buckwheat (seed), bovine prostate, flax seed oil extract, ascorbic acid, oat flour, soy bean lecithin, and mixed tocopherols. (Standard Process, Inc.)

Chickweed. A mild herb. Some use it to provide nutrients that must be present for the body's metabolism-balancing functions.

It contains vitamins A and C, some B vitamins, calcium, phosphorus, potassium, and zinc. (Nature's Sunshine Products)

Chromiun GTF. A trace mineral that plays a role in regulating blood sugar levels. Each "glucose tolerance factor" (GTF) molecule, a hormone-like compound, requires chromium as its central atom. GTF works with insulin to transport glucose from the blood into the cells. When this function is not working properly, the cells resist insulin and do not properly absorb the glucose needed for energy. The liver also needs chromium to manufacture fatty acids, lecithin, cholesterol, and lipoproteins. Without chromium, blood fats tend to rise because the liver cannot filter them out. Processing destroys much of the chromium content in foods. Each tablet of GTF-chromium contains amino acid chelate and chromium nicotinate in a base of horsetail herb, red clover tops, and yarrow flower. (Nature's Sunshine Products)

Drenamin. A special combination formula that supplies a wide variety of nutrients derived from its principal ingredients of vacuum-dried bovine adrenal and bovine adrenal PMG™ extract. The adrenal glands are involved in a number of physiological functions in the body. They are involved in pulmonary function, blood sugar metabolism, and carbohydrate metabolism. The adrenal glands play an important role in helping the body respond appropriately to changes caused by stress and different emotions. Drenamin is a proprietary blend of defatted wheat (germ), nutritional yeast, bovine liver, bovine adrenal, porcine stomach, bovine adrenal PMG extract, choline bitartrate, oat flour, dried buckwheat (leaf) juice, buckwheat (seed), alfalfa flour, magnesium citrate, mushroom, bovine bone, allantoin, bovine brain, carrot (root), soybean lecithin, veal bone meal, peanut (bran), and mixed tocopherols. (Standard Process, Inc.)

Dulse Liquid. Dulse, *rhodymenia palmate,* is a red seaweed that grows on rocks at the low tide line in the North Atlantic and Northwest Pacific oceans where currents are strong and the bottom is clean. The liquid extract of this plant provides several essential minerals, protein, and trace elements that help support thyroid gland activity and function. Dulse provides a natural source of iodine, an essential trace mineral that is needed by the thyroid gland to maintain proper metabolism. Iodine helps the body regulate temperature, blood cell production, muscle and nerve function, and other bodily functions. (Nature's Sunshine Products)

Iodomere.® Iodine is an integral part of the thyroid hormones and helps the thyroid gland to function properly. Iodomere is one of three iodine products offered by Standard Process, and falls between Allorganic Trace Minerals–B12® and Organic Iodine™ in iodine. This is a proprietary bend of conch (strombus gigas), carrot (root), bovine liver, and echinacea (root). (Standard Process, Inc.)

Kelp. Commonly referred to as seaweed, kelp grows along coastlines around the world. It is a rich source of natural vitamins and minerals, including essential trace minerals. Kelp is especially high in iodine, which must be present for proper glandular function and metabolism. It also contains iron, sodium, phosphorus, and calcium, as well as magnesium and potassium. Kelp is a source of vitamins A, B1, B2, C, D and E, plus amino acids. Because the plant's nutrients come in a natural form, they are easily assimilated by the body. (Nature's Sunshine Products)

Licorice Root. Licorice has been used by traditional herbalists as a general tonic and supports the liver. It is included in most Chinese herb combinations to balance the other herbs and promote vitality. It has a reputation for bringing the entire body into balance (particularly helpful to women who menstruate) and promoting well-being. Licorice contains triterpenoid saponins, flavonoids, isoflavonoids, magnesium, silicon, sodium, and other beneficial constituents. (Nature's Sunshine Products)

Nopal. Particularly useful in providing nutrients to the pancreas and liver that support digestion and help maintain blood sugar balance. Nutritional factors in Nopal may act in the bowel to prevent fat and excessive sugars from entering the bloodstream. (Nature's Sunshine Products)

Pro-pancreas. Contains 14 herbs that provide nutrients vital to the proper function of the pancreas. This formula is a natural source of many trace minerals, including chromium, iron, manganese, and selenium. It contains golden seal root, juniper berries, uva ursi leaves, cedar berries, mullein leaves, garlic bulb, yarrow flowers, slippery elm bark, capsicum fruit, dandelion root, marshmallow root, nettle herb, white oak bark, and licorice root. (Nature's Sunshine Products)

Super GLA Oil Blend. Provides generous amounts of essential omega-6 fatty acids (both linoleic and gamma-linolenic acid) from evening primrose, black currant, and borage oils. In the body, these can be converted into eicosanoids. This group of hormone-like compounds regulates many important bodily functions and processes. These include maintaining blood pressure and platelet aggregation levels that are already within normal ranges, supporting immunity, and regulating gastric secretions and hormonal responses to nerve impulses. *In addition, eicosanoids play a role in increasing lean muscle mass and decreasing body fat.* Three important eicosanoids are prostaglandins, thromboxanes, and leukotrienes.

Super GLA provides nutritional support to the female reproductive system, particularly before menstruation when mild mood changes, breast tenderness, cramps, and swelling can occur. It also plays a role in proper nerve development and function and helps maintain proper liver function. Each capsule contains gamma-linolenic acid from evening primrose, black currant, and borage oils. (Nature's Sunshine Products)

SugarReg.® A formulation of eight nutrients that support proper glandular function. Specifically, this combination helps support the body's effort to achieve balance between blood sugar and insulin. Many of the herbs in this formula (banaba leaf, gymnema, nopal, and bitter melon) have a history of successful use in supporting the glandular system. Bilberry provides antioxidant action and helps protect delicate eye blood vessels from the ravages of free radicals. Nopal nourishes the liver and promotes digestion. Chromium, a trace mineral, is essential for maintaining blood sugar levels already within the normal range. SugarReg contains banaba leaf (standardized to 1% corosolic acid), gymnema extract, bitter melon, nopal fruit, bilberry fruit, fenugreek herb, chromium, and vanadium. (Nature's Sunshine Products)

Cholester-Reg® II. If maintaining cholesterol balance is an issue, this product can be of assistance. It is a natural formula that helps maintain cholesterol levels that are already within the normal range. (Nature's Sunshine Products)

Target TS11. Designed to help meet the nutritional needs of the glandular system — the pituitary, thyroid, and hypothalamus glands in particular. Target minerals zinc and manganese are chelated to the amino acids glutamine, proline, and histidine, making them more readily absorbed. Cell growth and repair are highly dependent on zinc, which is also key to enzyme reactions. The herbs in this formula provide a rich source of iodine, necessary for proper thyroid function. (Nature's Sunshine Products)

Thyroid Activator. Nourishes the thyroid gland and contains many trace minerals lacking in the average Western diet. The combination is a natural source of iron, magnesium, iodine, potassium, selenium, sodium, zinc, and vitamin A. Thyroid Activator contains Irish moss plant, kelp plant, black walnut hulls, parsley herb, watercress herb, and sarsaparilla root. (Nature's Sunshine Products)

Thyroid Support. A blend of nutritional and herbal supplements specially designed to nourish the thyroid gland and support the actions of the thyroid hormones. The thyroid hormones regulate many body functions, including oxygen use, basal metabolic rate, cellular metabolism, growth and development, and body temperature. Contains L-tyrosine, kelp, zinc, copper citrate, pyridoxal-5 phosphate, protease, stinging nettle, manganese, and thyroid and brain glandular substances from certified BSE-free cows from New Zealand. (Nature's Sunshine Products)

Thytrophin PMG.® The thyroid gland of the endocrine system secretes hormones that have a profound effect on calcium metabolism and on the entire body's metabolic rate. Bovine thyroid PMG™ helps maintain the thyroid tissues in a good state of repair to support healthy thyroid function. Thytrophin PMG contains bovine thyroid PMG extract (processed to remove thyroxine) and magnesium citrate. The thyroid gland is an endocrine gland consisting of a large number of follicles that contain thryroglobulin. Thyroglobulin is an iodine-containing protein from which thyroxine and triiodothyronine are derived. Thyroxine, a principal hormone secreted by the thyroid gland, enhances the capability of all food types for energy production and increases the rate of protein synthesis in most tissues. (Standard Process, Inc.)

GLANDULAR SUPPORT FOR WOMEN

DHEA-F. Contains 25 mg DHEA per capsule in a synergistic herbal base of wild yam, false unicorn, and chaste tree (the "F" indicates that this formula is for females). Nature's Sunshine developed this supplement especially for women to help optimize vitality and fight the damaging effects of free radicals — unstable molecules believed to be prime culprits in the aging process. DHEA (dehdroepiandrosterone) is a hormone precursor produced by the adrenal glands. It is converted to essential hormones in the body. After about age 25, the body's production of DHEA declines, leading many experts to believe that DHEA plays a role in the aging process. (Nature's Sunshine Products)

Monthly Maintenance.® Provides nutrients that may be especially beneficial just before and during a woman's monthly cycle. A daily intake of 18 capsules comes in a base of Chinese herbs: dong quai root, peony root, burpleurum root, hoelen plant, atractylodes rhizome, codonopsis root, alisma bark, licorice root, magnolia bark, ginger root, peppermint leaves, moutan root, gardenia fruit, and cyperus rhizome. (Nature's Sunshine Products)

Natural Changes. Around the age of 50, many women experience troublesome symptoms due to a gradual decrease in hormone levels. Natural Changes combines nutritional supplements for mature women in easy-to-use packets. The finest herbs, essential fatty acids, and antioxidant nutrients nourish the body naturally to help balance hormone levels and cope with changes. Each packet contains two capsules of C-X (black cohosh root, blessed thistle herb, Siberian ginseng root, false unicorn root, sarsaparilla root), one skeletal strength, one wild yam with chaste tree, one flax seed oil (provides essential fatty acids), and one Nutri-Calm (excellent source of vitamins B and C). (Nature's Sunshine Products)

Symplex F. A special combination formula containing Protomorphogen™ extracts from bovine ovary, adrenal, pituitary, and thyroid glands. The ovaries secrete several female sex hormones, including estrogen and progesterone. These hormones function in a feedback system balancing female sexual functions. Symplex F contains Protomorphogen extracts which are uniquely derived nucleoprotein-mineral extracts that support cellular health. Bovine ovary, adrenal, pituitary, and thyroid PMG™ extracts help maintain the healthy function of these corresponding organs and glands. A proprietary blend of magnesium citrate, bovine ovary PMG extract, bovine adrenal

PMG extract, and bovine thyroid PMG extract (processed to remove its thyroxine). (Standard Process, Inc.)

GLANDULAR SUPPORT FOR MEN

DHEA-M. Contains 25 mg of DHA (dehydroepiandrosterone) per capsule in a synergistic herbal base of sarsaparilla, saw palmetto, damiana, pumpkin seed, and panax ginseng (the "M" indicates that this formula is for males). The herbal base provides dietary factors that are uniquely valuable to men. Saw palmetto has been shown to support healthy prostate function. Pumpkin seed contains zinc, essential to male reproductive health. Sarsaparilla and damiana have been used by men for centuries, and the unique, energizing herb panax ginseng is known the world over for its contribution to optimal well-being. DHEA is a hormone precursor produced by the adrenal glands. After about age 25, the body's production of DHEA declines, leading many experts to believe that DHEA plays a role in the aging process. (Nature's Sunshine Products)

Symplex® M–PMG. A special combination formula containing Protomorphogen™ extracts from bovine orchic, adrenal, pituitary, and thyroid glands. The testes secrete several male sex hormones called androgens. These hormones function in a feedback system balancing male sexual functions. Simplex M contains Protomorphogen extracts which are uniquely derived nucleoprotein-mineral extracts that support cellular health. Bovine orchic, adrenal, pituitary, and thyroid PMG™ extracts help maintain the healthy function of these corresponding organs and glands. (Standard Process, Inc.)

KIDNEYS, THE URINARY SYSTEM

Kidney Activator. Nutritionally supports the urinary system, specifically bladder and kidney health. Parsley supports the functions of the kidneys and bladder and aids overall urinary health. Uva ursi supports urinary health and digestive health.

Juniper berries support the urinary system (especially the kidneys), helping the body's efforts to maintain proper fluid balance. Berries contain resin, tannins, vitamin C, B vitamins, phosphorus, sodium, selenium, and zinc. This combination is an herbal source of iron, manganese, potassium, sodium, vitamin A, and riboflavin. It contains juniper berries, parsley herb, uva ursine leaves, dandelion root, and chamomile flowers. (Nature's Sunshine Products)

Kidney Activator, Chinese. A Chinese combination of 14 herbs designed to support the urinary and lymphatic systems. A stressed water element causes swelling in the body and may lead to inflammation and burning. Kidney Activator is called *qu shi*, meaning "to get rid of dampness." It promotes kidney function and helps clear retained water from the body, which may positively affect joints. Its primary herbs include morus, areca, hoelen, alisma, and astragalus. The formula contains hoelen plant, chaenomeles fruit, astragalus root, alisma rhizome, areca peel, atractylodes rhizome, magnolia bark, polyporus plant, cinnamon twig, citrus peel, ginger rhizome, pinellia rhizome, and licorice root. (Nature's Sunshine Products)

Kidney Drainage. Provides the kidneys with the nutritional support they need to meet the constant stress placed on them. Every day the kidneys filter 200 liters of fluid from the bloodstream. They excrete toxins, metabolic wastes, and excess ions, and reabsorb necessary metabolic byproducts. These two bean-shaped structures also regulate the volume and chemical composition of the blood. Good nutrition and fluid intake support kidney function and promote proper waste removal and healthy tissue. Kidney Drainage contains asparagua officinalis to increase the rate of cellular activity and urine production, and plantain leaf to help relieve fluid buildup in the kidneys. Juniper berries support the urinary system as it works to maintain proper fluid balance. Goldenrod increases the production of urine without reducing levels of important electrolytes. (Nature's Sunshine Products)

Uva Ursi. The leaves of this mountain bush contain a substance known as arbutin, which is a helpful nutritional aid for the urinary system. Uva ursi contains vitamin A, iron, and manganese. It is also so high in tannin content that it has been used to tan leather. (Nature's Sunshine Products)

Urinary Maintenance. The nutrients in this herbal formula support the urinary system organs and help maintain the body's delicate fluid and mineral balance controlled by the kidneys. If the urinary system fails to function properly, the whole body feels the effects. As toxins accumulate, all body systems are subjected to a higher risk of intoxication. Urinary Maintenance supports the blood vessels and promotes urine flow. It may also help sanitize the urinary tract and boost the immune system. This key product for the urinary system incorporates the benefits of watermelon seed powder, asparagus, and dandelion leaf, making it an efficient diuretic.

Watermelon seed powder contains cucurbiatcins, which have been shown to possess remarkable properties. Watermelon seed also contains citrulline and arginine, both of which are thought to increase urea production in the liver, thus promoting the flow of urine.

Asparagus contains asparagine, which is a strong diuretic. It is also useful in helping to flush waste products accumulated in the joints of the body.

Dandelion leaf has diuretic, bile-flow stimulating, and blood-purifying properties. It promotes urine flow and facilitates the removal of toxins from the body through the kidneys. (Nature's Sunshine Products)

LIVER CLEANSING AND SUPPORT

A-F Betafood.® Contains beet juice which is a good source of betaine. Betaine has been shown to be an effective lipotrophic agent. Lipotrophic agents promote the transportation and use of fats, helping to prevent the accumulation of fat in the liver. Vitamin A has an important and specific effect on lipid metabolism. Vitamin F complex has been shown to be important in the metabolism of blood fats. This is a proprietary blend of carrot (root), dried beet (leaf) juice, beet (root), oat flour, calcium lactate, defatted wheat (germ), magnesium citrate, bovine prostate, nutritional yeast, bovine liver, bovine kidney, alfalfa flour, bovine orchic extract, bovine liver fat extract, flax seed oil extract, mixed tocopherols, and soy bean lecithin. (Standard Process, Inc.)

Dandelion. A member of the sunflower family. Herbalists consider this plant one of the most nutrient-rich in the plant kingdom. The whole plant is edible—the flowers, leaves, and roots. Dandelion supports digestion and nourishes the liver. The herb is a source of potassium, calcium, iron, manganese, magnesium, silicon, phosphorus, and sodium. The leaves are a richer source of vitamin A than carrots and contain some B, C and D vitamins. (Nature's Sunshine Products)

Livaplex®. Helps support the complex and countless functions of the liver and contains the complete vitamin A complex in addition to more than ten other important nutrients for liver support. Livaplex combines exclusive animal tissue extracts, such as the bovine liver fat extract yakriton, with additional supportive nutritional concentrates from whole food sources.

The liver, the largest organ in the body, is the site of numerous metabolic functions. The liver plays a vital role in digestion, carbohydrate and fat metabolism, the storage of nutrients, and detoxification. Livaplex is primarily a liver support product. Proprietary blend of bovine liver PMG™ extract, Spanish black radish (root), bovine liver, calcium lactate, beet (root), carrot (root), tillandsia usneoides, dried beet (leaf) juice, betaine hydrochloride, magnesium citrate, choline bitartrate, soy (bean), oat flour, bovine kidney, bovine prostate, bovine adrenal Cytosol™ extract, defatted wheat (germ), bovine liver fat extract, bovine orchic extract, ascorbic acid, flax seed oil extract, and mixed tocopherols. (Standard Process, Inc.)

Liver Cleanse Formula. Consists of herbs historically used to cleanse, detoxify, and nourish the liver and provide support to the gastrointestinal tract. The combination is an herbal source of calcium, iron, magnesium, phosphorus, potassium, silicon, sodium, riboflavin, and vitamin A. This combination contains red beet root, dandelion root, parsley herb, horsetail herb, yellow dock root, black cohosh root, birch leaves, blessed thistle herb, angelica root, chamomile flowers, gentian root, and goldenrod herb. (Nature's Sunshine Products)

Liver Formula (LIV-J). The liver is a filtering organ. LIV-J is an herbal blend specially formulated to support digestion, support and cleanse the digestive system, and nourish the liver and spleen. These herbs are rich in essential vitamins and minerals, including chromium, iron, magnesium, potassium, silicon, sodium, and vitamin A. LIV-J contains dandelion root, barberry bark, rose hips, fennel seeds, horseradish root, parsley herb, and red beet root. (Nature's Sunshine Products)

Liver Balance, Chinese. A Chinese combination of 12 herbs designed to support the needs of a stressed wood constitution. The Chinese call this formula *tiao he*, which means "harmonizing." This formula supports both the digestive and nervous systems, optimizing liver health and reducing stress. Its primary herbs — scute, peony, bupleurum, and atractylodes — help normalize the nervous system during mental agitation and normalize the upper digestive system during tension and distress. It contains bupleurum root, peony root, pinellia rhizome, cinnamon twig, dang gui root, fushen plant, scute root, zhishi fruit, atractylodes rhizome, panax ginseng root, ginger rhizome, and licorice root. (Nature's Sunshine Products)

Milk Thistle Combination. Provides nutrients that must be present for the liver to perform its 500 or more functions. This longtime favorite boasts the same liver-protecting and free-radical-fighting ingredients, plus N-acetyl-cystine. N-acetyl-cystine optimizes the production of glutathione in the liver. Glutathione is used in the breakdown and elimination of toxins in the body. N-acetyl-cystine is also a powerful antioxidant that helps support the liver and eyes, prevents nerve degeneration, and protects against oxidative damage.

Milk thistle helps protect the liver from the toxins it collects and breaks down. It contains a constituent called silymarin, which has been the subject of numerous studies. Silymarin helps liver cells regenerate and stabilizes liver cell membranes. It actually changes the structure of the outer liver cell membrane, preventing toxins and poisons from entering the cell. Vitamin A and vitamin C are mixed in a base of milk thistle extract (80% silymarin), N-acetyl-cysteine, dandelion root, choline bitartrate, and inositol. (Nature's Sunshine Products)

Milk Thistle Time-Release. Provides a consistent supply of silymarin (a constituent of milk thistle) to the liver, giving it nourishment and protection against ingested toxins. The liver performs 500-plus functions, including filtering and destroying toxins in the body. Providing it with proper nutrients allows this essential organ to function at top capacity. Silymarin has shown remarkable ability to help liver cells regenerate and to stabilize liver cell membranes. Research shows that it actually changes the structure of the outer liver cell membrane, preventing toxins and poisons from entering the interior of the cell. It also stimulates protein synthesis in liver cells, which generates DNA and RNA. This helps regenerate damaged liver cells. As an antioxidant, silymarin is at least ten times more powerful that vitamin E. (Nature's Sunshine Products)

Tiao He Cleanse.® A ten-day nutritional program designed to help the body achieve *tiao he*—balance and harmony. It combines Chinese nutritional and Western herbal experience. *Tiao He Cleanse* is designed to support the cleansing mechanisms of the body by targeting the intestinal, digestive, and circulatory systems. Each packet contains one capsule each of Chinese Liver Balance, All-Cell Detox, LBSII, psyllium hulls, burdock root, and black walnut hulls. (Nature's Sunshine Products)

LYMPHATIC SYSTEM CLEANSING

Lymph Gland Cleanse. Provides nutrients that help strengthen and improve glandular function and promote optimal immunity. Parthenium has often been confused with echinacea because both herbs have similar immune-boosting properties. Lymph Gland Cleanse provides an herbal source of chromium, cobalt, manganese, selenium, silicon, and zinc. It's also high in riboflavin and vitamin C. Lymph Gland Cleanse contains parthenium root, goldenseal root, yarrow flowers, and capsicum fruit. (Nature's Sunshine Products)

Lymph Gland Cleanse–HY. Helps meet the nutritional needs of a stressed immune system and is particularly helpful to the lymphatic and respiratory systems. The herbal components provide a natural source of chromium, cobalt, manganese, selenium, silicon, zinc, and varying amounts of riboflavin and vitamin C. It consists of parthenium root, yarrow flowers, myrrh gum, and capsicum fruit. (Nature's Sunshine Products)

PARASITES

Artemisia Combination. Combines all the herbal components of Nature's Sunshine's former Elecampane Combination with two species of artemisia — wormwood and mugwort. These herbs contribute to a friendly environment for intestinal flora. Add to them elecampane root, clove flower buds, garlic bulb root, ginger root, spearmint herb, and turmeric root, and you have a more powerful product. Artemisia is used in China, Europe, and the U.S. (Nature's Sunshine Products)

Black Walnut. A rich source of the trace mineral chromium and is also high in iodine. The ancient Greeks used the hulls to support the intestinal system and to treat skin infections. Herbalists classify black walnut as an astringent because it is rich in tannin, a toning substance. Black walnut's fame in folk medicine is due to its cleansing properties. The unripe hulls of the black walnut are high in vitamin C. (Nature's Sunshine Products)

Clear Combination.™ This is an ancient herbal recipe that has been documented as being used for over 600 years. This is a clinically tested combination currently being used by physicians, veterinarians, health professionals, and colon specialists throughout the U.S. and Canada. It contains green hull/black walnut, black seed, cloves, cramp bark, fennel seed, hyssop, pumpkin seed, peppermint leaves, gentian root, thyme, grapefruit seed, and bee pollen. (Awareness Corporation)

Garlic. Garlic is a member of the family that includes onions, leeks, and shallots. This prized herb possesses antibiotic, antiviral, antibacterial, and antifungal properties. Garlic is a source of selenium, which must be present in the body for proper immune response. (Nature's Sunshine Products)

Herbal Pumpkin. This herbal combination helps make the intestines inhospitable to foreign invaders. Pumpkin, black walnut, and chamomile help create this inhospitable environment, while the other five herbs help cleanse and lubricate the colon to optimize intestinal function and health. Herbal pumpkin contains varying amounts of magnesium, phosphorus, selenium, and zinc, and is a source of vitamins A and C. It contains pumpkin seeds, black walnut hulls, cascara sagrada bark, violet leaves, chamomile flowers, mullein leaves, marshmallow root, and slippery elm bark. (Nature's Sunshine Products)

Para-Cleanse, Chinese. A ten-day program designed to support the efforts of the intestinal system in removing unwanted guests. This carefully formulated herbal combination supports an intestinal environment that is not hospitable to foreign invaders. Each packet contains six capsules total, with: two capsules of herbal pumpkin combination (a blend of pumpkin seeds, black walnut hulls, cascara sagrada bark, violet leaf, chamomile flowers, mullein leaves, marshmallow root, and slippery elm bark); two capsules containing caprylic acid in a base of black walnut hulls, red raspberry leaves, and elecampane root (enterically coated for proper absorption); and two capsules of Elecampane Combination (a blend of elecampane bark, spearmint leaf, turmeric root, garlic bulb, ginger root, and clove bud). (Nature's Sunshine Products)

Verma and Para Systems. Used for over ten years throughout the world, the Verma and Para Systems are the number one choice by doctors, colon hydrotherapists, acupuncturists, iridologists, and health care practitioners. The Verma and Para lines have been specifically designed to eliminate *all* stages of parasitic infestation (from cysts to larvae to full-fledged parasites) throughout the body, not just the intestinal tract.

Verma capsule contains black walnut, wormwood, balmony, wormseed, cascara sagrada, slippery elm, garlic, cloves. *Verma tincture* contains black walnut, wormwood, centaury, male fern, orange peel, cloves, and butternut. *Para capsules* contains cranberry concentrate, grapefruit seed extract, artemisia annua, garlic cayenne, slippery elm, and bromelain. *Para tincture* contains black walnut, artemisia annua, prickly ash bark, quassia, cloves, and cranberry concentrate. (Uni-Key)

STRESS SUPPORT FOR THE NERVOUS SYSTEM

Exhilarin.® Designed for a healthy stress response. Exhilarin is a blend of standardized Ayurvedic herbs traditionally used as adaptogens that support a healthy stress response and adrenal function. (Metagenics)

Mood Elevator (Chinese Formula). Composed of 18 herbs traditionally used as a "fire-enhancing" combination to regulate and untrap *chi* (vitality). Its two key ingredients, bupleurum root and cyperus rhizome, support and nourish the liver, the organ (according to Chinese philosophy) that plays an integral role in mood. When the liver is functioning at its peak, mood may be improved. (Nature's Sunshine Products)

Spirulina. A blue-green algae that grows in warm, alkaline fresh waters around the world. Spirulina is 65 to 71% complete protein, compared to beef's 22% protein. The algae is a source of all eight essential amino acids, as well as chelated minerals, natural plant sugars, trace minerals, and enzymes. Spirulina is easily assimilated by the body. It contains potassium, calcium, zinc, manganese, selenium, iron, and phosphorus. It is also rich in chlorophyll. Spirulina can be used as a pre-meal supplement. It is one of the few plant sources of vitamin B12—a teaspoon supplies 2½ times the daily value—making it an excellent nutritional supplement for vegetarians whose diets usually lack vitamin B12. (Nature's Sunshine Products)

Stress-J. This anti-stress formula provides nutrients that must be present for proper functioning of the nervous system. The formula contains one of the most favored herbs of Europe, chamomile, which is known as the calming herb. This combination is designed for occasional stress relief. It is high in chromium, magnesium, and vitamins A and C. Stress-J works well with other supplements like B-complex vitamins, bee pollen, and extra vitamin C. It contains chamomile flowers, passion flowers, fennel seeds, feverfew herb, hops flowers, and marshmallow root. (Nature's Sunshine Products)

Stress Pack. When exposed to physical stress, the body uses more of certain nutrients like the B-complex family and vitamin C. That's why Stress Pack contains Nutri-Calm,® a supplement rich in both of these nutrients. Stress Pack combines herbs and vitamins to nourish the body under physical stress.

30 individual packets. Each packet contains:

◆ *Stress-J* (2 capsules). Contains chamomile flowers, passion flowers, hops flowers, fennel seeds, marshmallow root, and feverfew herb.

◆ *Suma Combination* (2 capsules). Contains suma root, astragalus root, Siberian ginseng root, ginkgo leaves, and gotu kola herb.

◆ *Nutri-Calm* (1 tablet). Contains vitamin C, B1, B2, B6, B12, folic acid, biotin, niacinamide, and panthothenic acid in a base of schizandra fruit, choline bitartrate, PABA, wheat germ, bee pollen, valerian root, passion flower, inositol, hops flowers, and citrus bioflavonoids.

◆ *Hops Concentrate* (1 capsule). Standardized to 5% alpha bitter acid. Each capsule contains hops concentrate plus hops herb. (Nature's Sunshine Products)

Stress Relief (Chinese formula). A Chinese combination of 16 herbs and natural substances designed to support emotional balance and calm a stressed fire constitution. The Chinese call this formula *an shen,* which means "to pacify the spirit." These herbs nourish the nervous system and subsequently help improve gastric function and strengthen the urinary system. Its primary nutrients — polygonum, dragon bone, oyster shell, haliotis shell, and fushen — help normalize mental function and strengthen the cardiovascular system. Stress Relief contains dragon bone, oyster shell, albizzia bark, polygonum stem, fushen plant, acorus rhizome, curcuma root, haliotis shell, panax ginseng root, polygala root, saussurea root, zizyphus seed, coptis rhizome, cinnamon bark, ginger rhizome, and licorice root. This formula is commonly used in conjunction with vitamin B complex, vitamin C, passion flower herb, chamomile flowers, skullcap herb, and hops flowers. (Nature's Sunshine Products)

VITAL NUTRITIONAL SUPPORT

Cellular Energy. Contains vitamins, minerals, amino acids, and other co-factors involved in vital processes that regulate normal energy production and cellular metabolism. In addition to their nutritional value, the ingredients in Cellular Energy exert reasonable antioxidant effects that may help address some of the metabolic issues that affect energy production. The B vitamins in Cellular Energy perform important functions in cellular energy metabolism. Manganese and magnesium support muscular and skeletal systems, while zinc universally supports all body systems—either as an integral part or as a component of enzymes, hormones, and body fluids. People who experience fatigue, reduced stamina, feelings of weakness, or who need an energy boost for prolonged physical activity could benefit from supplementing their diet with Cellular Energy. It provides the most bioavailability forms of the vitamins and minerals needed to boost cellular metabolism. Cellular Energy contains vitamins B1, B2, E, niacin, pantothenic acid, zinc, manganese, magnesium, ferulic acid, alpha lipoic acid, alpha-ketoglutaric acid, L-carnitine, coenzyme-Q10, and dimethyl glycine. (Nature's Sunshine Products)

Colloidal Minerals. Helps meet your body's need for active enzyme systems, chemical balance, maintenance and repair of all body systems, and minerals to act with the body's many metabolic regulators. NSP Colloidal Minerals is made with the finest particle-size colloids that are ready for assimilation into the body, providing enhanced mineral supplementation in an economical, great-tasting lemon-lime flavor. These minerals come from ancient plant deposits; minerals are balanced by nature. It contains a full spectrum of macro and trace minerals, many of which are required for daily cell function and structure. pH balanced for maximum benefit. (Nature's Sunshine Products)

Coral Calcium. Designed especially for those who battle to keep their acidity levels within a normal range. Because Coral Calcium has a natural pH range of 10 to 11, it has an alkalizing effect on the body, which can be of great support to those who need to offset acidity levels. Plus it provides essential calcium to help maintain bone integrity and health. Scientific studies show that regular exercise and a healthy diet with adequate dietary minerals, such as those contained in Coral Calcium, can promote bone health. (Nature's Sunshine Products)

Super Algae. Packs all the benefits of the three most popular algae supplements on the market today. Algae is a super-food bursting with easily assimilable nutrients, including protein. Spirulina is often added to food for its nutritional value. Chlorella is a freshwater green algae noted for its chlorophyll content. The blue-green algae comes from pristine Klamath Lake in Oregon. Super Algae maximizes protein, amino acid, chlorophyll, and beta-carotene content of each algae species, providing a balanced, nutritional formula. Super Algae also boosts the immune system by stimulating macrophage activity. (Nature's Sunshine Products)

Super Supplemental Vitamins and Minerals. Augments any diet. Balanced nutrients are often in short supply during periods of physical stress or convalescence, or in a diet consisting of mostly processed foods. Supplementing your diet with Super Supplemental can help fill the void. This supplement is contained in a base of alfalfa herb, asparagus powder, barley grass juice, broccoli powder, cabbage powder, hesperidin, lemon bioflavonoids, rutin, rose hips, wheat germ, and kelp. (Nature's Sunshine Products)

Target Endurance Formula. A caffeine-free nutritional supplement to support the physiological needs of the body during strenuous activity. Organic target minerals are chelated to specific amino acids, making them more readily absorbed by the body. In this formula, copper, potassium, and zinc are chelated to the amino acids arginine, leucine, and glycine, all of which are required to produce energy in the cells. Copper and zinc are balanced for optimal use in the body. Potassium is important in the transmission of nerve impulses, muscle contractions, and blood pressure regulation. Zinc is stored in rather large amounts in the bones and muscles as well as the prostate and retina. It appears to be easily depleted and is important for many enzyme functions. The target minerals have been combined with a unique blend of bee pollen, Siberian ginseng root, gotu kola herb, capsicum fruit, licorice root, glutamine, and choline bitartrate. (Nature's Sunshine Products)

Ultimate GreenZone.® By combining protein-rich ingredients like amaranth seeds, brown rice, millet, and spirulina, with vitamin-rich food stuffs including carrots, broccoli, acerola fruit, and lemon bioflavonoids, NSP has created Ultimate GreenZone, a meal that is easily absorbed and metabolized into energy that you can feel almost instantly. It offers suitable meal replacement for dieters and provides additional nutrients and energy for people who are always on the go. Its fiber content helps your body maintain normal-range cholesterol levels and promotes bowel evacuation along with a healthy colon. Ultimate Green-Zone also provides digestive enzymes to support proper digestion. (Nature's Sunshine Products)

Vitamin C. An antioxidant that performs many functions involving the immune system and tissue development. It is involved in iron absorption and in the synthesis of enzymes, hormones, and proteins. The adrenal glands need large amounts of this nutrient. Water-soluble, it is easily washed from the body and needs to be replaced constantly. Without vitamin C, the body cannot make collagen, the substance that holds the body's cells together. It works best with attending bioflavonoids. Time-release formulations offer the advantage of a more consistent and efficient use of the vitamin by the body. (Nature's Sunshine Products)

WEIGHT LOSS

Cellu-Smooth® with Coleus. Provides nutrients that combine to support circulation, mobilize fat and lymph stores for better distribution, and protect against free radical damage to structural skin proteins. Coleus forskohlii root extract causes a shift from a more fatty body mass to a more lean body. The effect can be measured by decreases in the waist-hip ratio and the body mass index.

Cellu-Smooth also contains bladderwrack, which nourishes the thyroid gland with iodine, thereby supporting metabolism; milk thistle, which acts as an antioxidant, detoxifying the liver and aiding elimination; ginkgo leaves, known free radical scavengers; rhodiola root extract, which may improve strength and stamina; and rhododendron root, a powerful antioxidant that promotes microcirculation. (Nature's Sunshine Products)

Collatrim Plus® Liquid. Provides nutrients that help burn fat, promote energy, and increase lean muscle mass. This comprehensive formula boasts conjugated linoleic acid (CLA), which increases metabolic rate and reduces fat storage. It also promotes the burning of fat in fat cells and the building of lean body mass. Collatrim Plus also contains collagen, which is broken down into amino acids, which are used to build lean muscle mass. Collagen also helps support cartilage, tendons, and heart muscle tissues, and improves skin texture. Another ingredient, L-carnitine, boosts energy, helps reduce the accumulation of lactic acid in the muscles, and is good for heart health.

Garcinia cambogia contains hydroxycitric acid, which inhibits an enzyme that helps the body synthesize fat for storage in adipose tissue. Hydroxycitric acid also promotes energy, lowers the rate of production of cholesterol, and has an appetite-suppressing effect. It also contains aloe vera juice, citric acid, and natural flavoring. (Nature's Sunshine Products)

Carbo Grabbers.™ Now you can partially block the digestion of dietary starches with all-natural Carbo Grabbers. Carbo Grabbers contains an amylase inhibitor derived from phaseolus vulgaris, northern white kidney beans. It naturally and safely prevents the digestion of starchy carbohydrates and reduces the available calories your body may otherwise covert to fat. Carbo Grabbers helps prevent weight gain from carbohydrate (starch) intake. Because carbohydrate breakdown is mostly blocked, undigested starches are carried into the intestinal tract where the body can eliminate them.

Recent studies have shown that the equivalent of two capsules of this white bean extract effectively blocks 50% of the carbohydrates in a meal. Another study showed a ten-pound-per-month weight loss without any change in diet or exercise. In these studies, the amylase inhibitor also reduced after-meal increases in plasma concentrations of glucose and insulin. (Nature's Sunshine Products)

Fat Grabbers.® An ideal product for anyone wanting to absorb less fat from their everyday diet. No stimulants, no questionable ingredients — just wholesome nutritional substances that won't disrupt normal body processes. Fat Grabbers combines the high-quality fiber found in guar gum and psyllium hulls with chickweed and lecithin for a unique formula that traps fat molecules inside the intestinal tract before they can get into the bloodstream. Extensive research on guar gum and psyllium hulls indicates their effectiveness in minimizing the absorption of fat. Lecithin is a nutrient that works to break down fat, making it easier for the fibers to trap it. Chickweed contains saponins that also act as fat emulsifiers. Using Fat Grabbers in conjunction with a sensible dietary plan will help you create an effective overall weight-management program. All elements of Fat Grabbers provide nutrients to help maintain cholesterol levels already within the normal range and absorb less dietary fat, and they all enjoy a long history of safe use. (Nature's Sunshine Products)

Garcinia Combination. Boasts garcinia cambogia fruit as its chief ingredient. Numerous studies show that garcinia can be beneficial for weight management. Research on hydroxy citric acid (garcinia's key component) shows three benefits for weight management. It (1) decreases appetite, (2) inhibits the conversion of excess carbohydrates into fat, and (3) increases stores of the body's energy fuel (glucose). Nature's Sunshine combines garcinia with chickweed (offers nutritional support for weight management), L-carnitine (helps in the transport of long-chain fatty acids), and chromium (plays a key role in regulating blood sugar levels already within the normal range). The garcinia in this combination has been standardized to 50% hydroxy citric acid. (Nature's Sunshine Products)

Nature's Cleanse. A safe, convenient cleansing program for those who want to promote natural, healthy elimination; support normal glandular function; nourish the liver and digestive system; and get the most nutrition out of their food. Nature's Cleanse contains fiber, herbs, and other nutrients. Nature's Cleanse contains Bowel Detox, Master Gland Formula, Enviro-Detox, Liver Cleanse Formula, LBSII, SF,® and chromium. (Nature's Sunshine Products)

Nature's Syner-Slim (ephedra-free). Developed to help burn excess fat without the use of ephedra. It promotes increased thermogenesis, helps the body lower its weight set point, eliminates excess fat from the diet, decreases appetite, slows the conversion of carbohydrates into fat, and encourages the removal of trapped toxins under the skin. The products contained in this prepackaged formula are Slim-chi, 7-Keto,™ Fat Grabbers, Cellu-Smooth, and Garcinia Combination. (Nature's Sunshine Products)

7-Keto.™ A safe metabolite of dehydroepiandrosterone (DHEA). It is produced naturally by the adrenal glands, but levels of 7-Keto decline significantly with age. 7-Keto boosts the level of T3 thyroid hormone, which has the greatest effect on the body's metabolic rate. It is needed to help the body lower its fat storage set point, which governs the body's efforts to maintain ideal weight. The body works to meet this fat set point daily. 7-Keto also helps prevent muscle atrophy and boosts immune function. Clinical tests indicate that 100 mg of 7-Keto taken twice a day significantly lowered body fat over an eight-week study period. People who participated in the study group lost about three times as much fat as those in the control group. It is important to note that unlike other metabolites of DHEA, 7-Keto is not converted to sex hormones (either androgens or estrogens). (Nature's Sunshine Products)

Caution: Those with hyperthyroidism should consult their health care professional prior to use of 7 Keto™ capsules. 7 Keto™ is a trademark of the Humanetics Corporation, Patent No 5,296,481.

SF®–Skinny Formula. Designed to support the body's weight control mechanisms, it also benefits the urinary and digestive systems. SF® provides chromium, fiber, iron, magnesium, manganese, silicon, and zinc. Natural fibers, oils, enzymes, and vitamins add to the nutritional value of this product. SF contains chickweed herb, cascara sagrada bark, licorice root, safflower flowers, black walnut hulls, parthenium root, gotu kola herb, hawthorn berries, papaya fruit, fennel seeds, and dandelion root. (Nature's Sunshine Products)

◆ ◆ ◆

I am not diagnosing or prescribing to you. Many of these herbs and supplements can be ordered on your own and many are only available through health practitioners. Please consult the resource guide for information on obtaining any of these company's products.

All growth is a leap in the dark,
a spontaneous, unpremeditated act
without benefit of experience.

– Henry Miller

Putting It All Together: Let the Magic Begin

*Let's dare to be ourselves, for we do
that better than anyone else can.*

– Shirley Briggs

To be nobody but myself, in a world which is doing its best night and day to make me everybody else, means to fight the hardest battle which any human being can fight and never stop fighting.

– E.E. Cumings

CHAPTER 24

■ ■ ■ ■ ■ ■ ■ ■ ■ ■

On the Lighter Side ...

I have been on a constant diet for the last two decades. I've lost a total of 789 pounds. By all accounts I should be hanging from a charm bracelet.

— Erma Bombeck

You, too, have made a career of dieting and exercising. It is time to lighten up a little and break the tension. It's time to laugh at ourselves, it gets our endorphins going. I do not want to offend anyone here; this is all in good fun. I use my past behaviors to springboard us into the outrageous and absurd.

With my love of the theater and outrageous flair for comedy, I have always used humor to deal with issues in my life. This is where the silly-nilly mischievous little girl in me comes out to play. As Tony Robbins would say, "She always plays *full out.*"

I have created a persona, Greta Carbo,™ who is the queen of extreme! She is a 1940s vamp carbo addict (and proud of it), and has major attitude. Greta sings and writes songs about food and her favorite pastime: *eating!* She makes a complete mockery of the advice to eat healthy and exercise. As a matter of fact her motto is: "Donuts are a girl's best friend—life is too short to diet and exercise." Following are some excerpts of her soon-to-be world-famous book and CD by the same name.

Greta has used this diet successfully with herself and all her friends to keep them big, beautiful, and oh-so-sexy. It has taken her years of intense study of just the right food combinations for optimal weight gain. Oh, and by the way, if your man wants a Kate Moss model type, Greta says she has a song especially for him. It goes like this: *Hit the road Jack, and don't ya come back no more, no more, hit the road Jack, and don't ya come back no more!*

GRETA'S DREAM DIET*

Breakfast
+ ½ fresh pink grapefruit
+ 6 oz. of skim milk
+ 1 cup of Special Z cold cereal

Mid-morning snack
+ ½ protein bar

Lunch
+ 3½ oz. of broiled fish (no butter)
+ 1 cup steamed vegetables
+ 1 cup of green salad (nonfat dressing)
+ 3 Moreo cookies
+ Unsweetened herb tea

Mid-afternoon snack
+ Rest of the bag of *Moreos* cookies
+ ½ of leftover pizza right out of the carton
+ One quart of Bob & Gerry's Fudge Ripple low-fat frozen yogurt
+ One container of whipping cream

* Please consult with your physician before starting any new diet program.

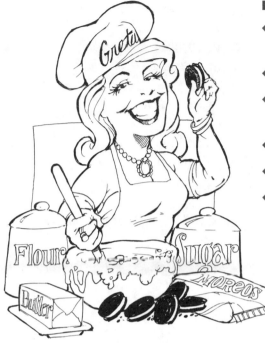

Dinner

◆ Large bucket of country fried chicken

◆ 1 loaf of garlic bread

◆ 1 large container of potato salad

◆ 4 cobs of corn

◆ 4 biscuits with gravy

◆ 1 large diet soda

Bedtime snack

◆ 1 diet soda

◆ 4 chocolate glazed donuts

DONUTS ARE A GIRL'S BEST FRIEND©

Lyrics written by Loree Taylor Jordan and sung to the tune of "Diamonds Are a Girl's Best Friend."

A kiss on the hand may be quite continental
But donuts are a girl's best friend
A kiss may be grand, but it won't cure the munchies
In those times of stress, or help you with that PMS
Men grown cold as girls grow fat
and we all lose our charms in the end
But large thighs or pear shape, we girls will lose our shape
Donuts are a girl's best friend
There may come a time when a lass tries to diet
but donuts are a girl's best friend
There may come a time when a well-meaning boyfriend
thinks you're awful fat,
get on that scale,

He'll leave you flat
He's your guy when weight is low
but beware when the scale starts to climb
That's why us lasses, have got big huge assets
Donuts are a girl's best friend
I've heard of affairs that are strictly low calorie
But donuts are a girl's best friend
and I think affairs that you must keep low calorie
are better bets, if little pets get big donettes
Time rolls on and youth is gone and you can't straighten up
when you bend
but stiff back or stiff knees you'll stand straight at . . . bakeries
Donuts . . . donuts . . .
I don't mean broccoli
But donuts are a girl's best . . . best friend.

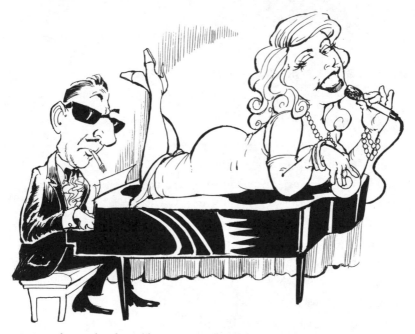

*Greta shamelessly self-promotes her glamorous vamp collection
of original songs such as "Donuts Are a Girl's Best Friend"©
with many personal appearances!*

KIDS: DON'T YOU JUST LOVE THEM?

I was in a clothing dressing room, and I had both of my sons with me. I was trying to squeeze into a pair of jeans; they were giving me a run for my money. *Squeeze* was the operative word here. I was panting and groaning, trying unsuccessfully to get the zipper up. The problem was that there was a jiggly jelly-belly (courtesy of childbirth—two C-sections) in the way. I was breaking out in a sweat because I was not, I tell you, *not* going to buy a bigger pant size. *No way José!*

The sales clerk came over to ask if I needed help. "No thank you," I gasped. *Maybe an oxygen mask or a paramedic standing by for me when I pass out from holding in my stomach!* I thought.

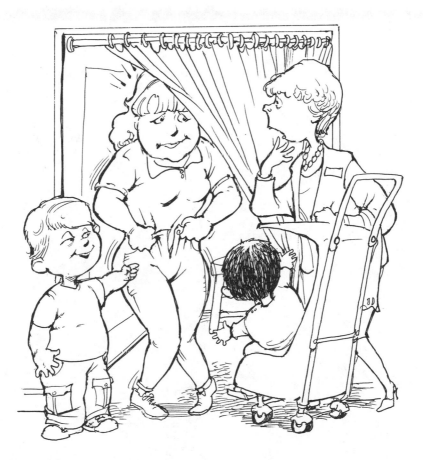

"Would you like to purchase those jeans ma'am?" she asked.

My older son, all of about three years old, emphatically stated to the sales clerk, complete with gestures, "My mommie can't wear those pants, because she is *too fat!*"

Thank you . . . Brandon!

◆ ◆ ◆

For more information about Greta's new lifestyle book and CD collection of her original songs, please see the resource guide at the end of this book.

Our entire life, with our fine moral code and our precious freedom, consists ultimately of accepting ourselves as we are.

– Jean Anouth

CHAPTER 25

■ ■ ■ ■ ■ ■ ■ ■ ■ ■

I Love ME!
Self-Honoring Behaviors

My previous marriage was give and take.
I gave . . . my husband took!

— Loree Taylor Jordan

Your kids have every toy or CD known to mankind, but when was the last time you took time out for a manicure or pedicure or both? When was the last time you just hung out and had a robe day? (For those of you unfamiliar with this term I coined, it is simple: hang out all day in your robe— don't get dressed). When was the last time you said yes when asked to do something that you didn't want to do, but if you didn't you would feel guilty?

Part of healing any disorder, whether it is emotional or physical, is an investment. An investment in yourself. There can be no payoff if the investment is never made. Use this chapter to take an inventory and see how you have fared with your "I love me" investment portfolio.

PERSONAL RELATIONSHIPS

Hopefully, you have not been and are not presently in a relationship that leaves you feeling emotionally bankrupt. If you are, I hope you will honor yourself enough to say, *"Next!"* Then move on. These behaviors will help motivate you to pack your suitcase or his or her suitcase—whichever the case may be.

Never love anyone else more than yourself. The affirmations that follow are designed for you to "fill your own cup" with positive and nurturing behaviors.

- I have loving, nourishing, supportive family members.

- I have healthy, intimate relationships with friends.

- I have at least one friend with whom I can share almost anything.

- I ask for help and support when I need it.

- I don't feel guilty if I set boundaries for myself with others.

- I express my feelings openly and honestly when appropriate.

- I don't feel guilty if I don't share the opinion of someone else.

- I realize that what you think of me is none of my business.

- I don't engage in codependent behavior.

- I love people for who they are and not who I think they should be.

- I don't allow others to verbally or physically abuse me.

- I am generous with myself and others.

- I generously tell others what I appreciate about them.

- I don't try to control others.

- I know that I alone can control my actions.

EMOTIONAL/FEELINGS

- I own my own feelings.

- I experience a wide range of emotions.

- I look for the humor in challenging situations.

- I laugh freely at myself.

- I allow myself fun time to just play at least twice a week.

- I maintain a realistic attitude and positive self-image.

- I rarely allow myself to experience jealousy of others.

- I readily forgive others for their mistakes.

- I readily forgive myself for my mistakes.

- I regularly donate money, food, my time, and other items to those less fortunate.

- I acknowledge myself as a spiritual being.

PHYSICAL/FITNESS

- I drink eight to ten glasses of purified water daily.

- I get seven to nine hours of restful sleep every night.

- I abstain from coffee, cigarettes, and recreational drugs.

- I limit alcohol to one or two times a week.

- I participate in exercise daily for at least 30 minutes.

- I take the stairs instead of the elevator.

- I regularly engage in physical activities I enjoy, such as yoga, meditation, and aerobics.

◆ I have a trainer or exercise buddy to help hold me accountable.

◆ I take my vitamins and supplements every day.

◆ I get a massage regularly to de-stress and take care of my body.

◆ I regularly see my dentist for prophylaxis (cleaning) and checkups.

◆ I regularly get chiropractic adjustments for structural support.

This following contract is good when you are making positive behavior changes. Make one up on your computer and tape a copy of it everywhere to remind yourself of the new pattern you are establishing.

My health/fitness contracts reads as follows:

> *I experience joy and serenity*
> *as I take a leisurely walk with Briggs and First*
> *Officer Riley.*
> *I commit to walking both dogs every day.*
>
> *Loree Taylor Jordan*

Your health/fitness contract:

I experience _____

as I _____ .

I commit to _____ .

Signed _____

Date _____

CONFIDENCE BOOSTERS

Many of you have allowed your excess weight or critical remarks by others to tug at your confidence and self-esteem. I know you are the same wonderful human being, whether you are dressed to the nines or in a T-shirt and jeans. However, when you feel better about how you look, it helps your confidence soar. I want your confidence to soar above the clouds, my friend.

- ◆ Recognize that you have unique qualities and deserve only the best in life. If you need to be reminded of your positive attributes, ask your friends and family to help you. Put your positive attributes on 3×5 cards and post them on your mirror to remind yourself how wonderful you truly are.

- ◆ Ladies, if you are not happy with your looks, change them. Get a new haircut, hairstyle, or color. Go to the mall and get a makeover or try some different makeup tips. Let your stylist or makeup artist assist you with styles and colors that will bring out your best. You will be magazine-cover perfect when they get done with you.

- ◆ Gentleman, if you need your confidence boosted, get a new haircut. Ask the women at the salon to help you look like the stud muffin that you are!

- ◆ Pamper yourself. Have a facial, or get a manicure and pedicure (I say all three). This can apply to men also. Personally guys, I think you should pass on the wild nail polish colors, but having your nails and cuticles manicured says you care about yourself. My suggestion, ladies, is that you put a date for salon services on your calendar and, barring an act of God, you need to make those appointments. If I leave the salon and say I will call for my next appointment, I get so busy that it gets shoved to the background. If your fingernails, toes, and face are well taken care of, it says, "I care about myself."

♦ Get a regular massage. This is a must. Schedule it regularly on the calendar in pen, and don't miss, cancel, or skip. It does a body good! I am a certified massage therapist and I know all the benefits to your body systems, lymph, circulation, and well-being that massage evokes. Besides, it feels so good!

♦ Try something new and daring to boost your self-confidence. Start taking kickboxing or tai kwon do, or learn to ski. Get your body moving in a way it has never experienced.

♦ Eliminate toxic people or associates who don't give you the appreciation you deserve. Who needs people around who are tearing you down, when you are trying so hard to build yourself up? What's wrong with them—don't they see how wonderful you are? *Lose them!*

♦ Look in the mirror at the most beautiful smile in the world . . . yours!

Show appreciation and gratitude for everything and everyone in your life. It is not selfish to love and take care of yourself. If you have tremendous love and respect for yourself and practice these behaviors, you will be an example to those around you.

Life is short and it is very fragile. You never know if life will grant you another day. Be grateful for another day of life and live it to the fullest.

CHAPTER 26

■ ■ ■ ■ ■ ■ ■ ■ ■ ■

Follow the Yellow Brick Road

*When you get to the end of your rope, tie a knot
and hang on. And SWING!*

– Leo Buscaglia

Believe me, from the bottom of my heart, we have all walked a mile in each other's shoes! Something in *Fat and Furious* spoke to you when you picked it up . . . something told you there is something here for you . . . some hope, some answers, something valuable to you. That is why you have embarked on this journey.

TOTO, WE'RE NOT IN KANSAS ANYMORE

You'll find like Dorothy did in *The Wizard of Oz*, you have the power to go home any time you choose—you just didn't know it. Dorothy didn't know clicking her ruby heels three times would get her back home to Kansas. Dorothy took a long, treacherous journey—just as many of you have—only to find out the great Wizard of Oz was an imposter (like your physician in the God-almighty white coat).

I wish I could tell you to just click your heels three times and you will be a size 10, but who would I be kidding? It won't be as instantaneous as clicking your heels or a magic wand passing over your head, but now you have the tools and the missing puzzle pieces to put together. Because you are unique, you will have your own combination of pieces that will make this all fit. The good news is, if you follow the yellow brick road you will come home to yourself. You may have been missing much longer than you were aware of.

TAKE A LEAP OF FAITH

Nothing can bring you peace, but yourself.

– Ralph Waldo Emerson

I have covered so many different scenarios in this book you may be a little overwhelmed. But my suggestion is that you start at the beginning. Start with your heart—that is where it all begins for us as human beings. If your heart is wounded, take a leap of faith and go into the dark. If you think all your issues are handled, but you see yourself in these mind games you can play with yourself (mentioned in the beginning of the book) or find yourself compulsively eating, trust me—your issues are there like cobwebs deep in your soul. It's time to do some deep soul-searching.

First and foremost, be gentle with yourself. You have been living in shame long enough. If you have used food as a way of coping with your emotions in the past, so be it. Don't be ashamed anymore of who you are. As a child, food was what was available to you when life got hairy and you did not know what to feel. It was the only anesthetic that was available to you.

You have to take the attitude: "I did the best I could with what I knew then. Now I have better information." That was then, now is now; the past does not equal the future.

I have opened my heart to you, and shared some very personal and painful pieces of my life, and those of others, so you can see what complex and emotional beings we truly are. In Chapter 3, Feelings Buried Alive Never Die, I shared some of my painful family issues that kept me emotionally immobilized for many years. Now that we have come to the end of our time together, I want to share with you the healing that can come from such a tremendous emotional catharsis.

When I came home from the John Bradshaw Center in Los Angeles I felt that I had left all that emotional baggage behind. When I walked in the door to the home I shared with my husband and two sons, I did not want the pain from the past to haunt me any longer. I wanted to be emotionally available to my family. I had healed, but I wanted to share my experience with the only living person still available to me, my father.

Months after I returned from Los Angeles my dad had come from Florida for a visit. I asked him to take a walk with me to the park so we could talk privately. I looked at him (with softness, not accusation) and said, "Dad, there are some things I need to share with you about what I experienced in my life growing up with you and Mom."

The first thing he said was, "Kiddo, I can tell you that I am not an alcoholic."

I said, "Dad, my experience has taught me that I grew up in an abusive alcoholic family."

"Dad," I said, "I am not here to put blame on anyone. I'm past that, but what I want is for you to hear my experience of certain events in my life that involve you and how it has affected me."

I gained a newfound respect for my dad that day. What I proceeded to tell him would not be easy for anyone to hear. The tone in my voice was soft and gentle—not accusatory or emotional. You have to understand that once you discharge the emotional pain of an event you can speak of it without all the emotionalism that was once attached to it. I told him some of the events that I experienced in our family from his abuse and his volatile temper when he was drinking.

The look on his face was like that of a little boy—very sad and ashamed. He honestly did not remember these incidents. His drinking had caused a lot of blackouts, which is common in alcoholism.

My goal was not to shame him but just speak my truth to him from my heart. Rather than get defensive and argue that these events did not occur, he expressed extreme regret and gently said, "Honey, I am so sorry."

"I know you are, Dad—no one wants to intentionally hurt his family," I said. "But the disease of alcoholism can take on a life of its own and tear up everyone in its path. Your drinking hurt me. It hurt our family."

He then admitted that he knew he had a drinking problem and had actually sought counseling in the years after my mother and he divorced. I feel grateful that he took care of himself to heal his wounds with a counselor.

My dad and I came to a healing that day out in the park and in the fresh air. Father and daughter shared thoughts and feelings that had been locked up for what seemed like a lifetime. I forgave my dad that day. I forgave my dad, as my father, a man who carried his wounded inner child deep within his heart.

As I shared with you earlier in the book, my dad recently passed away from colon cancer. As I write this book, he's now been gone a year. I'm grateful that we had those last days together to get closure and laugh about our lives as father and daughter. Yes, I wish had grown with the Ozzie and Harriet family, but I didn't, and forgiveness is a powerful tool.

LOVE YOURSELF NOW ... LIVE YOUR LIFE NOW ... STOP WAITING UNTIL ...

This is the hardest trap to avoid—waiting to feel good about yourself until you lose weight. You are beautiful or handsome right now . . . *today!* Not tomorrow, when you lose another half a pound (or in our case, an ounce if we're lucky!)— but now!

If you saw the movie *About Schmidt,* you saw a perfect example of a woman who is comfortable in her own skin and not a raving Hollywood model-type beauty, and that is Kathy Bates in the role of Roberta.

A showstopper in the movie comes in a hot tub scene featuring Kathy Bates, who has been the target of fat jokes in just about every one of Joan Rivers' Oscar-night fashion preview shows. Roberta (Bates) strips out of her caftan and plunks down naked next to Jack Nicholson in the hot tub. When I saw the movie, the theater exploded into applause as Roberta flashed her corpulence at Nicholson before submerging herself in the tub and leering at him.

Women were yelling and cheering "You go, girl!" but some of the loudest cheering came from the men. One fiftyish guy behind me said to his companion, "Now there's a *real* woman!" If you want real excitement, nothing beats Kathy Bates making Jack Nicholson very nervous in the hot tub.

I am not saying you should go flashing unsuspecting people in hot tubs, but you can learn something from Roberta—and that is *not* to apologize for who you are. One thing I've learned from being in the singles world is that there are lots of men (like the guy in the audience) who prefer—yes, I said *prefer*—more voluptuous, buxom, curvy type women. (I personally am going for the Marilyn Monroe or Greta Carbo look!)

I had the belief that if I did not weigh 115 pounds (and was not a size 4) I would never have a date. *Ever!* This was a limiting negative belief I had to let go of! It was limiting because I feared I would become a spinster living out my days writing books with rescued dogs and hundreds of screaming cats. Not true. I am never lacking for male attention and admiration because I have a great personality and choose to look and feel my best no matter what the scale says. It was an acquired skill not to beat myself up mercilessly; it did not happen overnight.

I feel healthier at a lower weight, as you might also, so I am continuing to work on balancing my hormonal system for optimal health, *not* to look like a magazine cover model. I addressed this issue in Chapter 5, The Shame Game, but it bears repeating. Never, I mean never, try to lose weight to please someone else. You are already fighting your biochemistry; you don't need to defend yourself against someone else's agenda.

BE WILLING AND OPEN TO THE PROCESS OF SUPPORT

Be willing to enroll in counseling, group therapy, or what-ever it takes to open yourself to hidden issues. You will have to tackle your weight issue on many levels. I suggest that you enroll a health care team to unravel all the missing pieces to get you on the road to weight loss success. You have got to find a physician who is willing to help you get to the root of your metabolic and emotional issues without using shame as a tool to get there.

If you are willing and open to the process, the weight will take care of itself. What you focus on, you get more of! If you focus and obsess on your weight, you will draw more of it. If you start looking at other positive things in your life, you will *feel* lighter. If you dwell in the negative (your weight) you will feel heavy, *heavy* on the inside. This is a delicate balancing act. You are so much more than a number on your scale. *Believe it!*

Many of you may not be food addicts, and all your issues *are* metabolic. In that case, some of this inner work may not apply to you. I mean no offense to anyone. It has just been my experience working with myself and others, that where there is smoke there is fire!

SEARCHING FOR DR. RIGHT!

Instead of the doctor interviewing you, *you* interview the doctor and his staff! Like the doctors who have contributed to this book, there are competent physicians and health professionals who can help you get to the root of your weight issues.

Here is a list of criteria for choosing a doctor or health care professional:

- Is he or she compassionate and caring?

- Does he or she show you respect?

- Can the doctor or staff show you measurable results with other patients facing metabolic challenges?

- Are appointments scheduled with adequate time to address all your questions and concerns? Does he or she *really* listen to you?

- Does he or she show genuine interest in viewing your health journal (remember the one you are keeping with all your statistics: food diary, moods, sleeping habits, exercise etc.)?

- Is he or she open to nutritional remedies rather than just prescriptions?

- Does he or she suggest another physician when your metabolic concerns are out of their field of expertise instead of having an ego and muddling their way through . . . at your expense?

Last but not least, trust your gut. Your gut feeling usually doesn't lead you astray. If you are feeling uneasiness for whatever reason, move on! It's, *"Next!"*

THIS TOO SHALL PASS

Hold your head high, stick your chest out. You can make it. It gets dark sometimes but morning comes . . . Keep hope alive.

– Jesse Jackson

When I was down to the finish line of this book (and revising another), everything that could go wrong, did! Plus more! My writing office is in my home, and one night I was sitting at my dining room table waiting for my dinner date to arrive (yes, even though I am writing books I still have to eat) when I heard this huge crash in my office! This was so loud I thought the three bookcases I had in there had toppled over. Well, that would have been good news compared to what I saw when I got the nerve to look. Half of the ceiling had collapsed with water pouring onto the floor (the air conditioning piping had come loose in the attic). The water was dousing the whole room, my reference books, bookcases, and my business equipment. I stood at the doorway in stunned silence, my mouth hanging open.

Well, you know what this means—insurance agents, filing claims, millions of phone calls, construction crews, pricing and replacing items—on and on and on it goes.

The office cave-in was on Wednesday and on Saturday (that same week) I had my gallbladder problem that had to be addressed with medical personnel in an emergency situation. The following week a water leak in my bathroom required the whole floor and shower to be ripped out. More construction crews, more insurance agents, pick out tile, paint, and shower doors—yada yada yada. All this *distraction* and *drama*. All this time I kept shouting in my head "No more, please . . . I am on two book deadlines! I have to concentrate! I can't take any more!" My friends keep telling me I should become a stand-up comedian because my life is such good material!

I finally got my *colon* out of a twisted knot from all this drama while I was trying to focus on finishing these two books. I had to put things in perspective. I still had a roof over my head and another usable bathroom. Yes, I had to go digging in sealed boxes to get to my reference material (packed from my office) while writing this book. Yes, it was annoying as hell to live in a construction site, but in the scheme of things, a minor bump in the road. It wasn't life or death, and it certainly wasn't a cancer diagnosis. I was grateful for what I have. So I told myself, Loree, *get over it!* And I did. Just more material for my new stand-up comedy routine or a new book!

And last but not least, *laugh!* I have used humor in this book because if we can laugh at ourselves and not take everything so seriously it lightens our load. Laughter is the best medicine. Remember, today's problems are good material to laugh about another day. I have always used silliness as a way to de-stress. Sometimes my sons look at me with that, "Okay . . . Mom has gone nuts" look, but by now they are used to it. They know who I am, and what are they going to do about it? Give me up for adoption?

ATTITUDE OF GRATITUDE

> *Attitude is everything. Mae West lived into her eighties believing she was twenty, and it never occurred to her that her arithmetic was lousy.*
>
> – *Soundings* magazine

As I was nearing the finish date for this book I will have to admit I was tired. I was working long hours and even longer days trying to make up for lost time. Like a marathon runner who has "hit the wall" everything started to blur together. I felt like I was only one step above a corpse! The fatigue started to make me question why I was expending all this energy writing this book.

Then I woke up one morning with just a few chapters left to write (coming to the finish line), and I got a surprise phone call. I stepped out of the shower to the sound of my cell phone ringing. As I bolted for the phone (naked as a jaybird) my only thought was, "Don't you dare slip and fall — you can't type with your arm in a cast!" (After all the drama I'd had in the last few months that would be the icing on the cake.)

The upshot of this incredible conversation was Tara (who is a colon therapist) was calling me from Oregon (I had not spoken with her for over a year) to tell me how much she appreciated me, and how grateful she was for the books I have written! She went on to tell me (for ten minutes) how much I "rocked her world" and what an inspiration I was to her. My book on detoxification, *Detox for Life,* was written to help colon therapists like her educate their clients. Tara's call reminded me that I am doing my soul's work, and why I put all my energy into writing books and educating others. I am also very grateful to Tara for her support and her loving spirit to step forward and share her appreciation of me. Wow! Timing really is everything!

It was her sincere and genuine gratitude for what I have brought to her life that pumped life into this corpse. You don't

> **Develop an attitude of gratitude.**
> **If you look to others for fulfillment,**
> **You will never truly be fulfilled.**
> **If your happiness depends on money,**
> **You will never be happy with yourself.**
> **Be content with what you have;**
> **Rejoice in the way things are.**
> **When you realize there is nothing lacking,**
> **The whole world belongs to you.**
>
> **— Lao Tzu**

THE GIFTS OF GRATITUDE

Gratitude unlocks the fullness of life.

It turns what we have into enough, and more.

It turns denial into acceptance, chaos into order, confusion to clarity . . .

Gratitude makes sense of our past, brings peace for today, and creates a vision for tomorrow.

– Melody Bettie

think I had energy and motivation to write like a whirlwind after a call like that?

When you experience a sense of gratitude, the more endorphins and the less adrenaline you will pump into your system, and you'll have a longer, healthier life. As you count your blessings and become grateful, you literally bathe yourself in positive healing hormones. Who can you tell today with all sincerity and gratitude how much they have contributed to your life? There is no time like the present to make that call.

I am grateful that I have all of you, and that we have each other, in support and healing. You are truly a miracle. Thank you for allowing me to share with you part of my heart and soul on my journey. If, in the process of this journey, I have lightened your load, brightened your spirit, given you hope, or made you laugh, I am truly blessed.

> *I believe in the sun even when it isn't shining.*
> *I believe in love even when I am alone.*
> *I believe in God even when He is silent.*
>
> – World War II refugee

Afterword

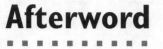

The alternative medicine approach does not focus exclusively on diet, but rather recognizes that obesity is caused by multiple factors that overload your body systems. Unlike conventional medicine, alternative medicine physicians know that it will be impossible to lose weight safely and permanently without first correcting any underlying imbalances. They set about to identify these factors—from colon and liver toxicity to an underactive thyroid or hormone imbalances—through precise, nontoxic tests. Once the underlying factors have been pinpointed, a treatment plan can be designed to address each one. Instead of another fad diet, alternative medicine goes to the root causes and so can provide a real and lasting solution to weight problems.

In this book, you have learned how alternative medicine physicians reversed weight problems using an individualized, holistic approach. You read success stories of people who finally found the answers to their weight problems after years of frustration with dieting and the conventional approach to obesity. You too can have successful weight loss. God bless.

– Burton Goldberg, publisher, *An Alternative Guide to Weight Loss, and Alternative Medicine Digest,* www.alternativemedicine.com

Resource Guide
■ ■ ■ ■ ■ ■ ■ ■ ■ ■ ■ ■ ■ ■ ■

ALTERNATIVE NUTRITIONAL AND METABOLIC HEALTH PROFESSIONALS AND PHYSICIANS

I want to mention that these health professionals were asked *by me* to provide all their contact information, websites, and book ordering information so you may contact them if you feel that they may be able to help you. My commitment to *you* is to assist you in finding the help you need. You never know—one of these professionals might be right around the corner from you!

American Association of Clinical   (904) 384-9490
   Endocrinologists   www.aace.com
2589 Park Street
Jacksonville, FL 32204

American Holistic Medical Association   (703) 556-9728
6728 Old McLean Village Drive   www.holisticmedicine.org
McLean, VA 22101

American Holistic Nurses Association   (800) 278-AHNA
P.O. Box 2130   www.ahna.org
Flagstaff, AZ 86003-2130

Joseph Debé, DC   (516) 829-1515
38 Great Neck Rd.   www.drdebe.com
Great Neck, NY 11021

    Dr. Joseph Debé is dedicated to helping you reach your health potential by combining cutting-edge scientific evaluation with holistic natural therapies. He is a chiropractor and board-certified nutritionist.

Dr. Debé is available for telephone consultations with those who cannot visit in person. Visit his website for articles on nutrition, metabolism, and health. Dr. Debé is the author of THE ULTIMATE CREATINE HANDBOOK: THE SAFE ALTERNATIVE FOR HEALTHY MUSCLE BUILDING.

Endocrine Society   (301) 941-0200
4350 East West Highway, Suite 500   www.endo-society.org
Bethesda, MD 20814

Howard E. Hagglund, MD   (405) 329-4457
1818 W. Lindsey, Suite #C-100   www.doctortalk.com
Norman, OK 73069

Dr. Hagglund is a respected authority on thyroid disease and has had many years of experience treating hypothyroid patients. Dr. Hagglund is also an author and broadcaster who works to educate physicians and patients about thyroid disease diagnosis and treatment.

He has been a practicing medical doctor in the field of family practice since 1976, specializing in allergies and metabolic diseases; and is sole owner of the Hagglund Clinic in Norman, Oklahoma.

He is the author of WHY DO I FEEL SO BAD (WHEN THE DOCTOR SAYS I'M O.K.?), which explains health in its broadest aspect; and is co-author of HELP! I FEEL AWFUL.

John Hipps, MD   (814) 486-2084
General Practice   fax (814) 486-2438
314 East Fourth Street   www.thecountrydoctor.com
P.O. Box 189
Emporium, PA 15834

Dr. John Hipps takes a common-sense, compassionate approach to medicine. He practices medicine with a caring *"country doctor" approach to health care problems related to the toxic environment of foods, air, water, home, and workplace. He devotes special expertise to victims with chronic pain and fatigue, and fibromyalgia, and has an active practice in Emporium, Pennsylvania, where he promotes the physical, psychological, and spiritual well-being of his patients.*

He also has an active public speaking schedule, and provides popular seminars on many aspects of modern and old-fashioned health care practices. He is the author of THE COUNTRY DOCTOR: ALIVE AND WELL. *For more information about Dr. Hipps and his books or other writings see contact information.*

Dr. Honeyman-Lowe   (303) 413-9100
Center for Metabolic Health   www.drlowe.com
1800 30th Street, Suite 217-A
Boulder, CO 80301

Dr. Honeyman-Lowe has specialized in metabolic rehabilitation of hypometabolic patients diagnosed with fibromyalgia, chronic fatigue, hypothyroidism, and thyroid hormone resistance since 1996. Besides clinical practice, she places a priority on public education about these disorders through lectures and radio interviews. Dr. Honeyman-Lowe is an active participant in ongoing clinical trials involving the metabolic rehabilitation of hypothyroid and thyroid hormone resistant patients. Dr. Honeyman-Lowe is the co-author of YOUR GUIDE TO METABOLIC HEALTH: A COMPANION BOOK TO THE METABOLIC TREATMENT OF FIBROMYALGIA *by Dr. John C. Lowe.*

YOUR GUIDE TO METABOLIC HEALTH may be ordered at www.McDowellPublishing.com or you can request that your local bookstore order it for you. Its companion book, THE METABOLIC TREATMENT OF FIBROMYALGIA *by Dr. John C. Lowe, can be found at the same site. You can also call McDowell Publishing Co. at (303) 570-7231 to place orders directly.*

Drs. Honeyman-Lowe and Lowe provide telephone consultations for patients and/or their local doctors so people who cannot visit their clinic can learn about metabolic rehabilitation. Their website, www.drlowe.com, has information about treatment and consulting options. Consultations are by appointment and may be scheduled through Diane Patterson, office manager.

Ralph J. Luciani, DO, MS, Ph.D.   (505) 298-5995
The Albuquerque Clinic   info@abqclinic.com
2301 San Pedro NE, Suite G
Albuquerque, NM 87110

Dr. Ralph Luciani graduated from Seton Hall University in 1963, and graduated as valedictorian from medical school at the College of Osteopathic Medicine in Kansas City, Missouri. He became board-certified in Family Practice in 1976. In 1973 and 1974 he studied Oriental Medicine both here and in the Orient and received a Ph.D. in Medical Acupuncture in 1974 for his research in pain and functional disorders.

Dr. Luciani is the founder and Medical Director of the Albuquerque Clinic. The clinic specializes in integrating alternative medical modalities with conventional medicine.

C. Richard Mabray, MD   (361)-574-9697
115 Medical Drive, Suite #202
Victoria, TX 77904

Dr. C. Richard Mabray is a board-certified obstetrician-gynecologist in private practice since 1972 in Victoria, Texas. He is a graduate of Howard Payne University in Brawnwood, Texas, and received his medical degree from Baylor College of Medicine in Houston.

He is a member of the American College of Obstetricians and Gynecologists, the Pan American Allergy Society, the American Society of Bariatric Physicians, and the American Academy of Environmental Medicine. He has published and presented several papers on topics ranging from obesity and allergy to endometriosis and hormone replacement therapy.

He is the author of LOSE WEIGHT, NOT YOUR HEALTH: LOOKING GOOD, FEELING GOOD, LIVING LONGER—WHAT GOD INTENDS FOR YOUR HEALTH AND LIFE.

Ron Manzanero, MD   (512) 343-6223
4412 Spicewood Springs Rd., Suite 1007
Austin, TX 78759

Dr. Ron Manzanero is a physician who works with both conventional and alternative therapies, using an integrative approach. He received his medical degree from the University of Texas Medical Branch in Galveston and completed a family practice residence at the University of Massachusetts Medical Center in 1990. He has practiced in Austin, Texas, since 1990. While recognizing the benefits of prescription drugs and surgery, Dr. Manzanero seeks to determine the root of a patient's problem from a holistic frame of reference. He is particularly interested in hypothyroidism, insulin resistance syndrome, and anti-aging and wellness therapies. Dr. Manzanero draws upon his specialty of family practice and his extensive education in alternative medicine to plan the appropriate treatment for each individual.

Dr. Joseph Mercola   www.mercola.com
author of *The No Grain Diet*

David Overton, PA-C, herbalist   (360) 357-8054
Natural Medicines & Family Practice   toll-free (888) 568-6067
4780 Capitol Blvd SE, #2   natmeds@cco.net
Tumwater, WA 98501

David Overton, Physicians Assistant and herbalist, received his degree in Family Practice Medicine from the University of California at Davis in 1983. He has been an active practitioner and teacher since. He maintains his private practice at Natural Medicines & Family Practice in Tumwater, Washington, under the supervision of Dr. Walck, MD.

You may arrange to have your blood chemistries reviewed and natural treatment recommendations made. You can also obtain saliva test kits (for adrenal, thyroid, male and female sex hormones), stool test kits (comprehensive stool and digestive analysis for parasites and food allergies), hair test kit (checks toxins and mineral deficiencies) mailed to you for a small fee. They use only state and federally licensed labs. Written consultation reports with supplemental treatment recommendations are provided. Contact them for details.

In addition to clinical practice, David teaches integrated and natural medicine concepts and protocols to health care providers and the public.

David Parrish, MD   (480) 991-1769
Advanced Therapeutics
Scottsdale Airpark
7418 E. Helm Drive, Suite 236
Scottsdale, AZ 85260

Dr. David Parrish is board-certified in neurology and psycho-pharmacology, with post-graduate training in endocrinology. He specializes in chronic fatigue, fibromayalgia, and adrenal and thyroid disorders.

David A. Ramsey, DC   (408) 371-5190
New Life Health Center   fax (408) 371-5128
900 E. Campbell Ave. Suite #1   www.biohealthscan.com
Campbell, CA 95008

David A. Ramsey is a Doctor of Chiropractic at the New Life Health Center in Silicon Valley. He believes that your failure to lose weight can be due to metabolic imbalances found in your body chemistry and symptom analysis. "Bio Health Scan" (urine and saliva testing) uncovers critical key factors missed by outdated traditional medical lab tests. New methods for testing thyroid and adrenal activity levels, free radical levels, pH, minerals, and other deficiencies, as well as malabsorption, can reveal the total solution to weight loss difficulties. Symptom Survey Analysis and Toxicity Evaluations provide a nutritional plan targeted at regenerating your body toward optimum health and weight loss success. Visit his website at www.biohealthscan.com.

Neal Rouzier, MD   (760) 320-4292
2825 Tahquitz Canyon Way   contact person: Carolyn
Suite B200
Palm Springs, CA 92262

Neal Rouzier, MD, is an innovator and educator in the research and development of a new medical specialty that involves replacing and adjusting natural hormones. Formally trained in Emergency Medicine and Family Practice at UCLA, he also specializes in the treatment of hormonal and nutritional deficiencies. In addition, he is instrumental in teaching physicians the art and science of diagnosing, treating, monitoring, and adjusting natural hormones for women and men. His physician training course is the most popular and successful instructional program in the U.S. Dr. Rouzier is a popular guest lecturer for professional medical organizations. His most recent publication is NATURAL HORMONE REPLACEMENT FOR MEN AND WOMEN: HOW TO ACHIEVE HEALTHY AGING.

He offers training courses for physicians and has trained more than 2,000 physicians in all aspects of natural hormones for both men and women. For assistance locating an enlightened physician in your area, send an e-mail to hormonedoc@earthlink. net. If you are interested in information about hormones, a consultation, or Dr. Rouzier's book, please contact Carolyn at his office listed above.

Richard L. Shames, MD   (415) 472-2343
Karilee H. Shames, RN, Ph.D.   www.Thyroidpower.com
Preventive Medicine Center
25 Mitchell Boulevard, Suite #8
San Rafael, CA 94903

Dr. Richard Shames is a graduate of Harvard and the University of Pennsylvania Medical School. A founding member of the American Holistic Medical Association, he has served as adjunct faculty of UCSF Medical Center and Florida Atlantic University, and is a general practitioner in Mill Valley, California, specializing in thyroid treatment and telephone thyroid coaching nationally.

Karilee H. Shames, RN, Ph.D., is a clinical specialist in psychiatric nursing and a certified holistic nurse. She is an assistant professor of nursing at Florida Atlantic University. A low thyroid person herself, Karilee has led thyroid recovery support groups for many years and works with Dr. Richard Shames, providing national telephone consultation and speaking at Thyroid Power conferences.

Drs. Richard and Karilee Shames are authors of THYROID POWER: 10 STEPS TO TOTAL HEALTH.

If you need further information to make sure a thyroid coaching session is right for you, call toll-free (866) 468-4979.

For organizations that offer highest quality nutritional products, the authors of THYROID POWER *recommend that you contact their constantly updated clearinghouse for thyroid information and treatment called ThyRx. You can call toll-free about products at (866) GO-THYRX or, for a listing of products and latest research, visit www.thyroidpower.com.*

Robban A. Sica, MD   (203) 799-7733
Center for the Healing Arts, PC
370 Post Rd.
Orange, CT 06477
e-mail: support@centerhealingarts.com

Dr. Robban A. Sica graduated magna cum laude from the University of Toledo and the Medical College of Ohio. She took courses in holistic medicine and psychotherapy, including an intensive holistic studies program. Dr. Sica has continued to pursue the study of alternative therapies; her experience encompasses an integrative approach to the endocrine system, environmental medicine, and longevity medicine. She is certified in Advanced Longevity Medicine and Clinical Metal Toxicology.

Dr. Sica founded an integrative multi-specialty private practice of natural and alternative medicine, The Center for the Healing Arts, PC, in Orange, Connecticut, where Dr. Sica and staff are dedicated to development of a new model for integrative practice. Dr. Sica has found that her integrative approach is very successful for patients with chronic health conditions as well as those wishing to prevent illness. She has frequently been sought out as a speaker on holistic and alternative medicine and has appeared on radio and television, speaking on a wide range of topics including holistic medicine, anti-aging, natural hormone replacement and endocrine problems, nutrition/vitamin supplementation including natural alternatives to medication, allergies and environmental medicine, heavy metal toxicity, chronic fatigue syndrome, and treatment of chronic illnesses from an integrative perspective.

COLONIC THERAPIES AND REFERRAL SERVICES

Colema Boards™   www.detoxforlife.net
P.O. Box 34710
North Kansas, MO 64116

For those of you not too keen on seeing a colon therapist, you can view different examples of Colema boards on my website. You can order a home colonic unit to use in the privacy of your own home.

The International Association of   (210) 366-2888
    Colon Hydrdotherapy   fax (760) 749-1248
P.O. Box 461285   www. i-act.org
San Antonio, TX 78246-1285
e-mail: IACT@Healthy.net

Contact them for a colon therapist in your area.

Specialty Health Products   (800) 343-4950
21636 14th Ave. #A-1   (602) 582-4950
Phoenix, AZ 85027

Contact them for a colon hydrotherapist in your area.

FOOD AND SELF-ESTEEM ISSUES

Deirdra Price, Ph.D.   (619) 230-1880
Diet-Free Solution   (800) 521-6067
2220 Fifth Avenue
San Diego, CA 92101

Deirdra Price, Ph.D., President and CEO of Diet-Free Solution, is a licensed psychologist, speaker, and seminar leader who conducts individual, group, and family therapy. She has facilitated groups for the National Association of Anorexia Nervosa and Associated Disorders, and has worked extensively in both in-patient and out-patient hospital-based eating disorder programs. Dr. Price has a private practice in San Diego, California, and is the author of HEALING THE HUNGRY SELF:

THE DIET-FREE SOLUTION TO LIFELONG WEIGHT MANAGE-
MENT.

Overeaters Anonymous   (505) 891-2264
OA World Service   www.overeatersanonymous.org
P.O. Box 44020   www.oa.org
Rio Rancho, NM 87174-4020
e-mail: info@oa.org

*You can find meetings in your area, literature, and member
support.*

HEALTH PRODUCTS

The BodyGem™ and Balance Log™   www.healthetech.com
HealtheTech, Inc.
523 Park Pont Drive, 3rd Floor
Golden, CO 80401

*The BodyGem™ by HealtheTech is a handheld indirect
calorimeter that measures resting metabolic rate (RMR), the
number of calories a person burns in a day at rest. You can find
a practitioner in your area from their website.*

Awareness Corporation   orders (800) 692-9273
25 S. Arizona Place   fax (800) 772-7112
Fifth Floor, Suite 500   sponsor ID #1090501
Chandler, AZ 85225   www.awarecorp.com

*For ordering the Clear™ products. Give the sponsor number
to order directly. You may view product information or you can
order directly from our website: www.detoxforlife.net.*

Metagenics®   (800) 692-9400
100 Avenida La Pata   www.metagenics.com
San Clemente, CA 92673

Natural Health Retreats and Services   (619) 464-3346
Optimum Health Institute of San Diego   (800) 993-4325
6970 Central Ave.   www.optimumhealth.org
Lemon Grove, CA 91945

They offer week-long programs that include wheatgrass juice, enemas, colonics, massage, and nutritional classes. (You may not bring your own herbs or supplements to their location.)

Nature's Sunshine Products   orders (800) 453-1422
P.O. Box 19005   www.naturessunshine.com
Spanish Fork, UT   sponsor ID #118691-2

You can order any of the products listed in Chapter 23, Nature's Pharmacy, from Nature's Sunshine directly at wholesale prices. You can also order the pH testing kits directly from Nature's Sunshine. If you give them the product name they will provide a stock number for ordering. You must provide my sponsor ID# to order.

Standard Process Products, Inc®   (800) 848-5061
Whole Food Supplements   www.standardprocess.com
1200 West Royal Lee Drive
P.O. Box 904
Palmyra, WI 53156-0904

These products can't be purchased at a health food store. You will have to contact them to find a holistic health practitioner/physician that uses their products. I highly recommend their supplements.

Uni Key Health Systems, Inc.   orders (800) 888-4353
P.O. Box 2287   cust. service (208) 762-6833
Hayden ID 83835   www.unikeyhealth.com

The Vera and Para Systems, as well as the Super GI Cleanse, are recommended in Ann Louise Gittleman's revised and updated GUESS WHAT CAME TO DINNER.

We Care Health Retreat (800) 888-2523
18000 Long Canyon Rd. www.wecarespa.com
Desert Hot Springs, CA 92241

Participate in a week-long fast and colon cleanse at this 13-room retreat center with a pool. They also offer colonics and massage.

NATURAL HORMONE TESTING

Aeron Lifecycles (800) 631-7900
1933 Davis St., Suite 310
San Leandro, CA 94577

Laboratory for saliva testing of hormones.

Broda Barnes, MD, Research Foundation (203) 261-2101
P.O. Box 98
Trumbull, CT 06611

Urine determination of thyroid status.

Corning-Nichols Diagnostic Laboratory (800) NICHOLS
33608 Ortega Highway
San Juan Capistrano, CA 92675

Special determinations for TSH antibodies.

Diagnos-Techs, Inc. (206) 251-0596
P.O. Box 58948
Seattle, WA 98138

Adrenal hormone testing.

Immuno-Diagnostics Laboratory (800) 888-1113
10930 Bigge Street www.salivatest.com
San Leandro, CA 94577

Excellent lab for routine and special blood thyroid tests.

THYROID INFORMATION AND PATIENT ADVOCATE

American Foundation of Thyroid Patients   (281) 855-6608
18534 N. Lyford
Katy, TX 77449

Endocrine Nurses Society   (503) 494-3714
P.O. Box 229
West Linn, OR 97068

Mary Shomon   www.thyroid-info.com
www.thyroid-about.com

Mary Shomon is a communications consultant and published author who has transformed her own struggle with thyroid disease into an award-winning website and national prominence as a thyroid patient advocate.

Mary is the author of the bestselling book, LIVING WELL WITH HYPOTHYROIDISM: WHAT YOUR DOCTOR DOESN'T TELL YOU . . . THAT YOU NEED TO KNOW, which was published in March of 2000 by HarperCollins.

Mary holds a BS degree from Georgetown University in Washington, D.C. She is the founder of www.thyroid-info.com and www.thyroid-about.com, and can be reached through her website.

From Mary Shomon: "Traditional medicine dismisses thyroid disease as a mundane 'take this pill and you'll be fine' disease, but sufferers know better. My motto is 'We're patients. . . not lab values!' I feel that information, empowerment, and support can take us all a long way in our continuing effort to achieve good health. This is my focus for the thyroid site here at About.com, and in my patient-oriented book and other writings on thyroid disease." Her patient advocacy focus brings much-needed attention to the underdiagnosed and often overlooked issue of thyroid disease.

WATER SOURCES

Penta-Hydrate ™   (858) 452-8868
Bio-Hydration Research Lab, Inc.   (800) 531-5088
6370 Nancy Ridge Drive #104   www.hydrateforlife.com
San Diego, CA 92121

Penta-Hydrate water is available in some health food stores or you can order directly from their website. In addition to retail outlets, the company's health practitioner program, headed by Dr. Norman Deithch, DC, provides Penta-Hydrate to more than 350 medical doctors, nutritionists, chiropractors, and other health care professionals across the U.S.

Recommended Reading

■ ■

LOREE'S FAVORITE MUST READS!

Alternative Medicine Definitive Guide to Weight Loss
by Burton Goldberg and editors of *Alternative Medicine*
Alternative Medicine.com Books
1640 Tiburon Blvd., Suite 2
Tiburon, CA 94920
www.alternativemedicine.com
ISBN 1-887299-19-X

Attitudes of Gratitude: How to Give and
Receive Joy Every Day of Your Life
by M.J. Ryan
MJF Books
Fine Communications
Two Lincoln Square
New York, NY 10023
ISBN 1-56731-372-8

Beyond Feast or Famine: Daily Affirmations
for Compulsive Eaters
by Susan Ward, MA, MSW
Health Communications, Inc.
3201 S.W. 15th Street
Deerfield Beach, FL 33442-8124
ISBN 1-55874-076-7

Codependent: An Original Jokebook
by Jann Mitchell
Andrews and McMeel
A Universal Press Syndicate Company
Kansas City
ISBN 0-8362-7998-0

*The Cortisol Connection: Why Stress Makes You Fat and
Ruins Your Health — and What You Can Do About It*
by Shawn Talbott, Ph.D.
Hunter House Publishers
P.O. Box 2914   (800) 266-5592
Alameda, CA 94501   fax (510) 865-4295
ISBN 0-89793-391-5   www.hunterhouse.com

Dare to Lose: Four Simple Steps to a Better Body
by Shari Lieberman, Ph.D., CNS, FACN
with Nancy Bruning
Avery
A Member of Penguin Putnam Inc.
375 Hudson Street
New York NY 10014
ISBN 1-58333-125-5

Well, of course I am going to suggest to you my other books:

*Detox for Life: Your Bottom Line —
It's Your Colon or Your Life*
by Loree Taylor Jordan, CCH, ID
Madison Publishing
P.O. Box 231   orders (800) 247-6553
Campbell, CA 95009   fax (419) 281-6883
www.DetoxforLife.net   www.bookmaster.com
ISBN 0-9679878-6-5

Donuts Are a Girl's Best Friend:
  Life is Too Short to Diet and Exercise
  by Greta Carbo,™ a.k.a. Loree Taylor Jordan
  Madison Publishing
  P.O. Box 231   orders (800) 247-6553
  Campbell, CA 95009   fax (419) 281-6883
  www.gretacarbo.com   www.bookmaster.com
  ISBN 0-9679878-8-1

Eat Fat, Lose Weight: How the Right Fats
  Can Make You Thin for Life
  by Ann Louise Gittleman, MS, CNS
  with Dina R. Nunziato, CSW
  Keats Publishing, a division of NTC/
     Contemporary Publishing Group, Inc.
  4255 West Touhy Avenue
  Lincolnwood, IL 60646-1975
  ISBN 0-87983-966-X

Fat and Furious: Overcome Your Body's Resistance to
  Weight Loss Now!
  by Loree Taylor Jordan, CCH, ID
  Madison Publishing
  P.O. Box 231   orders (800) 247-6553
  Campbell, CA 95009   fax (419) 281-6883
  ISBN 0-9677779878-9-X   www.bookmaster.com

The Fat Flush Plan
  by Ann Louise Gittleman, MS, CNS
  McGraw-Hill (2002)
  ISBN 0-07-138383-2

Fight Fat After Forty
> by Pamela Peeke, MD, MPH
> Penguin Books
> Penguin Putnam Inc.
> 375 Hudson Street
> New York, NY 10014
> ISBN 0-14-10-0181 X

Get the Sugar Out: 501 Simple Ways
> *to Cut the Sugar Out of Any Diet*
> by Ann Louise Gittleman, MS, CNS
> Three Rivers Press
> A division of Crown Publishers, Inc.
> 201 East 50th Street
> New York, NY 10022
> ISBN 0-517-88653-7

Heal Your Body: The Mental Causes for Physical Illness
> *and the Metaphysical Way to Overcome Them*
> by Louise L. Hay
> Hay House, Inc.
> P.O. Box 6204
> Carson, CA 90749-6204
> ISBN 0-937611-35-2

How to Lower Your Fat Thermostat: The No-Diet
> *Reprogramming Plan for Lifelong Weight Control*
> by Dennis Remington, MD; Garth Fisher, Ph.D.;
>   and Edward Parent, Ph.D.
> Vitality House International, Inc
> 1675 N. Freedom Blvd. #11-C
> Provo, UT 84604   (800) 637-0708
> ISBN 0-912547-01-4

An Alternative Healing Reference (ninth edition)
Healthy Healing Publications
by Linda Page, ND, Ph.D.
P.O. Box 436   (800) 223-8225
Carmel Valley, CA 93924   www.healthyhealing.com

Living Well with Hypothyroidism: What Your Doctor
Doesn't Tell You . . . That You Need to Know
by Mary J. Shomon
HarperCollins Publishers, Inc.
10 East 53rd Street
New York, NY 10022
ISBN 0-380-80898-6

The Metabolic Plan: Stay Younger Longer
by Stephen Cherniske, MS
Ballantine Books
New York   www.ballantinebooks.com
ISBN 0-345-44101-X

NSP from A to Z: Body Systems and Sales Aids
Nature's Sunshine Products, Inc.
P.O. Box 19005
75 East 1700 South
Provo, UT 84605-9005   (800) 223-8225
Stock # 2720.7

The pH Miracle: Balance Your Diet, Reclaim Your Health
by Robert O. Young, Ph.D. and Shelley Redford Young
Warner Books, Inc.
1271 Avenue of the Americas
New York, NY 10020
ISBN 0-446-52809-9

Syndrome X: The Complete Nutritional Program to
Prevent and Reverse Insulin Resistance

by Jack Challem, Burton Berkson, M.D, Ph.D.,
and Melissa Diane Smith
John Wiley & Sons, Inc.
ISBN 0-471-39858-6

The Schwarzbein Principle: The Truth About
Losing Weight, Being Healthy, and Feeling Younger

by Diane Schwarzbein, MD, and Nancy Deville
Health Communications, Inc.
3201 S. W. 15th Street
Deerfield Beach, FL 33442-8190   www.hci-online.com
ISBN 1-55874-680-3

The Schwarzbein Principle II, The Transition:
A Regeneration Process to Prevent and Reverse
Accelerated Aging

by Diana Schwarzbein, MD, with Marilyn Brown
Health Communications, Inc.
3201 SW 15th Street
Deerfield Beach FL 33442-8190   www.hci-online.com
ISBN 1-55874-964-0

Thyroid Power: 10 Steps to Total Health

by Richard L. Shames, MD, and
Karilee Halo Shames, RN, Ph.D.
HarperCollins Publishers, Inc.
10 East 53rd Street
New York, NY 10022
ISBN 0-06-008222-4

*The Thyroid Solution: A Mind–Body Program for Beating
    Depression and Regaining Your Emotional & Physical Health*
    by Ridha Arem, MD
    Ballantine Books
    New York
    ISBN 0-345-42920-6

Tired of Being Tired: Rescue–Repair–Rejuvenate
    by Jesse Lynn Hanley, MD, with Nancy Deville
    The Berkley Publishing Group
    A division of Penguin Putnam Inc.
    375 Hudson Street
    New York, NY 10014
    ISBN 0-425-18459-5

Water: The Foundation of Youth, Health, and Beauty
    by William D. Holloway, Jr. and Herb Joiner-Bey, ND
    IMPAKT Health
    1133 Broadway, 4th Floor
    New York, NY 10010   fax (646) 336-1927
    ISBN 1-890694-38-X

Your Body's Many Cries for Water
    by F. Batmanghelidj, MD
    Global Health Solutions
    P.O. Box 3189
    Falls Church, VA 22043   (800) 759-3999
    ISBN 0-9629942-3-5

The Zone: A Dietary Road Map
    by Barry Sears, Ph.D. with Bill Lawren
    ReganBooks
    HarperCollins Publishers, Inc.
    10 East 53rd Street
    New York, NY 10022
    ISBN 0-06-039150-2

References

■ ■ ■ ■ ■ ■ ■ ■ ■ ■ ■

Aihara, Herman. *Acid & Alkaline.* George Ohwawa Macrobiotic Foundation.

Batmanghelidj, F., MD. *Your Body's Many Cries for Water.*

Cabot, Sandra, MD. *The Liver Cleansing Diet.* 1996.

Challem, Jack. "Syndrome X: The Hidden Disease You May Already Have." *Let's Live,* 1997.

Challem, Jack; Berkson, Burton, MD; and Melissa Smith. *Syndrome X: The Complete Nutritional Program to Prevent and Reverse Insulin Resistance.*

Cherniske, Stephen, MS. *The Metabolic Plan.*

Gittleman, Ann Louise, MS, CNS. *Guess What Came to Dinner: Parasites and Your Health* (revised edition). 2001.

Gittleman, Ann Louise, MS, CNS. *The Fat Flush Plan.*

Gittleman, Ann Louise, MS, CNS. *Get the Sugar Out: 501 Simple Ways to Cut the Sugar Out of Any Diet.*

Gittleman, Ann Louise, MS, CNS. *Eat Fat, Lose Weight: How the Right Fats Can Make You Thin for Life.*

Goldberg, Burton. *Alternative Medicine Definitive Guide to Weight Loss.*

Hagglund, Howard, ND, with contributions from Mary Shomon. "Natural Thyroid in Practice." *Townsend Letter for Doctors & Patients,* February/March 2002.

Hay, Louise. *Heal Your Body.* 1988.

Hipps, John, MD. *The Country Doctor: Alive and Well.*

Honeyman-Lowe, Gina, DC. *Your Guide to Metabolic Health*

Howell, Edward. *Enzyme Nutrition: The Food Enzyme Concept.*

Jordan, Loree Taylor CCH, ID. *Detox for Life: Your Bottom Line— It's Your Colon or Your Life.* 2002.

Jordan, Loree Taylor CCH, ID. *Farfrompoopin: When Sh*t Doesn't Happen.* Collectors Edition 2000.

Lieberman, Shari, Ph.D., CNS, FACN, with Nancy Bruning. *Dare to Lose.*

Mabray, C. Richard, MD. *Lose Weight, Not Your Health.*

Marcus, Eric. *Pessimisms.*

Mitchell, Jann. *Codependent: An Original Jokebook.*

Nature's Sunshine. *pH Balancing Simplified and An Introduction to Natural Health.*

Nature's Sunshine. *A–Z Body Systems and Sales Aids.*

Overton, David, PA-C. *Functional and Nutritional Blood Chemistry: What the Numbers Really Mean.*

Page, Linda, ND, PhD. *Healthy Healing: An Alternative Healing Reference* (ninth edition). Healthy Healing Publications, 1992.

Peeke, Pamela, MD, MPH. *Fight Fat After Forty.*

Price, Deidra, Ph.D. *Healing the Hungry Self: The Diet-Free Solution to Lifelong Weight Management.* Plume, 1996.

Rouzier, Neal, MD. *Natural Hormone Replacement for Men and Women: How to Achieve Healthy Aging.*

Ryan, M.J. *Attitudes of Gratitude: How to Give and Receive Joy Every Day of Your Life.*

Santillo, Humbart, NH, ND. *Food Enzymes: The Missing Link.*

Shomon, Mary J. *Living Well with Hypothyroidism: What Your Doctor Doesn't Tell You . . . That You Need to Know.* HarperCollins, 2000.

Talbott, Shawn, Ph.D. *The Cortisol Connection: Why Stress Makes You Fat and Ruins Your Health and What You Can Do About It.*

Tilden, John. *Toxemia Explained.*

Truman, Karol Delmonte. *Feelings Buried Alive Never Die.*

Ward, Susan, MA, MSW. *Beyond Feast or Famine.*

Weiss, Jennifer and Vena Burnett. *Colon Cleansing: The Best-kept Secret.* 1989

Weiss, Jennifer and Vena Burnett. *Colon Cleanse the Easy Way.*

Young, Robert O., Ph.D., and Shelly Redford Young. *The pH Miracle: Balance Your Diet, Reclaim your health.*

Index
■ ■ ■ ■ ■ ■

Absorption, and digestion, 95

Abusing food, 200–201
and negative beliefs, 46–49

Acceptance, 61–62

Acid/alkaline balance
checking your pH, 294–296
high alkalinity in the body, 293–294
in weight loss, 291–293

Adrenal function. *See also Cortisol levels*
balancing, 91, 114
and fatigue, 168–171

Alcohol, as poison, 173–174

Alkalinity. *See Acid/alkaline balance*

Allergies, to foods, 96–98

Anti-X™ diet, 187

Appearance, 4–7, 80–104

Autointoxication, 195–197

Balance, 111–115
adrenal, 91
emotional, 116–118
metabolic, 105–131, 291–299

Beliefs
limiting, 8–11, 18–23
negative, 46–49

Biochemical individuality, 83, 98

Blood sugar, and glandular balance, 303–310

Blood type, and metabolic type, 98–101

Body chemistry, balancing for weight loss, 291–299

Body fat. *See Weight*

Body-mind connection, 101–104. *See also Beliefs*

Bowel, detoxifying, 195–209, 300–303

Carbohydrate addiction, 175–177, 186–188

Carbohydrate sensitivity, and insulin resistance, 84–85

Case studies, 132–149, 200

Child within, healing, 25–26, 36

Children, 337–338
sugar addiction and obesity in, 188–190

Chocolate, 172–192

Cholesterol deprivation, causing gallstones, 251–253

Chronic fatigue syndrome, 96

Cleansing
and cellulite, 244–245
the colon, 210–218
the kidneys, 242–243
the liver, 314–318
the lymphatic system, 243–244
power of water, 237–245

CleanStart®, 215–218, 301–302

Codependency, 50–52

Colon, death beginning in, 199–200

Colon cleansing, 195–218, 300–303
for bulimics, 213–214
denial over, 206–208
medical objections to, 208–209
for men too, 213
powerpooping, 214–218

Compassion, 54, 60–61

Confidence, boosting, 343–344

Constipation
defined, 202–203
primary causes of, 203–205

Cortisol levels, 91, 164–168

Death, beginning in the colon, 199–200

Denial, 26–27, 206–208

Deprivation diets, 82–83

Detoxification, 193–254
of the colon, 195–209, 300–303
of the liver and gallbladder, 249

Dieting, 288–290
to fit into your clothes, 80–104
not based on starvation or deprivation, 82–83
for physical mastery, 255–329
types of, xxiv, 80–82

Digestion, and absorption, 95

Dignity, 79, 145–148

Doctors
humiliating overweight patients, 52–57, 145–146
interviewing, 351

Doctors *(continued)*
    objections to colon
        cleansing, 208–209
    patient experiences,
        156–158
    professional opinions of,
        197–198

Eating
    taking responsibility for,
        38–41
    for the wrong reasons,
        13–18, 37–41
Encouragement, 64–65
Enzymes
    assisting the metabolic
        process, 296–297
    defined, 297–299
Exercise, 255–329
    and metabolism, 277–287

Faith, taking the leap of,
    346–348
Fat. *See Weight*
Fat people
    deserving dignity and
        respect, 60–65, 145–148
    humiliated by doctors,
        52–57
Fatigue. *See also Chronic
    fatigue syndrome*
    adrenal, 168–171

Feelings, 341
    about food, 13–18, 37–41
    burying, 24–36
    denying, 26–27
    healing the child within,
        25–26, 36
Female hormones, 91–93
    natural replacement of,
        158–163
Fiber foods, 201–202
Food, 85–89
    abusing, 46–49
    eating for the wrong
        reasons, 13–18, 37–41
    feelings about, 37–41
    high-fiber, 201–202
    taking responsibility for,
        38–41
Food allergies, 96–98

Gallbladder
    detoxifing, 249
    role of, 249
Gallstones, 249–251
    cholesterol deprivation
        causing, 251–253
Game-playing, 12–23
    and shame, 42–57
Glandular balance, and blood
    sugar, 303–310
Glandular support, 310–312

Gratitude, 353–355

Heart disease, and insulin resistance, 185

Herbs, from nature's pharmacy, 300–329

Hormones, 91–94, 160, 162
 balancing, 90–91, 111–114, 118–120, 134–145
 replacing naturally, 92, 150–165

Humor, 352–353

Hypoallergenic treatment, for hypothyroidism, 152–153

Hypothyroidism, 56, 127–129
 with normal TSH levels, 151
 treating naturally, 151–153

Individuality, biochemical, 83

Inner child, 57
 healing, 25–26, 36

Inner critic, silencing, 45–46

Insulin release, 177–178
 and carbohydrate sensitivity, 84–85
 and glucose transport disorder, 179–181
 and Syndrome X, 172–173

Kidneys, cleansing, 242–243, 312-314

Laboratory tests, "normal," 120–127

Leap of faith, 346–348

Limiting beliefs, 18–23

Liver
 cleansing, 246–254, 314–318
 detoxifing, 249
 fat burned by, 247
 metabolism in, 247–248

Loving yourself, 348–350

Lymphatic system, cleansing, 243–244, 318

Male hormones, 93–94, 160, 162

Menopause, natural solutions to, 158

Metabolic type, and blood type, 98–101

Metabolism, 67–192
 enzymes assisting, 296–297
 and exercise and training, 277–287
 imbalance in, 105–131, 279–280
 impaired, 105–111
 monitoring, 283–284
 rate of, 89–90, 129–130

Natural nutrition, xxix

Natural solutions, for perimenopause, 158

Natural thyroid, in practice,
153–155

Nature's pharmacy, 300–329
herbs and supplements
from, 300–329

Negative beliefs, and food
abuse, 46–49

Nervous system, supporting,
320–322

"Normal" laboratory tests,
122–127

Nutrition
holistic, xxviii–xxix
for physical mastery,
255–329

Nutritional abuse, 200–201

Nutritional support, 323–325

Overexercising, to lose body
fat, 284–287

Overweight, 120–122. *See also*
Fat people; Weight

Parasites, 219–220, 318–320
eliminating, 232–236
essential knowledge
about, 220–222
experiences with, 231–232
sources of infestation,
224–228

Parasites *(continued)*
tapeworms, 229, 231–232
testing for, 222–224
and weight gain, 219–236

Parents, as role models,
190–192

Perimenopause, natural
solutions for, 158

Physical fitness, 341–342

Physical mastery, exercise,
diet, and nutrition, 255–329

Powerpooping, 214–218

Relationships, xxix–xxxii,
339–340

Repressing feelings, 27–29

Respect, 62–64, 145–148

Self-esteem
recovering, 4, 58–65, 79
tools for, 60–65

Self-honoring behaviors,
339–344

Shame, 42–57
using as leverage, 49–52

Solutions, natural, 158,
300–329

Starvation, diets not based
on, 82–83

Stress and overweight,
164–171

Stress and overweight
(*continued*)

  supporting the nervous
    system, 320–322

Sugar, 173–174

  and insulin resistance,
    183–184

Supplements, from nature's
  pharmacy, 300–329

Support

  being open and willing to
    receive, 350

  glandular, 310-312

  for the liver, 314–318

  for the nervous system,
    320-322

  nutritional, 323–325

Syndrome X

  a hidden disease, 182–188

  and insulin resistance,
    71–76, 86, 172–173

Tapeworms, 232

Thyroid function, and metabolic rate, 89–90, 106–109

Toxicity, 37, 95–96

  emotional, 253–254

  internal, 199

Trace minerals, 94–95,
  119–120

Training, 257–276

  and metabolism, 77–78,
    277–287

Urinary system, 312-314

Water

  cleansing power of,
    237–245

  live vs. dead, 241–242

  not sodas, 239–240

Weight

  facing up to, 69–79

  overexercising to lose,
    284–287

  payoff for keeping, 3–11

  reasons for losing, 4–7

  reasons for not losing,
    8–10

Weight gain, removing
  parasites to reverse, 219–236

Weight loss, 326–329

  acid/alkaline balance in,
    291–293

  balancing body chemistry
    for, 291–299

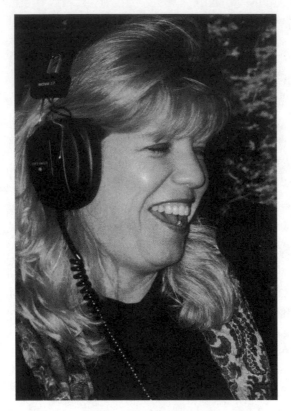

Loree Taylor Jordan

**For author interviews/speaking engagements,
call LTJ Associates: (408) 379-9488**

**For free reports, information, and newsletter
sign-up go to www.Loreetaylorjordan.com**

About the Author

Loree Taylor Jordan is a reformed dieting maniac, leading health expert in the holistic health field, and the most appropriate person to write this book. Her own personal struggle with sugar addiction, metabolic dysfunction, and the dieting yo-yo syndrome give her tremendous personal and professional credibility in the "weight game."

Ms. Jordan has 17 years of practical and professional experience as a colon hydrotherapist and holistic health educator. She graduated from the National Holistic Institute in Berkeley, California, and is an active member of the International Association of Colon Therapy, The National Speakers Association, and Toastmasters.

Ms. Jordan previously hosted a two-hour radio talk show in the San Francisco Bay Area. Her "don't-sugar-coat-it . . . tell-it-like-it-is" persona has given Loree almost a shock jock appeal that really makes people take notice. Her radio show was very successful and an extension of her kick-butt, no-holds-barred message.

Ms. Jordan has a tremendous love of the theater and an outrageous sense of humor. She has successfully written and produced stage productions of her health themes. Ms. Jordan has also created multiple personalities such as Greta Carbo™ and Marilyn Menopause™ to deliver her health message with humor. She is known for her hilarious parodies, such as "Donuts Are a Girl's Best Friend,"© complete with over-the-top costumes.

Ms. Jordan resides in the Bay Area, where she was born. She is an avid animal lover and lives with two dogs and six cats. She is the mother of two grown sons.

Praise for
Detox for Life...

Many alternative physicians abide by the maxim: disease starts in the colon. With today's polluted environment, combined with our diet of devitalized, additive-laden foods, detoxification is imperative to prevent and reverse chronic disease. A person who doesn't have two or three bowel movements a day is constipated. The information provided in Detox for Life *is comprehensive and vital for anyone interested in taking responsibility for their health.*

– Burton Goldberg, publisher, *An Alternative Medicine Definitive Guide to Cancer* and *Alternative Medicine Digest*

Detox for Life *is a very thorough, entertaining, and informative book on intestinal health. It should be read by everyone who is interested in preventing cancer and other long-term consequences of bowel toxicity. In caring for cancer patients using multiple modalities over the last 30 years, I have found that detoxification is an indispensable part of the treatment. Many cancer patients have a history of sluggish bowel function throughout their lives, and all have some degree of toxicity.*

– Douglas Brodie, MD, cancer specialist, Reno, Nevada

Detox for Life *is a powerhouse of information for anyone desirous of implementing their own tools and strategies for improved health. The guidance it provides can be easily integrated and incorporated into your daily routine.*

– Arthur E. Brawer, MD, Director of Rheumatology Monmouth Medical Center, Long Branch, New Jersey

Ms. Jordan has put together all the vital information necessary for detoxification in this era of environmental pollution. I congratulate her on a job well done!

– W. John Diamond, MD, co-author of *The Alternative Medicine Definitive Guide to Cancer*

Detox for Life is the most thorough book on colon cleansing I have ever seen. It gives excellent understanding about the importance of detoxification, proper digestion, and elimination, and is also an excellent manual for health care practitioners.

— Pamela Whitney, ND, Smithfield, Rhode Island

Detox for Life gives careful consideration to the balance of convenience, safety, and efficacy required for success in detoxification. This book is essential for anyone considering holistic cleansing.

— Mark Pederson, author of *Nutritional Herbology*

From the beginner to the pro, this book offers a motivating, entertaining, and informative look at detoxification and its beneficial effect on overall health. I highly recommend it to anyone interested in decreasing the cumulative effects of aging and its consequences.

— Diane Thorson, DC, BSN

Superb! Detox for Life is well laid out, very user friendly, and as informative as it could be. Ms. Jordan's concepts are easy to follow and essentially empirical for the cleansing and detoxification of the putrefied colon—the root of numerous diseases!

— Sharda Sharma, MD, Millburn, New Jersey

Colon therapy is not as American as hot dogs and apple pie, but it will do wonders for your health and life. The waste that exists in your poor, sick body can best be described as cancer that hasn't happened yet. This is a must read! Share it with everyone you care about.

— John Thomas, author of *Young Again!*
How to Reverse the Aging Process

Detox for Life is a winner, one of the best books written on the subject on colon cleansing and detoxification in the last 15 years. My clients laugh out loud, and say it's funny and very informative. Once they start reading they can't put it down.

— Gayle Marie Bradshaw, colon hydrotherapist

As a long-time recipient of colonics and practicing colon hydrotherapist, I am so grateful to be able to offer Detox for Life *to my friends, family, and clients. The reactions have been overwhelmingly positive. Loree's sense of humor makes it fun to read as well as an educational experience. I have decided to include this book as part of my client's first session. The information and tools are invaluable. Thanks Loree!*

– Sally Negus LMT, CT, Nashua, New Hampshire

I have never known Loree Taylor Jordan to be less than passionate about detoxification, while maintaining a healthy sense of humor about it. This book takes you through the entire process, from the basics of digestion to how to detoxify the whole body, in a very easy-to-understand format.

– L. Pataki, Ph.D., Cs.C.

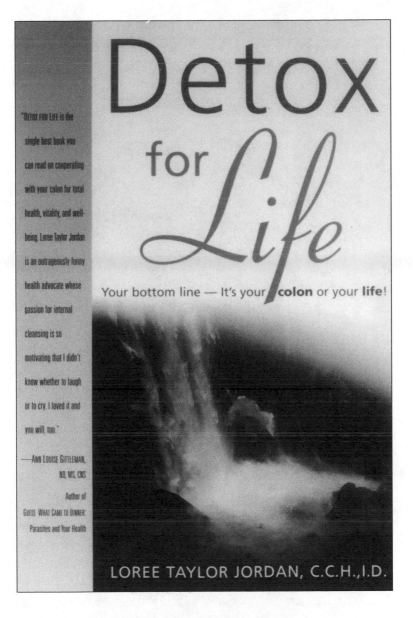

Detox for Life

for Life

Your bottom line — It's your colon or your life!

"DETOX FOR LIFE is the single best book you can read on cooperating with your colon for total health, vitality, and well-being. Loree Taylor Jordan is an outrageously funny health advocate whose passion for internal cleansing is so motivating that I didn't know whether to laugh or to cry. I loved it and you will, too."

——ANN LOUISE GITTLEMAN, ND, MS, CNS
Author of
GUESS WHAT CAME TO DINNER:
Parasites and Your Health

LOREE TAYLOR JORDAN, C.C.H.,I.D.

ISBN 0-9679878-6-5 $19.95

Available wherever books are sold. To order direct:
phone (800) 247-6553 ◆ fax (419) 281-6883
online: www.detoxforlife.net or www.bookmaster.com

DONUTS ARE A GIRL'S BEST FRIEND

Life is Too Short to Diet and Exercise

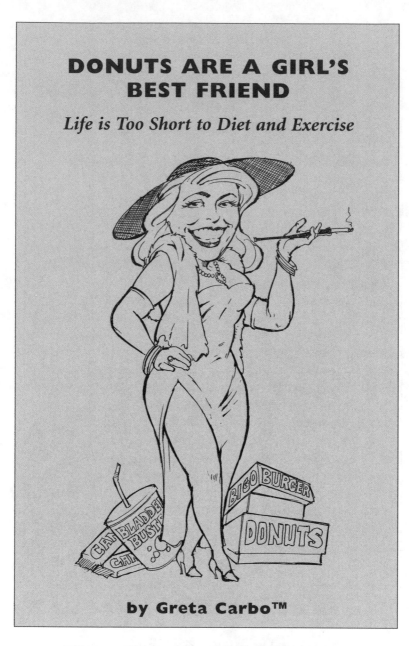

by Greta Carbo™

ISBN 0-9679878-8-1   Book with CD $19.95

Available at www.gretacarbo.com
www.bookmaster.com
or (800) 247-6553

Quick Order Form

Fax orders: (419) 281-6883. Send this form.

Telephone orders: (800) 247-6553. Please have your Visa or Master-Card ready.

E-mail orders: www.loreetaylorjordan.com

Postal orders: Bookmasters, P.O. Box 388, Ashland, OH 44805 (800) 247-6553.

❑ Please send the following books, tapes, or CDs:

_____

_____

Please send me FREE information about:

❑ upcoming books/tapes   ❑ Loree's products/programs

❑ speaking/seminars   ❑ consulting/health coaching

❑ Please add me to your mailing list.

Name _____

Address _____

City _____ State ____ Zip _____

Telephone (day) _____ (eve) _____

E-mail _____

Sales tax: Please add 8.25% for products shipped to California.

Shipping: $4.50 U.S. for the first book and $2 for each additional product. All books are shipped Priority Mail or UPS Ground (please specify).

Payment: ❑ Check   ❑ Visa   ❑ MasterCard

Card number _____

Name on card _____ Exp. _____

Do you have a success story to share?

Has *Fat and Furious: Overcome Your Body's Resistance to Weight Loss Now* helped you finally get to the root of your metabolic challenges and lose weight? If so, please write and tell us your story. We are looking for positive metabolic success stories. Share your experience, strength, and hope in an upcoming book, *Fat and Furious Too!*

Be sure to include all current contact information (name; daytime, evening, and cell phone number; e-mail address) so we can reach you for permission if we decide to publish your success story. Before-and-after photos are welcome!

Please submit your story to managing editor, care of:

Madison Publishing
P.O. Box 231
Campbell, CA 95009
(408) 379-6534
e-mail: Madisonpublish@aol.com

*If you have any comments to the author
we would love to hear from you!*